Ecological Research to Promote Social Change

Methodological Advances
from Community Psychology

Ecological Research to Promote Social Change

Methodological Advances
from Community Psychology

Edited by

Tracey A. Revenson, Senior Editor

*The Graduate Center of the City
   University of New York
New York, New York*

Anthony R. D'Augelli

*Pennsylvania State University
University Park, Pennsylvania*

Sabine E. French

*University of California
Riverside, California*

Diane L. Hughes

*New York University
New York, New York*

David Livert

*The Graduate Center of the City
   University of New York
New York, New York*

Edward Seidman

*New York University
New York, New York*

Marybeth Shinn

*New York University
New York, New York*

Hirokazu Yoshikawa

*New York University
New York, New York*

Kluwer Academic / Plenum Publishers
New York   Boston   Dordrecht   London   Moscow

ISBN 0-306-46727-5 (hardbound)
    0-306-46728-3 (paperback)

© 2002 Kluwer Academic / Plenum Publishers, New York
233 Spring Street, New York, New York 10013

http://www.wkap.nl

10 9 8 7 6 5 4 3 2 1

To our students—past, present, and future—
whose curiosity keeps our intellectual fires burning
and who are creating the interventions
and methods of the future

Contributors

Leona S. Aiken, Department of Psychology, Arizona State University, Tempe, Arizona 85287

W. Steven Barnett, Graduate School of Education, Rutgers University, New Brunswick, New Jersey 08901

Janette Beals, Division of American Indian and Alaska Native Programs, University of Colorado Health Sciences Center, Denver, Colorado 80220

Robert D. Caplan, Department of Psychology, George Washington University, 2125 G Street NW, Washington, D.C. 20052

William A. Corsaro, Department of Sociology, Indiana University, Bloomington, Indiana 47405

Claudia J. Coulton, Mandel School of Applied Social Sciences, Case Western Reserve University, Cleveland, Ohio 44106

Anthony R. D'Augelli, Department of Human Development and Family Studies, The Pennsylvania State University, University Park, Pennsylvania 16802

Kimberly DuMont, Department of Psychiatry, New Jersey Medical School, Newark, New Jersey 07107

Diane L. Hughes, Department of Psychology, New York University, New York, New York 10003

Jill E. Korbin, Case Western Reserve University, Cleveland, Ohio 44106

Douglas Luke, St. Louis University School of Public Health, St. Louis, Missouri 63108

Christina M. Mitchell, Division of American Indian and Alaska Native Programs, University of Colorado Health Sciences Center, Denver, Colorado 80220

Douglas D. Perkins, Department of Human and Organizational Development, Peabody College, Vanderbilt University, Nashville, Tennessee, 37203

Richard H. Price, Institute for Social Research, University of Michigan, Ann Arbor, Michigan 48106

Julian Rappaport, Department of Psychology, University of Illinois, Urbana, Illinois 61820

Tracey A. Revenson, Doctoral Program in Psychology, The Graduate Center of the City University of New York, New York, NY 10016-4309

Thomas A. Rizzo, 492 East Butterfield Road, Elmhurst, New York 60126

Edward Seidman, Department of Psychology, New York University, New York, New York 10003

Marybeth Shinn, Department of Psychology, New York University, New York, NY 10003

Mark Tausig, Department of Sociology, University of Akron, Akron, Ohio 44325

Ralph B. Taylor, Department of Criminal Justice, Temple University, Philadelphia, Pennsylvania 19122

Michael Todd, Department of Psychology, Arizona State University, Tempe, Arizona 85287

Amiram D. Vinokur, Institute for Social Research, University of Michigan, Ann Arbor, Michigan 48106

Stephen G. West, Department of Psychology, Arizona State University, Tempe, Arizona 85287

Preface

This volume was conceived during many long conversations among the editors as they were preparing *A Quarter Century of Community Psychology: Readings from the* American Journal of Community Psychology (Revenson, D'Augelli, French, Hughes, Livert, Seidman, Shinn, & Yoshikawa, 2002). For that volume, the editors were charged with the task of assembling a collection of the outstanding articles from the first 25 years of the *American Journal of Community Psychology* (*AJCP*), the premier journal of the Society for Community Research and Action. In reading and rereading the several hundred articles from the 25 years of the journal's existence, it became apparent that one of the crowning achievements of that quarter century of research was the development of innovative methods in the areas of intervention and prevention research, ecological assessment, and culturally anchored research.

With the support of our "midwife" at Kluwer Academic/Plenum Publishers, Eliot Werner, an editorial decision was made to produce twin volumes, one focusing on innovative theory and research and the other on imaginative methods. This gave us the opportunity to showcase the methodological advances of community psychology—advances that have found a place in sister disciplines as well.

This reader will be useful for scholars, researchers, and interventionists not only in community psychology but also in other subdisciplines of psychology and other social sciences, including:

- Developmental psychologists, whose research involves prevention programs, schools and neighborhoods
- Clinical psychologists and social workers who study community-based treatment
- Evaluation researchers
- Researchers in public health or behavioral medicine who design or evaluate community-based health programs and preventive trials.
- Social psychologists who have moved out of the laboratory to study real-world issues.
- Researchers in any discipline who understand the importance of culture in the study of contexts or interventions.

The material presented in this volume is sophisticated enough for researchers and professionals, yet comprehensible enough for master's-level and doctoral-level students. It can serve as one of the primary texts for a methods course or as a supplemental reader for master's- and doctoral-level graduate courses in community psychology, field research design, and public health. Above all, the volume is targeted toward researchers who want to understand and change social contexts to promote human health and welfare, and who want to be cognizant of some of the most sophisticated methods for doing so.

Our thanks again to Irwin Sandler and Christopher Keys, who, as Publications Chair and President, guided the Society for Community Research and Action (Division 27 of the American Psychological Association) as it embarked on this project, and to Jodi Kellar and Jenni Hoffman for their untiring help with "cataloguing" the hundreds of articles in the *American Journal of Community Psychology* during the two-year selection process. We are extremely grateful to Eliot Werner, our Executive Editor at Plenum, who made this book an easy labor.

We also want to pay tribute to the four editors of the American Journal of Community Psychology during the quarter century we reviewed: Charles Spielberger (1973–1976); John C. Glidewell (1977–1988); Julian Rappaport (1989–1992); and Edison J. Trickett (1993–1997), for there would be no content to this book without their mark on the field. Julian Rappaport and Ed Trickett, in particular, encouraged community psychologists to work on the development of new methods or the reformation and tailoring of existing ones, and by their choices of articles to be published, gave voice to methods based on different epistemologies.

TRACEY A. REVENSON
ANTHONY R. D'AUGELLI
SABINE E. FRENCH
DIANE L. HUGHES
DAVID LIVERT
EDWARD SEIDMAN
MARYBETH SHINN
HIROKAZU YOSHIKAWA

REFERENCES

Revenson, T. A., D'Augelli, A. R., French, S. E., Hughes, D. L., Livert, D. E., Seidman, E., Shinn, M., & Yoshikawa, H. (Eds), *A quarter century of community psychology: Readings from the* American Journal of Community Psychology. New York: Kluwer Academic/Plenum Publishers.

Contents

Ecological Research to Promote Social Change

Methodological Advances
from Community Psychology

Introduction

Tracey A. Revenson

During the past quarter century, community psychologists have worked to make more relevant contributions to human welfare in community settings and to effect social change. Community psychologists work in and with schools, neighborhood organizations, religious institutions, and government agencies on social issues including discrimination, violence, educational achievement, and health. Using a social ecological paradigm as their guiding framework, community psychologists focus on the interactions between persons and their environments, cultural diversity, and local empowerment for understanding organizational, community, and social change.

In conducting their research and in evaluating preventive interventions and social action programs, many community psychologists found that traditional research methods were inadequate to deal with multilayered social and community problems—problems that stemmed as much from a lack of fit between persons and their environments as they did from individual deficits. Community psychology always has relied on multiple methods in its toolbox, including field experiments and quasi-experiments, ethnography, needs assessment, epidemiology, cost-effectiveness analysis, program evaluation, and time-series analyses. But more often than not, community psychologists have had to articulate new methodologies or to adapt existing ones.

In order to understand a central theme of the field—the study of persons in ecological context—existing approaches have been used in innovative ways. For example, Shinn and Rapkin (2000) tackled the notion of cross-level research, which involves relationships among variables at more than one level of analysis. Alternatively, cluster analysis has been used to develop profiles of persons in their settings, allowing us to examine the relationships of person-setting units to individual and community-level outcomes

Tracey A. Revenson • Doctoral Program in Psychology, The Graduate Center of the City University of New York, New York, New York 10016-4309.

Ecological Research to Promote Social Change: Methodological Advances from Community Psychology, edited by Tracey A. Revenson et al. Kluwer Academic/Plenum Publishers, New York, 2002.

1

(e.g., Kuhn & Culhane, 1998). For primers on statistical techniques that are becoming more commonly used in community psychology, we recommend the following pieces: Durlak and Lipsey (1991) on meta-analysis, Luke (1993) on survival analysis, and Rapkin and Luke (1993) on cluster analysis. In addition, special issues of the *American Journal of Community Psychology* (AJCP) have been devoted entirely to specific methodological topics, such as prevention research (Seidman, 1993); culturally anchored methodology (Seidman, Hughes, & Williams, 1993), ecological assessment (Shinn, 1996), and qualitative research (Miller & Banyard, 1998).

An explicit emphasis on methodology is fairly recent for community psychology, but the past decade has been one of rapid and complex growth. Indications are that it will continue to grow, as we became more vocal about requiring approaches that emphasize contextual awareness, ecological validity, and the rich variation in people's lives. Signaling a possible methodological paradigm shift in the field, feminist and qualitative methodologies are gaining a greater voice because of the potential for their results to be translated into social change (e.g., Cosgrove & McHugh, 2000; Miller & Banyard, 1998; Stewart, 2000).

The chapters in this volume reflect the sophisticated techniques and thorny issues that surround investigators doing real-world research. What research designs should be used for comparing the efficacy of different preventive interventions or different components of a multi-component intervention? How do we assess the cost-effectiveness of such programs? How can we ensure validity in ethnographic research? How can one use quantitative methods and still conduct research that is culturally sensitive? Each of the chapters reflects advances in methodology that help us to study the linkages between persons and environments, or to uncover the unique aspects of culture that help us understand a set of findings.

The first section of this volume, *Design Issues in Intervention Research*, focuses on distinctive methodological concerns that arise out of doing social intervention, e.g., evaluating which component of a multicomponent intervention "works," assessing to what degree nonparticipation or dropout during an intervention biases the findings, and evaluating the cost-effectiveness of an intervention. These issues are relevant not only for the evaluation researcher, but for those who design preventive intervention programs as well.

The second section, *Ecological Assessment*, focuses on a number of issues that are critical in order to collect and analyze data across multiple settings. Chapters in this section address: measuring the influences of social settings (in this case, neighborhoods) on behavior, using network analysis to quantify the web of social services and the interactions among its components, examining ecological influences on behavior from a set of ethnographic studies, and using complex behavioral observation systems to understand social interactions within existing social organizations.

The final section, *Culturally Anchored Research*, tackles the issue of how diversity and culture have been "translated" in basic and intervention research, and how they can and need to be integrated into all phases of the research process. The readings in this section provide both a blueprint for and examples of research that integrate the cultural context into all aspects of the research process.

These readings focus on methodological advances over the past decade that address concerns central to community psychology. However, with the rising prominence of feminist and qualitative methodologies as well as dynamic, longitudinal, quantitative methods, we can expect another such volume in the next decade.

REFERENCES

Cosgrove, L., & McHugh, M. (2000). Speaking for ourselves: Feminist methods and community psychology. *American Journal of Community Psychology, 8*, 815–838.

Durlak, J. A., & Lipsey, M. (1991). A practitioner's guide to meta-analysis. *American Journal of Community Psychology, 19*, 291–332.

Kuhn, R., & Culhane, D. P. (1998). Applying cluster analysis to test a typology of homelessness by pattern of shelter administration: Results from the analysis of administrative data. *American Journal of Community Psychology, 26*, 207–232.

Luke, D. A. (1993). Charting the process of change: A primer on survival analysis. *American Journal of Community Psychology, 21*, 203–246.

Miller, K. E., & Banyard, V. (Eds.) (1998). Qualitative research in community psychology. [Special Issue]. *American Journal of Community Psychology, 26*(4).

Rapkin, B. D., & Luke, D. A. (1993). Cluster analysis in community research: Epistemology and practice. *American Journal of Community Psychology, 21*, 247–277.

Seidman, E. (Ed.) (1993). Methodological issues in prevention research. [Special Issue]. *American Journal of Community Psychology, 21*(5).

Seidman, E., Hughes, D. L., & Williams, N. (Eds.) (1993). Culturally anchored methodology. [Special Issue]. *American Journal of Community Psychology, 21*(6).

Shinn, M. (Ed.) (1996). Ecological assessment. [Special Issue]. *American Journal of Community Psychology, 24*(1).

Shinn, M., & Rapkin, B. (2000). Cross-level research without cross-ups in community psychology. In J. Rappaport & E. Seidman (Eds.), *Handbook of Community Psychology* (pp. 669–695). New York: Kluwer Academic/Plenum Publishers.

Stewart, E. (2000). Thinking through others: Qualitative research and community psychology. In J. Rappaport & E. Seidman (Eds.), *Handbook of Community Psychology* (pp. 725–736). New York: Kluwer Academic/Plenum Publishers.

I

Design Issues in Intervention Research

Anthony R. D'Augelli

Research design in intervention historically has focused on two broad classes of change processes: psychotherapy/counseling and human service programs. Both psychotherapy research and evaluation research have provided rich perspectives on construct articulation, theoretical frameworks, research designs, and analytic strategies that have informed larger-scale intervention research. In addition, community psychology has profoundly altered the way we think about intervention theory with its ecological, multi-level model of change that centers attention on relationships between people and the diverse settings of their lives (Yoshikawa & Shinn, 2002). Such a model of change is directly helpful in designing and evaluating interventions designed to prevent mental health problems and to enhance development in particular populations and communities.

The three papers in this section focus on distinctive methodological concerns that arise for intervention researchers. These examples not only reveal how researchers can develop methodological solutions to vexing issues related to implementing and evaluating particular programmatic efforts, but also show how these solutions can lead to social change grounded in real-life circumstances. A dynamic blend of rigor and relevance emerges from a reading of these reports—a balancing of the need for scientific precision with a deep respect for the exigencies of social interventions in actual community settings (Jansen & Johnson, 1993).

In the first paper, West, Aiken, and Todd (1993) provide ample evidence that prevention research has evolved in to a position of considerable sophistication. Understanding that prevention programs are highly complex social activities involving many components that influence change among many participants, West and his colleagues endeavor to clarify ways

Anthony R. D'Augelli ● Department of Human Development and Family Studies, The Pennsylvania State University, University Park, Pennsylvania 16802.

for evaluators to determine which program components are crucial and which are, in their words, "inert" (p. 572). In addition, they argue that there are two other pressing questions facing prevention researchers: Whether the program represents the optimal use of available resources, and what processes explain why a program works. West and his colleagues extrapolate suggestions from psychotherapy research design to answer these questions for prevention researchers, and note the strengths and limitations of traditional designs when attempted in field settings. They wisely describe the importance of fractional designs, which, in contrast to factorial designs, selectively test different combinations of program components. Finally, they describe the crucial importance of mediational analysis in prevention research. Indeed, mediational analyses—which seek to understand the powerful factors that lead to program success or failure—are crucial to an ecologically valid evaluation of an intervention project. Given the complexity of most social interventions and the communities in which they operate, such an analysis is paramount if evaluators wish to confidently recommend the widespread dissemination of a particular prevention program.

It was as a result of such a specifically targeted preventive intervention to assist unemployed workers that Vinokur, Price, and Caplan (1991) conducted the study reprinted here. Showing the careful pragmatism of field researchers, Vinokur and his colleagues investigated the status of the many people who were approached to participate in the intervention but did not participate, as well as those who agreed to participate but never showed up. Carefully designed intervention experiments are often threatened when differential participation or dropout destroys randomization. Given the time, commitment, and funds required by preventive interventions, as well as program developers' strong bias in favor of their program's usefulness, what can we say of those who do not complete an intervention? Nonparticipation is a serious obstacle in making conclusive statements about the efficacy of programmatic efforts; the possibility that self-selection may lead to the overestimation of a program's impact can thwart the implementation of an effective intervention. Vinokur, Price, and Caplan provide an elegant solution to this problem. Their study's results demonstrate that those who actually completed the program showed considerable benefit whereas those who did not choose to participate were able to change without program involvement. This paper illustrates the power of intervention to inform social policy. There were very real consequences of this study, most pointedly the recommendation that additional resources should not be allocated to attracting more people to the program or to retaining those who started. Instead, it would be more cost-effective to spend resources on replications of the program, as self-selection apparently engaged those people who would, in fact, be helped.

Barnett and Escobar (1989) tackle the issue of cost-effectiveness of early intervention in more depth. Relatively few studies of efforts to enhance the development of children in less-advantaged situations have focused on long-term consequences, even though such longitudinal research is of paramount importance. Barnett and Escobar argue that such long-range evaluations must incorporate an economic analysis of costs and benefits to society. Beyond an understanding of how different intervention components contribute to a program's success (West, Aiken, & Todd, 1991), or how issues such as self-selection affect practical decisions about resource allocation (Vinokur, Price, & Caplan 1991), Barnett and Escobar provide examples of why a cost–benefit analysis is essential to determining if an intervention is worth the investment. They also note the difficulties of drawing conclusions for policy decisions from studies that do not use sophisticated research designs or economic analyses. Their conclusion— that a wide variety of early childhood interventions "work"—is a reassuring one, given the social and fiscal resources invested in these efforts. Importantly, they note that one could hardly do ecologically valid intervention research without cost-effectiveness information, yet most researchers do not. Without knowing whether an intervention for young children and their families really deserves the time and commitment required for participation, it may be presumptuous to recommend these activities. And to know if these programs are valuable demands a broad, yet rigorous, review of many factors speaking to impact, including an economic cost–benefit analysis (see Durlak & Wells, 1997, for a meta-analytic review of crucial issues for intervention researchers).

The three papers in this section show the seriousness with which the fundamental question of the effectiveness of social intervention must be approached. Each paper provides a unique strategy for designing projects to answer the same question: Do our efforts to help people actually matter? The suggestions contained in these papers provide a variety of ways to answer that question, in ways that are distinctly suited to real-world decision-making about intervention in community settings.

REFERENCES

Barnett, W. S., & Escobar, C. M. (1989). Research on the cost effectiveness of early educational implications for research and policy. *American Journal of Community Psychology*, 17, 677–704.

Durlak, J. A., & Wells, A. M. (1997). Primary prevention in mental health programs for children and adolescents: A meta-analytic review. *American Journal of Community Psychology*, 25, 115–152.

Jansen, M. A., & Johnson, E. M. (1993). Methodological issues in prevention research. [Special Issue]. *American Journal of Community Psychology*, 21(5).

Vinokur, A. D., Price, R. H., & Caplan, R. D. (1991). From field experiments to program implementation: Assessing the potential outcomes of an experimental intervention program for unemployed persons. *American Journal of Community Psychology, 19*, 543–562.

West, S. G., Aiken, L. S., & Todd, M. (1993). Probing the effects of individual components in multiple component prevention programs. *American Journal of Community Psychology, 21*, 571–606.

Yoshikawa, H., & Shinn, M. (2002). Facilitating change: Where and how should community psychology intervene? In T. A. Revenson, A. R. D'Augelli, S. E. French, D. L. Hughes, D. Livert, E. Seidman, M. Shinn, & H. Yoshikawa (Eds.). *A quarter century of community psychology: Readings from the* American Journal of Community Psychology (pp. 33–49). New York: Kluwer Academic/Plenum Publishers.

1

Probing the Effects of Individual Components in Multiple Component Prevention Programs

Stephen G. West, Leona S. Aiken, and Michael Todd

Assessing the contributions of individual components in multi-component interventions poses complex challenges for prevention researchers. We review the strengths and weaknesses of designs and analyses that may be useful in answering three questions: (1) Is each of the individual components contributing to the outcome? (2) Is the program optimal? and(3), Through what processes are the components of the program achieving their effects? Factorial and fractional factorial designs in which a systematically selected portion of all possible treatment combinations is implemented are used to address question 1. Response surface designsin which each component is quantitatively scaled are explored in relation to question 2. Mediational analysis, a hybrid of experimental andcorrelational approaches, is considered in relation to question 3. Design enhancements are offered that may further strengthen some of thesetechniques. These techniques offer promise of enhancing both the basic science and applied science contributions of prevention research.

Originally published in the *American Journal of Community Psychology, 21*(5) (1993): 571–605.

Ecological Research to Promote Social Change: Methodological Advances from Community Psychology, edited by Tracey A. Revenson et al. Kluwer Academic/Plenum Publishers, New York, 2002.

INTRODUCTION

Recent reviews have called for multiple component interventions to prevent complex social, health, and mental health problems (Hawkins, Catalano, & Miller, 1992; Shaffer, Phillips, & Enzer, 1989; Weissberg, Caplan, & Sivo, 1989). These reviews have highlighted the multiple pathways that exist between early risk factors and the later development of significant problems. Responding to these calls, recent prevention programs have included multiple components, each of which is targeted toward one or more of the pathways believed to underlie the development of the problem. To cite but two examples, Flay (1985) reviewed school-based social influences smoking prevention programs and concluded that the successful programs were of extended duration and were characterized by six components: media material with similar age peers, information on immediate physiological effects of smoking, correction of misperceptions about the prevalence of smoking, discussion of family and media influences on smoking and methods of dealing with them, explicit learning of behavioral skills, and a public commitment procedure. Wolchik et al. (1993) describe a program for custodial mothers of children of divorce involving five components: the custodial parent–child relationship, the noncustodial parent-child relationship, discipline strategies, reduction of stressful events, and support from nonparental adults. Each of these programs has been evaluated in randomized trials comparing the intervention with a control group. Each program has shown some degree of success in producing its desired final outcome of reducing the prevalence of adolescent smoking and decreasing the children's symptoms, respectively. However, continued demonstrations of success will give rise to a new set of questions related to the multi-component nature of these programs.

THREE QUESTIONS ABOUT MULTI-COMPONENT PROGRAMS

The process of the development and evaluation of multi-component programs raises questions for both basic and applied scientists. The source of these questions for basic scientists is their concern with maximizing the informativeness of the results of the randomized trial of the intervention for basic psychological theory; the source of these questions for applied scientists is their concern about maximizing the effectiveness of the program in producing the desired outcomes. These concerns result in three intertwined questions that may be raised about multi-component programs and that will be considered throughout this article.

1. *Is each of the individual components of the program contributing to the outcome*? Basic scientists seek to show that each component of the program is producing the desired outcome in the service of establishing the construct validity of the independent variables (Cook & Campbell, 1979; Higginbotham, West, & Forsyth, 1988). Applied scientists may be interested in the effectiveness of individual components for more pragmatic reasons. Some components may have been included that in fact reduced the effectiveness of the overall intervention package in producing the desired outcome. Or, inert components may have been included that are neither harmful or helpful, but that are costly to include in the program package. In such cases, applied scientists would desire to identify and delete such ineffective components from the overall program.

2. *Is the program optimal*? Program developers may wish to combine several promising components to develop a new program, to add promising components to an existing program, or to fine tune a successful program to achieve maximal effectiveness. Or, a program developer may have to operate within the constraints of a fixed amount of program time or program budget and wonder about how to allocate these resources to each of the components of the overall program. In each case, the program developer is seeking to identify the combination of components that produces the optimal outcome.

3. *Through what processes are the components of the program achieving their effectiveness*? Basic scientists are interested in understanding the processes through which each component may be achieving its effect on the outcome of interest. A new generation of prevention programs is explicitly being created based on psychosocial theory and research on the development and maintenance of the targeted problem (Caplan, Vinokur, Price, & Van Ryn, 1989; Sandler et al., 1992). Careful study of the processes through which preventive interventions achieve their effects potentially provides the strongest information possible to inform basic researchers about the development of psychopathology in children and adults (Coie et al., 1993). In addition, information about the processes through which the program operates may be critical in making appropriate modifications that help make the program successful in new sites.

The purpose of this article is to consider the strengths, weaknesses, and areas of application of a variety of designs that have been proposed to answer these three questions about multi-component programs. We begin by considering the often neglected background issue of statistical power, an issue that can place serious limits on the range of intervention designs that can be realistically considered. We then review traditional intervention designs discussed in the psychotherapy research literature. These designs have been adapted and used in the majority of randomized prevention trials reported in current psychological literature and can be considered to represent current practice. Turning to the statistics literature, we show that these traditional psychotherapy designs can be considered to be special cases of factorial and fractional factorial designs. Insights from the statistics literature are used to refine our understanding of what we can learn from the traditional psychotherapy designs and to address question 1 and question 2 in more depth. We then consider response surface designs that may suggest more sophisticated methods of addressing question 2 (program optimality). Finally, we consider strategies of examining mediation that combine experimental design and correlational approaches, addressing question 3 by providing an understanding of the process through which each component contributes to the outcome.

SOME IMPORTANT BACKGROUND: STATISTICAL POWER

For a randomized trial to be worth doing, it must have adequate statistical power to detect differences among intervention conditions. Following Cohen (1988), norms have been developed in the social sciences defining small, moderate, and large effect sizes as corresponding to a difference between treatment and control groups means of .20, .50, and .80 standard deviation units, respectively. A .80 or higher probability of detecting a specified effect size at $\alpha = .05$ is typically defined as adequate statistical power. Rossi (1990) reviewed articles in the 1982 volume of the *Journal of Consulting and Clinical Psychology* and found that mean power to detect small, moderate, and large effects was .17, .57, and .83, respectively. Other reviewers (e.g., Sedlmeier & Gigerenzer, 1989; West, Newsom, & Fenaughty, 1992) have reached similar conclusions about the power of statistical tests in other areas of psychological research. The implication of these results is that, with the exception of large effect sizes, the probability of detecting true differences between treatment conditions is virtual coin flip or worse in the typical study in psychology.

Many researchers continue to be unaware of the number of participants required to detect differences between treatment conditions with adequate power (see Aiken, West, Sechrest, & Reno, 1990). For example, in a randomized trial comparing an intervention and control group in which there are an equal number of participants in each condition, 52 total participants (n = 26 per cell) would be needed to detect a large effect, 126 participants would be needed to detect a moderate effect, and 786 participants would be required to detect a small effect on the outcome measure with .80 power and $\alpha = .05.$[1] User friendly statistical software (e.g., Borenstein & Cohen, 1988, Woodward, Bonett, & Brecht, 1990) is now available to provide *a priori* estimates of statistical power for commonly used intervention designs.

The work on statistical power holds several intriguing implications for the design of studies of the individual components of interventions. First, moderate to large sample sizes will be required to detect the moderate or small effects that apparently characterize many current preventive interventions (Durlak, Wells, Cotten, & Lampmann, 1993). These sample size requirements have little practical effect on large scale school-based or community-based primary prevention programs;[2] however, such requirements may restrict the complexity of the designs that may be contemplated for preventive interventions addressing more limited populations, notably populations with identified risk factors (e.g., bereaved children; Sandler et al., 1992). Second, initial comparisons of a full, multi-component program with a no treatment control will nearly always yield larger effect sizes than comparisons involving the effect of the inclusion of a single component over and above the effect of other components in an intervention package. Larger sample sizes will be needed in these latter designs to detect small effects. Third, developing efficient designs with contrasts focused on detecting the theoretically most important effects will have more power than omnibus comparisons of several treatment conditions to detect differences when, in fact, they do exist. To the extent such contrasts can be constructed to have equal sample sizes, their statistical power will be further enhanced.

CURRENT PRACTICE: TRADITIONAL PSYCHOTHERAPY RESEARCH DESIGNS

Kazdin (1980, 1986) has reviewed traditional intervention designs from the psychotherapy research literature. Below, we identify and review

---

[1] These sample size requirements can be lowered by design improvements. The inclusion of a pretest measure that has a .5 correlation with the outcome measure in the above example lowers the total number of participants required to 19, 61, and 584 to detect large, moderate and small effect sizes, respectively, with .80 power.

[2] Issues of the proper unit of analysis (Higginbotham et al., 1988; Shadish, 2002) may be raised for many large scale studies since they involve the assignment of units such as classrooms, schools, or communities to intervention conditions. These issues can be addressed through the use of hierarchical linear models (Bryk & Raudenbush, 1992; Kreft, 1992) if outcome data are collected from individual participants. These models adjust for the amount of dependency among cases within each unit, giving proper estimates of treatment effects.

several approaches which have been adapted and used in nearly all randomized preventive trials. The first two of the designs are relatively common, whereas the latter three are currently only infrequently used in published prevention trials. An example of each approach is provided from the prevention literature where possible and from the clinical treatment literature when no instances of the approach could be located.

   1. *Treatment Package Strategy*. In this approach, the effectiveness of the total treatment package is contrasted with that of an appropriate comparison group. For example, Wolchik et al. (1993) randomly assigned custodial mothers sampled from county divorce records to receive either the full intervention program or a delayed intervention (control group) begun after posttest data were collected. The full intervention package consisted of 13 group and individual sessions containing components that addressed each of the areas identified above (see p. 572). Such designs are ideal for determining whether the program works and is worthy of further research. Indeed, Sechrest, West, Phillips, Redner, and Yeaton (1979) have argued strongly for the use of this strategy to test initially what program developers believe is the strongest possible version of the program. However, this design by itself provides little information about the effectiveness of individual treatment components or the processes through which they operate.

   2. *Comparative Treatment Strategy*. In the comparative treatment strategy, two or more alternative interventions are directly compared. An additional no treatment comparison group is often included in the design to enhance the interpretability of the results (Kazdin, 1986). The goal of this strategy is to choose the most effective single intervention from the set of alternative interventions under consideration. For example, Hansen, Johnson, Flay, Graham, and Sobel (1988) randomly assigned 84 school classrooms to receive one of three intervention conditions: (a) the social influences drug abuse prevention program, (b) an affective education program emphasizing stress management, values clarification, decision making, goal setting, and self-esteem building, or (c) no intervention (control). Such comparative designs can identify the most efficacious of a set of interventions as they were implemented in a particular randomized trial.[3]

   Although Hansen et al. compared entire programs, the comparative design can also be applied to compare the effectiveness of potential components of a larger intervention package. When the design is used in this latter

---

[3] More general interpretations about the relative efficacy of the interventions depend on meeting several important assumptions: The interventions should be of equal strength relative to the ideal treatment of that type, be implemented with equal fidelity, and should be expected to affect the same outcome variables (Cooper & Richardson, 1986; Sechrest et al., 1979).

manner, it provides information about the unique effectiveness of each separate individual component. Such information can be useful to program developers in the design of a multi-component intervention package.

3. *Dismantling Strategy*. In the dismantling strategy (also termed the subtraction design) the full version of the program is compared with a reduced version in which one or more components have been eliminated. Criteria for selecting the component(s) to be deleted from the treatment package vary; however, they are often based on theory or other empirical work suggesting that the deleted component(s) may be inert or reduce the effectiveness of the retained components. Component(s) that are expensive or very difficult to deliver may also become candidates for deletion. Dismantling designs often add a third no treatment comparison group to enhance interpretability.

Pentz et al. (1989) provide an illustration of the use of this design to study the effectiveness of combinations of entire intervention packages. They designed a comprehensive community drug abuse prevention program from four component programs: (a) a school-based social influences program as one component (see p. 572), (b) a component training parents in positive parent–child communication skills, (c) a component training community leaders in the organization of a community drug prevention task force, and (d) mass media coverage. The comprehensive program was compared with a reduced, lower cost version that only included components (c) and (d). To the extent that the reduced version of the program produced outcomes that did not differ from the comprehensive program, but did differ from a no treatment comparison group, the researchers would be justified in concluding that the addition of programs components (a) and (b) did not add to the effectiveness of the comprehensive program *over and above* that of the reduced program comprised of components (c) and (d).[4]

4. *Constructive Research Strategy*. In the constructive research strategy, one or more components are added to a base intervention. The base intervention may be a single component or it may be an entire program package. Added components that increase the effectiveness of the base intervention are retained by program developers, whereas those that do not

---

[4] As will be discussed in section below on factorial and fractional factorial designs, this comparison is not informative about the effectiveness of components A, B, or A + B considered alone. The effect of the full program reflects the main effect of each component taken separately plus all possible interactions among the components. The effect of the reduced version of the program only reflects the main effects and interactions among the components that are present in the reduced program.

improve or which decrease effectiveness relative to the base intervention are discarded.

To illustrate, Perri et al. (1988) examined the effects of several components designed to help maintain weight loss in obese adults. All participants received the base intervention, a 20-week behavior therapy program [B]. Participants were then randomly assigned to receive one of four combinations of weight loss maintenance components or a fifth, control condition consisting of no additional maintenance components. The four maintenance interventions examined were (a) bi-weekly therapist contact [C], (b) bi-weekly therapist contact plus a social influence component [S] designed to enhance the participant's motivation, (c) bi-weekly therapist contact plus aerobic exercise component [A], and (d) bi-weekly therapist contact plus social influence component plus aerobic exercise component. Thus, the five conditions of this constructive research study can be described as B, BC, BCS, BCA, BCAS.

Like the dismantling strategy, the constructive strategy can provide information about the effectiveness of adding individual intervention components over and above a base intervention. Indeed, in the minimal versions of these designs that are presently represented in the literature (e.g., comparing an intervention comprised of component A with one comprised of components A and B), the designs can be distinguished only by whether the researchers take A (constructive) or A + B (dismantling) as the base comparison group. The information about the effectiveness of individual components provided by the constructive strategy depends on the theoretical rationale for the selection of components, the number of components that are added in each comparison, and the particular combinations of components that are selected relative to the full set of possible combinations.

5. *Factorial Designs.* Complete factorial designs have long been among the most commonly used designs in laboratory experiments in psychology; they have also attracted modest attention in the psychotherapy research literature (Kazdin, 1980). In these designs, interventions representing all possible combinations of the levels of one component (factor A) and the levels of a second component (factor B) are created. For example, Webster-Stratton, Kolpacoff, and Hollinsworth (1988) randomly assigned parents of conduct problem children to one of four conditions in a 2×2 factorial design: (a) videotape modeling of parenting skills plus group discussion, (b) videotape modeling only, (c) group discussion only, and (d) a waiting list control group. This design permits separate estimates of the effects of the videotape modeling component (factor A), the group discussion component (factor B), and their interaction.

Factorial designs potentially represent a powerful approach to the examination of the separate and combined effects of treatment components.

However, virtually all of the factorial designs in the published literature on intervention trials are limited to 2×2 designs involving the presence vs. absence of two intervention components. The use of factorial designs in the investigation of more complex multi-component interventions would appear to be a natural extension of such previous research. However, as will be discussed in the next section, the complexity of the resulting designs, the difficulty in mounting the large number of treatment combinations, and the large number of participants required for adequate statistical power have thus far limited the use of full factorial designs.

INSIGHTS FROM THE EXPERIMENTAL DESIGN LITERATURE

The review of traditional intervention research designs has provided several insights about how the first two questions posed in the introduction can be addressed. Additional insights can be gleaned from a consideration of new and recycled ideas from the experimental design literature in statistics and in psychology (Box & Draper, 1987; Box, Hunter, & Hunter, 1978; Mead, 1988; Myers, Khuri, & Carter, 1989; Pilz, 1983; Steinberg & Hunter, 1984; Woodward, Bonett, & Brecht, 1990). Two areas are of particular interest. First, we initially limit our consideration to designs in which components can only be included or not included in an intervention package. For these designs the work on factorial and fractional factorial designs allows us to extend and refine the insights from the traditional psychotherapy research literature in answering the first two questions outlined in the introduction. Second, we consider the possibility that the strength of the intervention components can be quantitatively scaled so a range of strengths of each component can be considered. For this case ideas from work on response surface designs that may provide particularly strong answers to question 2.

Factorial and Fractional Factorial Designs

We have previously noted the problem that complete factorial designs in which each component is separately manipulated rapidly become too complex to implement. To illustrate this problem, consider developing a factorial design for the Wolchik et al. (1993) custodial parent-based program for children of divorce which involved five components (see p. 572). Each of the five components would be independently manipulated to be present or absent in the treatment condition. This strategy gives rise to a 2^5 ($2 \times 2 \times 2 \times 2 \times 2$) factorial design with 32 treatment conditions. The design would be analyzed with analysis of variance (ANOVA) giving rise to five main effects (corresponding to the main effect of each separate component), ten two-way interactions, ten three-way interactions, five four-way interactions, and one five-way interaction. Such a design would typically not be practical because of both the difficulty in implementing the large number of intervention conditions and the very large number of participants that would be required to achieve adequate statistical power for the tests of the interactions. Further, the design is likely to be inefficient since researchers almost never have theoretical or empirical expectations that the higher order (three-way, four-way, and five-way) interactions will be significant.

Considerable work in the statistics literature indicates that these complex full factorial designs may be simplified to fractional factorial designs in which only a systematically selected portion of all possible treatment combinations are implemented. Such simplification requires that the researcher be willing to assume that certain effects, typically higher order interactions, are negligible. Indeed, all of the traditional intervention designs from the psychotherapy research literature discussed above can be considered to be special cases of fractional factional or full factorial designs. This fact helps clarify the assumptions underlying the traditional designs as well as providing a basis for suggesting improvements to the traditional designs.

We illustrate the use of three of these simplified fractional factorial designs to investigate three of Wolchik et al.'s (1993) five intervention components: (a) custodial parent–child relationship, (b) discipline strategies, and (c) stressful events. In Table I, we show the combinations of conditions that constitute the design; these combinations are always a subset of the eight (2^3) unique combinations of the complete factorial design that could be created from the three intervention components. In keeping with our focus in this section on designs in which each program component can only be either present or absent in the intervention package, we designate those components that are present in the package with "yes" and those that are excluded with "no." For example, A = yes, B = no, and C = yes means that the custodial parent–child relationship and the stressful events, but not the discipline strategies components were included in the intervention package.

The first example of a fractional factorial design is illustrated in Table I (A). This design addresses question 1, comparing a set of intervention conditions, each comprised of a different single component, with a no treatment comparison group. Note that we have reduced the full factorial design to a comparative treatment design (see p. 576) that contrasts

Table I.

A. Comparative treatment strategy including no treatment control group

Condition	A	B	C
1	no	no	no
2	yes	no	no
3	no	yes	no
4	no	no	yes

B. Constructive research strategy including no treatment control group

Condition	A	B	C
1	no	no	no
2	yes	no	no
3	yes	yes	no
4	yes	yes	yes

C. Two fractional factorial designs that permit main effect estimates

	Block 1				Block 2		
Condition	A	B	C	Condition	A	B	C
1	no	no	no	5	no	no	yes
2	no	yes	yes	6	no	yes	no
3	yes	no	yes	7	yes	no	no
4	yes	yes	no	8	yes	yes	yes

components A, B, and C with a control group. This design provides unbiased estimates of the effect of each component separately, but *only in the absence of any of the other components*. Without making assumptions that all two-way and three-way interactions are negligible, predictions cannot be made about the effectiveness of combinations of treatment components.

A second fractional factorial design is illustrated in Table I(B). This design adds each component sequentially to the treatment package. A no treatment control group is compared with groups receiving only component A, components A and B, and components A, B, and C. This design is identical to the most commonly used version of the constructive strategy (see p. 577) with three components. Recall in this design, each test reflects the contribution of the new component *over and above* the components that are already included. For example, the comparison of the A + B + C intervention with the $A + B$ intervention tests the effectiveness of what component C adds, given that A and B are already present in the treatment package. This design does not provide tests of the unique effect of each component unless it is assumed that the three two-way and one three-way interactions among the components are negligible.

A third fractional factorial design illustrated in Table I(C) is unfamiliar to most intervention researchers in psychology. Two different examples (Block 1; Block 2) of this type of design known as the $2^3 - 1$ design (half fraction; Box, Hunter, & Hunter, 1978) are presented in the left and right halves of Part C of the table. This design provides unbiased estimates of main effects of each treatment component if we assume that all interactions are negligible. Given this assumption, the four conditions in *either* Block 1 or Block 2 provide unbiased estimates of the main effects of each of the three components.

Readers should recognize that the three fractional factorial designs described above answer different questions and have different strengths and weaknesses. Design A provides an answer to question 1 in that it informs us about the unique effects of each component; however, it provides no information about the effectiveness of intervention packages comprised of combinations of the components unless it is assumed that the components do not interact. This deficiency can be partially remedied in the general case by adding a fifth condition to the design, A = yes, B = yes, C = yes. This added condition provides information about whether the sum of the three two-way and one three-way interaction effects is 0.

Design B provides a partial answer to question 2. This design informs us about one specific sequence of building up the intervention components; however, it does not provide information about the effects of individual components unless it is assumed that they do not interact. Further, other non-examined intervention packages (e.g., A = no; B = yes; C = yes) could potentially be even more effective than any of the set of interventions that were examined. There is no guarantee that the set of tested combinations of components will include the program representing the optimal combination of components.

Design C offers a higher level of statistical power in testing question 1 than does Design A. However, its interpretation requires the strong assumption that the components do not interact. An interesting feature of this design is that the two versions illustrated are complementary. If Block 1 of Design C were used in the initial intervention trial and Block 2 were used in a replication, the full factorial design is constituted across the two studies in an economical manner. The Block (replication) effect in this case is unconfounded with all main effects and two-way interactions. If there were a main effect of Block stemming, for example, from the use of a healthier population in study 2 than study 1, the only effect estimate that would be biased is the three-way interaction.

More generally, fractional factorial designs can be constructed to permit economical tests of a specific set of effects of interest given the assumption that all other effects are negligible. For example, if a researcher were interested in testing the main effects of components A, B, and C and the A × B interaction, the five condition design illustrated in Table II provides unbiased tests of each of these effects. Box, Hunter, and Hunter (1978) describe general methods for constructing fractional factorial designs that provide unconfounded estimates of main effects and two-way interactions if higher order interactions are assumed to be zero; Anderson and McLean (1984) provide a cookbook of these designs. These sources should be consulted to develop customized designs that permit tests of the specific effects of interest to the investigator. Many of the designs are very economical relative to the full factorial designs. For example, consider the social influences smoking prevention programs described earlier which has six components. Box et al. (1978) describe a 16 cell design (quarter fraction) that provides unbiased estimates of all main effects all and two-way interactions for six factors, each having two levels, assuming all three-way and above interactions are negligible. This design is distinctly more feasible than the full 2^6 factorial design which requires 64 cells. At the same time, prevention researchers will rarely be able to mount large enough trials to permit even 16 intervention combinations to be investigated. Even these reduced designs can become impractical if several main effects and two-way interactions are of interest.

Comment. Each of the fractional factorial designs adequately addresses a version of either question 1 or question 2. However, since these are not complete factorial designs, additional assumptions must be made in each case to answer more general questions, particularly those involving component combinations not included in the design. If these assumptions are not reasonable, the estimates of effects of interest will be biased because they will be confounded by higher order interactions. This same

Table II. Fractional Factorial Design: Estimates A, B, and C Main Effects and A × B Interaction

Condition	A	B	C
1	no	no	no
2	no	yes	no
3	yes	no	no
4	yes	yes	no
5	no	no	yes

issue applies to the first four traditional intervention designs reviewed in the previous section. Researchers need to be attentive to the possibility that nonzero interactions among components have the potential to alter their conclusions.

The examples of factorial and fractional factorial designs discussed in this section have all involved only two levels of each component. This design decision implicitly makes the assumption that each of the treatment components can only have linear effects on the outcome variable (Aiken & West, 1991). Fractional factorial designs can be extended to address factors having more than two levels (Anderson & McLean, 1984; Box, Hunter, & Hunter, 1978), again at a cost of requiring a large number of intervention combinations.

Dose Response, Response Surface, and Optimal Designs

Another class of potentially useful design approaches is applicable for researchers interested in addressing question 2, if each component can be scaled on a *continuum* of strength relative to the ideal version of the component. This strategy is often followed in drug research in which the outcomes produced by conditions representing three (or more) levels of dosage of the drug (typically including a no dosage placebo control) are compared. For example, Whalen et al. (1987) compared the social behaviors of hyperactive children who had received a placebo, a low dose, or a high dose of methylphenidate. Such designs can identify components that have a optimal strength beyond which further increases in strength lead to either decreases or no further increases in effectiveness.

Sechrest et al. (1979) have proposed that many types of interventions could also be scaled on a dimension of treatment strength and have suggested methods for doing this. To cite a straightforward example, Shure (1988) has argued that a session of her school-based interpersonal cognitive problem solving (ICPS) intervention for young children should be delivered daily for approximately 12 weeks duration to achieve maximum effectiveness. Other researchers have used markedly shorter versions of the program with far less impressive outcomes. An experiment could be designed in which the duration of the program was varied, leading to a dose-response curve relating program duration to outcome. The selection of the levels of the strength of the treatments that are compared would depend on theory or prior empirical work. For example, if researchers expected the dose response curve to be linear and wanted to run four conditions, they might use 0 (no treatment control), 4 weeks, 8 weeks, and 12 weeks. On the other hand, if they had a strong expectation that the curve would be of an exponential form in which the outcome initially increases very quickly followed by a tapering off of the rate of increase with additional sessions, they might consider using 0 weeks, 1 week, 2 weeks, 4 weeks, and 12 weeks.[5] Of course, other cost-related or practical criteria (e.g., what length program is the school willing to consider?) could be used in the design of the dose–response intervention trial.

Dose response experiments can also be generalized to more than one dimension of treatment. This generalization requires that each of the intervention components be scaled on a continuum of treatment strength. If we construct several interventions representing a number of combinations of different levels of strength of each treatment component and plot the outcome for each combination, the resulting figure would be known as a response surface. To illustrate the response surface design, imagine that the school-based component now represents only the first component of the ICPS program, which may be administered for varying lengths of time up to 30 weeks. The second component consists of a home-based program in which parents also train their children in ICPS skills for up to 12 weeks. The response surface representing the relation between each possible combination of durations of (a) the school-based component, and (b) the home-based component to the level of the child's outcome on a measure of adjustment can be plotted. Figure 1 represents several *hypothetical* response surfaces. In Fig. 1a, the effectiveness of the home-based program increases linearly with the duration of the program, whereas the school-based program has no effect. In Fig. 1b the duration of both the school-based and home-based programs are linearly and additively related to child adjustment. In Fig. 1c both programs have positive effects when each is presented separately, but they have a negative interaction when combined such that the combined effect substantially is less than the effects of either component when delivered separately. Finally, Fig. 1d represents curvilinear (quadratic) effects such that the maximum effectiveness is obtained for an 18-week school-based component combined with an 8-week home-based component. These hypothetical response surfaces clearly illustrate a few of the complexities that potentially may arise when treatment components are combined in a program.

---

[5] If the program content is generally uniform, repeated measures designs provide more efficient estimates of the dose response curve. However, if the program involves several sequential phases with the duration of the program being determined by the amount of time spent on each phase (e.g., amount of practice), between subjects designs may be preferable (see Greenwald, 1976). Response surface methods applied to programs with generally uniform content are probably best implemented as mixed between-within designs.

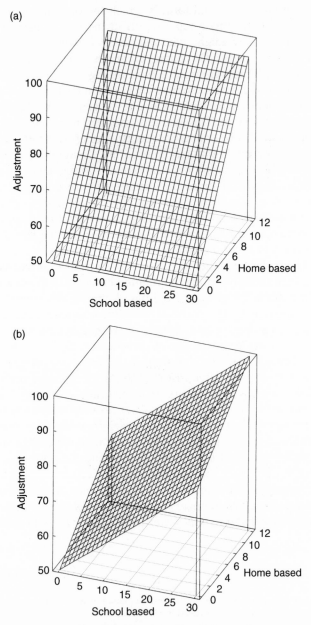

Figure 1. Four hypothetical response surfaces. Each hypothetical response surface represents the level of adjustment of children receiving various combinations of the school-based (0–30 weeks) and the home-based (0–12 weeks) program. (a) represents a linear effect of only the home based program. (b) represents linear effects of both the school-based and home-based programs.

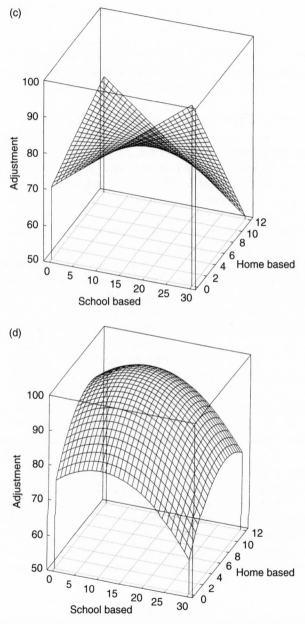

(c) represents a negative interaction between the school based on home-based programs. (d) represents curvilinear effects of both the school-based and home-based programs.

Response surface methodology (Box & Draper, 1987; Myers, Khuri, & Carter, 1989) provides an approach to identifying which combination of components produces the optimum outcome. This approach is also useful for studying the tradeoffs in outcomes that occur when the resources allotted to each program component are varied within an intervention package in which the total duration or the total costs of the program are fixed. As is illustrated by Fig. 1c, conducting separate dose response experiments on each component often may not identify the intervention package that includes the combination of components that produces the maximum outcome. Box, Hunter, and Hunter (1978, pp. 510–513) present an extensive illustration of the limitations of individual dose response experiments in the identification of the optimal combination of components.

Returning to our example, assume that the duration of the school-based (component A) and home-based (component B) components may have linear or quadratic relations to adjustment. Further, the two components may interact so long as the form of the interaction is linear by linear. Under these constraints, the researchers might use the four corners plus central point design illustrated in Table III, which can probe each of these effects. Note that the levels of each of the duration variables listed in Table III are simply called low, medium, and high. If a prior empirical or theoretical basis existed for describing the response surface, then optimal values for the durations of each component in each of the five conditions to maximize the power of the test of each potential effect can be statistically specified (see Atkinson, 1985; Pilz, 1983; Silvey, 1980). In the absence of prior knowledge, the five conditions could be placed at the extreme values for each component (A = 0, B = 0; A = 0, B = 12; A = 30, B = 0; A = 30; B = 12) and the approximate midpoint of the two components (A = 15; B = 6). The response surface can then be plotted, permitting the researcher to provide a preliminary estimate of the combination of levels of components under which the maximum (or minimum) response should occur.[6]

An interesting feature of response surface methodology as it has been applied in engineering and applied biology is that the initial answer is considered to be only preliminary (Mason, Gunst, & Hess, 1987). The statistical theory prescribes methods for designing a sequence of experiments to help pinpoint the combination of levels of the components that produce the maximum point on the response surface (optimum intervention).

---

[6] Researchers studying a positive outcome such as self-esteem or social competence would have interest in the maximum point, whereas researchers attempting to decrease a negative outcome such as symptoms would search for the minimum point. For ease of presentation, we assume the researcher is interested only in the maximum point in our discussion.

Table III. Four Corners Plus Center Design[a]

		A. Duration of cognitive problem solving		
		Low	Moderate	High
B. Duration of parent training	Low	yes	—	yes
	Moderate	—	yes	—
	High	yes	—	yes

[a] Yes = treatment condition is included in design; — treatment condition is omitted from design.

However, given the current stage of development of prevention research, the use of these sophisticated statistical procedures is premature. But, three lessons from response surface methodology are potentially very important. (a) Increasing the strength of a component does not always lead to corresponding increases in effectiveness. Similarly, combining two individually effective components may lead to a program that is either more or less effective than the individual components. (b) Programs can be improved sequentially through refinement of each of the individual components and the study of their combined effects. Development of an optimal program is an evolutionary process. (c) In addition to studying programs whose effectiveness is at the apparent maximum of the response surface, it is also sometimes useful to contemplate interventions representing areas of the response surface that have not actually been studied. If there is a strong theoretical rationale for a specific combination of components and the plotted theoretical response surface appears to be increasing around the particular combination of interest, then there is a reasonable chance that the new combination of components may produce optimal or near optimal effectiveness.

Comment. Response surface methodology is the best method for identifying the optimal combination of a set of treatment components which have been quantitatively scaled. Difficulties may arise in attempting to quantitatively scale many intervention dimensions. In addition, interventions often have multiple outcomes which may vary in their degree of positivity. That is, different packages of intervention components may produce the optimal result on each of several different outcome measures. Or, the outcomes from different treatment packages may differ over time with intervention A showing the best result at immediate posttest, whereas intervention B produces the best result at 1-year followup. Such issues can be addressed by selecting the single most important criterion of outcome, by defining a single aggregate outcome measure, or by choosing a set of weights to represent the importance of each outcome measure (see also Myers et al., 1989). Although the most sophisticated applications of response surface methodology are beyond the current stage of development of prevention research, many of the concepts from this methodology provide presently useful design insights. For example, the Four Corners plus Center design shown in Table III offers a good initial picture of a variety of response surfaces including all those depicted in Fig. 1. The concept of the evolution of designs based on prior theory and data permits us to fine tune a program to achieve optimal effectiveness. These basic concepts underlying response surface methodology have occasionally been used in prevention research with considerable success. For example, Tharp and Gallimore (1979; see also Fienberg, Singer, & Tanur, 1985 for statistical commentary) describe a successful 10-year project in which they developed an early educational intervention program for native Hawaiian school children based on adaptations of several of the fundamental concepts underlying response surface methodology.

MEDIATIONAL ANALYSIS

Mediational analysis provides an economical, but less definitive approach to question 1 than factorial and fractional factorial designs. It also provides an excellent method of addressing question 3, the process through which each component has its influence.

In mediational analysis, the researcher articulates what Lipsey (1992; see also Wolchik et al., 1993) terms a "small theory" that specifies the processes that are targeted by each component of intervention. The relation of each of these processes to the outcome(s) of interest is then specified. Reliable measures of each of the processes (putative mediators) and each of the outcome variables are included in the design. Through statistical techniques such as structural equation analyses the researcher has some ability to probe the contribution of each of the putative mediators to the outcome.

To understand mediational analysis, it is useful to consider initially the case of a simple, one component program. Imagine that a hypothetical training program is expected to improve children's social skills and that these improved social skills, in turn, are expected to reduce the children's level of aggressiveness. Figure 2a depicts this set of relations which represent the small theory of this simple program. The researchers conduct a randomized trial comparing program participants with a no treatment control group. Each child's level of social skills and aggressiveness are assessed after completion of the program.

Following Judd and Kenny (1981a), three conditions must be met to demonstrate that social skills mediated the outcome.

1. The program must cause differences in the putative mediator, here the measure of social skills. This can be tested with a simple two group Analysis of Variance (ANOVA) or equivalently by regression analysis with a binary predictor (intervention, no intervention), which, if significant, shows that the program affected the mediator. The standardized regression coefficient from such an analysis is the path coefficient a in Fig. 2a.

2. The program must cause differences in the outcome, here aggressiveness. Again, this can be tested with ANOVA or with regression analysis, yielding the path coefficient b in Fig. 2b.

3. The links from intervention to social skills to aggressiveness (paths a and c in Fig. 2c) represent mediation. When these paths are controlled,

2a. Mediational analysis for test of small theory.

(1). Condition 1: Effect of treatment on mediator.

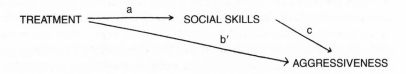

(2). Condition 2: Effect of treatment on outcome.

(3). Condition 3: Complete model with mediational path.

2b. Alternative Model of Program Outcomes (no mediation)

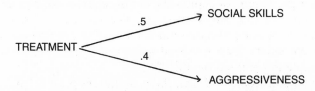

Figure 2. Mediational analysis of small theory of a program.

the magnitude of path b' must be significantly reduced. If path b' does not differ from 0, then social skills may be inferred to be fully mediating the effect of the program on aggressiveness. If the magnitude of path b' is significantly reduced relative to its value (b) in the test of condition 2, social skills only partially mediate the effect of the program on aggression. This result suggests that at least one other mediator that affects the outcome is also affected by the training program. This other mediator may represent other unmeasured skills taught by the program or other unmeasured effects such as the child's relationship with the intervenor. This third condition can be tested using multiple regression or structural equation modeling (see Baron & Kenny, 1986).

Conditions 1 and 2 are straightforward and have long been tested by researchers with mediational hypotheses. A few researchers have also tested what may appear to be an alternative to condition 3, namely that the putative mediator must be correlated with the outcome variable. This condition, in fact, must hold true if mediation is taking place. However, results in which mediation is *not* taking place can also meet this alternative condition. To illustrate, consider the result depicted in Fig. 2d in which the program has two *independent* effects: an increase in social skills and a decrease in aggression. This result passes conditions 1 and 2. Further, since social skills and aggression share the common third variable of program status, they will be correlated: $r = .20$ in this example (see Duncan, 1975). Only by imposing condition 3 can we rule out this and some other possibilities that are not consistent with the small theory of the program.

Mediational analysis is illustrated in a study by Harackiewitz, Sansone, Blair, Epstein, and Manderlink (1987) who compared the effectiveness of four smoking cessation program packages: (a) nicotine gum plus a self-help manual with an intrinsic motivational orientation; (b) nicotine gum plus a self-help manual with an extrinsic motivational orientation; (c) intrinsic self-help manual only; (d) a brief booklet containing tips for stopping smoking (control). Measures of one putative mediator, attributions for success or failure in quitting smoking, were collected 6-weeks after intake; follow-up measures of smoking status were collected at regular intervals up to 1 year after intake. The results were consistent with Judd and Kenny's (1981a) three conditions and suggested that intrinsic attributions for success partially mediated successful maintenance of nonsmoking status.[7]

---

[7] Complications in this conclusion arise because of the focus of the analysis only on those participants who had successfully quit 6 weeks after intake and the nature of the outcome measures (smoker vs. nonsmoker; duration of nonsmoking status [time to failure]). The latter problem can be addressed through the use of alternative analysis strategies to test conditions 2 and 3 (see MacKinnon & Dwyer, 1993).

The extension of mediational analysis to multiple component intervention programs raises new issues, particularly ones associated with the simultaneous investigation of the effects of more than one putative mediator. The small theory of the intervention typically becomes considerably more complex. Exactly how to apportion variance among competing mediational paths becomes less definitive. The statistical tests of the model also increase in difficulty and the impact of problems in study design or measurement of the mediators becomes more serious.

To illustrate some of these issues, we consider partial data from a trial of the second generation of an educational program originally developed by Reynolds, West, and Aiken (1990) to increase the incidence of screening mammography. In this trial Aiken and West (1993) exposed eligible women to an intervention package that included components designed to influence the participants' *perceptions* of four putative mediators proposed by the Health Belief Model (HBM): susceptibility to breast cancer, severity of breast cancer, benefits of screening mammography, and barriers to screening mammography. Each of these putative mediators, in turn, was expected to influence the participants' intentions to get a screening mammogram. Eligible women ($n = 135$) were assigned to intervention or control groups, and their level on each of the four putative mediating variables and the outcome variable of intentions to get a screening mammogram were assessed immediately after the presentation of the program.

Applying the three conditions of Judd and Kenny (1981a) to these data, we observe the following results (see Fig. 3).

1. In the test of the relations of intervention to the mediators (see Fig. 3a), the intervention package led to higher perceptions of two of the putative mediators, susceptibility to breast cancer, $\beta = .27$, $F(1,132) = 10.80$, $p < .005$, and benefits of screening mammography, $\beta = .27$, $F(1,132) = 10.32$, $p < .005$. Neither perceived severity of breast cancer, $\beta = .04$, nor perceived barriers to screening mammography, $\beta = -.10$, were significantly affected by the intervention.

2. The intervention package led to a significant increase in the outcome variable, intentions to get a screening mammogram, $\beta = .51$, $F(1,132) = 43.99$, $p < .001$ (see Fig. 3b).

Three of the putative mediators, perceived susceptibility to breast cancer, $r = .18$, perceived benefits of screening mammography, $r = .52$, and perceived barriers to screening mammography, $r = -.23$, showed significant relations with intentions to get a screening mammogram. Perceived severity of breast cancer was not significantly related to intentions, $r = -.02$, ns. The results of these initial analyses suggest that perceived susceptibility and perceived benefits are candidate mediators of the effect of the intervention on intentions.

3. To test the third condition proposed by Judd and Kenny (1981a), we constructed the structural equation model depicted in Fig. 3c. In this model the intervention had indirect paths through each of the four putative mediators specified by our small theory as well as a direct (unmediated) path to intentions. In addition to the paths that are depicted, we allowed the errors of measurement between each pair of putative mediators to be correlated. The initial test of the just identified model indicated that *none* of the putative mediators had even a marginally significant ($p < .10$) path to intentions. However, note also that the effect of the intervention on intentions

3a. Condition 1: Effect of treatment on mediators.

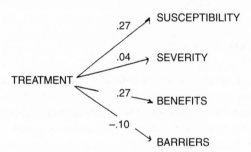

3b. Condition 2: Effect of treatment on outcome.

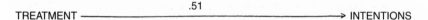

3c. Condition 3: Complete model with mediational paths
   (correlated errors omitted from figure for clarity).

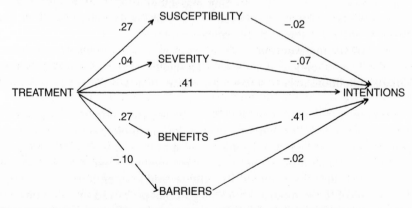

Figure 3. Sequence of models used to examine mediation of outcomes in multicomponent program. Note: Correlated errors between putative mediators are omitted from figure.

3d. Final Reduced Mediational Model

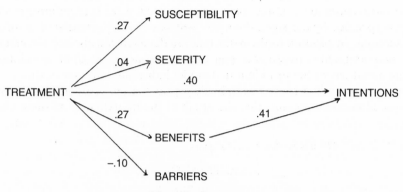

Figure 3. Continued.

was also no longer significant, $\beta = .41$, ns. This result illustrates one complexity that can arise in probing the effects of multiple putative mediators: None of the putative mediators demonstrated a significant path to outcome, yet the effect of the intervention was substantially reduced suggesting that partial mediation may be taking place.

To understand these results further, we tested a reduced model that omitted the four paths from the mediators to the outcome. This model permits only a direct effect of the intervention on intentions. A χ^2 difference test (Bentler & Bonett, 1980) comparing the model depicted in Fig. 3c and this initial reduced model showed that the addition of the paths from the four putative mediators to the outcome improved the fit of the model, $\chi^2(4) = 14.50$, $p = .005$. This analysis suggests that mediation is occurring through the set of measured mediators, but does not identify which of the mediators are accounting for the effect.

To explore this question further, we tested two models in which the path from one of the two candidate mediators (perceived susceptibility; perceived benefits) identified above to the outcome was added to the model. In these models the intervention has its effect on intentions only through the direct path and the single indirect path through the putative mediator under consideration. The chi-square difference tests were $\chi^2(1) = 2.34$, ns for perceived susceptibility and $\chi^2(1) = 13.04$, $p < .001$, for perceived benefits. Of interest, the final reduced model including the indirect path through benefits to intentions depicted in Fig. 3d provided an adequate fit to the data, $\chi^2(3) = 1.46$, ns, CFI = 1.00. The path from perceived benefits to intentions was significant, $\beta = .41$, $p < .05$; and the path from the intervention to intentions to get a mammogram was marginal, $\beta = .40$,

$p < .10$. These results are consistent with an interpretation of partial mediation in which benefits is the only putative mediator that meets all conditions for mediation. However, caution must be exercised in interpreting these results: Other models, for example, involving interactions between program components are *not* ruled out by these analyses.

The above example illustrates the extension of mediational analysis to the probing of multiple potential mediators between the intervention and the outcome variables. Mediational analysis can also be extended to test small theories that propose longer causal chains between the intervention and the outcome variable. For example, Judd and Kenny (1981b) outline a mediational analysis of the Stanford Heart Disease prevention project (Maccoby & Farquhar, 1975) in which (a) mass media and personal interventions were expected to (b) increase knowledge about diet and heart disease. This increased knowledge, in turn, was expected to change (c) participant's dietary behavior, which in the long run was expected to lead to (d) lowered physiological indicators of risk for heart disease (blood cholesterol and triglyceride levels). Although the logic of this extension is straightforward, to the authors' knowledge no examples of the actual mediational analysis of preventive trials expected to operate through longer causal chains are currently available in the literature (but see Aiken, West, Woodward, Reno, & Reynolds, 1994, for an example).

Comment. Mediational analysis provides an economical method for probing the contributions of individual components and the processes through which they operate to produce the outcome. Such analyses have now been used successfully for this purpose in several preventive intervention trials (Aiken et al., 1994; MacKinnon et al., 1991; Wolchik et al., 1993). At the same time, the limitations of this technique need to be clearly recognized.

Mediational analysis as applied in preventive trials is a hybrid between experimental and correlational (structural equation) approaches. Judd and Kenny's (1981a) conditions 1 and 2 are experimental tests whose interpretation is predicated only on the success of the random assignment to the intervention groups. The test of condition 3 is at its heart correlational; its interpretation depends on meeting a number of assumptions associated with the use of structural equation models.

1. Measurement error in any of the putative mediators can bias the results of a mediational analysis. If the "true" mediator is unreliably measured in a simple one mediator model (e.g., Fig. 2), the importance of that mediational path will be underestimated. Measurement error has much more complex effects when measurement error exists in multiple putative mediators in models such as that depicted in Fig. 3c. We are not guaranteed that the direction of bias will be downward (underestimating mediation).

When measurement error exists in one of a set of correlated mediators, then the coefficients of all of the mediators may be biased (see discussions of measurement error in Aiken & West, 1991; Duncan, 1975; Kenny, 1979). This problem can be overcome by the use of structural equation models using multiple indicators of each of the measured constructs (Judd & Kenny, 1981b), though often at a cost of requiring a much larger sample size to achieve proper estimation of the more complex model.

2. A mediational analysis requires the specification of a small theory of the intervention. Mediational analysis presumes that small theory of the intervention is correct and examines the fit of the model implied by the small theory to the data. However, if the small theory is not correct (a condition known as a specification error), biased results may occur. Three potential problems are of special note. (a) The intervention may affect an important unmeasured third variable, which, in turn, causes both the mediator and the outcome. (b) The mediator(s) and the outcome may mutually influence each other (bidirectional causality). (c) The presence of one of the mediators may be a necessary condition for the operation of a second mediator. For example, the mediational analysis presented above based on data from Aiken et al. (1994) indicated that perceived benefits was the only variable that appeared to mediate the effect of the intervention on intentions to get a screening mammogram. However, these results may be misleading; a plausible alternative hypothesis is that women would be unlikely to be motivated to get an expensive screening mammogram unless they also perceived that they were susceptible to breast cancer. The perceived susceptibility component may be a necessary condition for perceived benefits to have its impact.

Each of these three potential problems can lead to serious misestimates of the role of the putative mediators in the model. Techniques for detecting some forms of specification errors in mediational analysis are discussed in James and Brett (1984). Design enhancements discussed below can also address some of these problems.

3. The test of condition 3 may include several putative mediators as well as the intervention in a regression equation predicting the outcome variable, as illustrated in Fig. 3c. Even when the model is correctly specified, multicollinearity among the set of mediators and the intervention will be created, particularly when the intervention has relatively strong effects on the mediators. The mediators and the intervention serve as predictors of the outcome variable in the regression equation; with high inter-predictor correlation there are difficulties in apportioning unique variance to the mediators and the intervention, large standard errors of the path coefficients, and low statistical power for the tests of mediation. Larger sample sizes can help alleviate this problem. Alternatively, the use of factorial or fractional factorial

designs which include intervention components designed to target specific mediators can reduce the multicollinearity among the mediators.

4. Mediational analyses can be extended to investigate several forms of interactions that may occur. Tests of interactions of an intervention with the participant's level on a pretest measure (e.g., initial level of symptoms) can be accomplished with straightforward extensions of the techniques described above (see Baron & Kenny, 1986; James & Brett, 1984 for techniques; Wolchik et al., 1993 for an empirical example). More problematic are two other forms of interactions: (a) interactions between treatment components, and (b) interactions between mediators. These two forms of interactions often cannot be effectively probed when the prevalent treatment package strategy or the comparative treatment strategy designs are used in the randomized trial.

To illustrate, reconsider the hypothesis raised earlier that perceived susceptibility to breast cancer is a necessary condition for perceived benefits of mammography to have an impact on intentions to get a screening mammogram. This hypothesis predicts an interaction between perceived susceptibility and perceived benefits such that perceived benefits will be related to intentions only with perceived susceptibility is high. To the extent the intervention is effective, the level of both these putative mediators will be relatively high in the intervention condition and low in the control condition. This means that there will be few participants for whom perceived susceptibility is high, but perceived benefits are low or perceived susceptibility is low, but perceived benefits are high. The existence of such "off diagonal" cases is absolutely essential if stable estimates of interaction effects are to be produced. Strong tests of such interactions require that additional intervention conditions containing components that target only one of the two mediators be added to the design.

Despite these potential limitations, mediational analysis remains a promising, efficient method of probing the processes through which treatment components exert their effects on the outcome variable. These techniques can be applied to prevention trials involving more than two intervention conditions, multiple mediators, and extended causal chains. Theoretically, these techniques can also be extended to cases in which curvilinear relations among variables are expected. When the assumptions are met, these techniques provide strong tests of the small theory of the intervention and may have the potential to enhance the contribution of intervention trials to basic psychosocial research. Limited techniques exist for investigating the extent to which the assumptions are violated and in some cases for correcting for effects of these violations. In addition, several features may be added in the design of the intervention trial that can help minimize several of these potential problems.

CONCLUSION

At the beginning of this article we raised three questions about the results of trials of multicomponent interventions that are of concern to researchers. Question 1, identification of the influence of each component on the desired final outcome, is best addressed through the use of factorial designs, or fractional factorial designs if certain effects can plausibly be assumed to be negligible. The primary drawback in the application of these designs to interventions with multiple components is that large sample sizes may be required for adequate statistical power if higher order interactions between components are of interest. Question 2, identifying the combination of components that produces the optimal outcome tentatively appears to be best addressed by response surface methodology. Sample size requirements to achieve adequate statistical power may limit the applicability of this approach for multicomponent interactions. Further, the rarity of published examples raises issues about the success with which components can be scaled for treatment strength, a requirement of response surface methodology. Nonetheless, some adaptation of the basic approach of initially estimating the form of a response surface and then investigating that surface through sequential experimental trials would seem to hold considerable promise. Finally, question 3, the processes through which each component achieves its effect on the final outcome, is addressed through the use of mediational analyses. Such analyses require the specification of a small theory of the intervention which is rarely a feature of current reports of intervention trials. However, clear specification of the likely path(s) of influence of each component hold considerable promise for enhancing the basic science contribution of the results of intervention trials. Mediational analyses do have important potential limitations because of their correlational base, but many of these features can be addressed through focused analyses (e.g., statistical correction for error of measurement) or design enhancements (e.g., multiple indicators of each construct) to address specific problems.

A theme that clearly underlies nearly all of the topics discussed in this paper is the necessity to articulate clearly the effects that are of interest in both the design and analysis of the intervention trial. The use of only two levels of an intervention in the design strongly presumes that only a linear effect can occur; more than two levels are required to detect curvilinear effects. Similarly, the failure to include higher order (e.g., quadratic) components in regression or structural equation analyses means that only linear effects can be detected. Likewise, many of the techniques discussed in this article make strong assumptions about the nature of the effects of the components that are of interest. If these assumptions are seriously violated, the techniques will yield biased estimates of these effects. At the same time, readers should recognize that the traditional psychotherapy research designs such as the comparative and constructive designs also make strong assumptions that have rarely been articulated by researchers. Interventions representing combinations of components may be more or less than the sum of individually effective components. Researchers need to use the best technique to address their specific questions of interest and to state clearly the assumptions that have been made. However, designs and analyses should be developed to the extent possible to be capable of probing the plausibility of the assumptions that have been made, particularly if they are compatible with other competing theoretical viewpoints (Coie et al., 1993).

Because of space limitations in this article, we have not explored a number of hybrid design and analysis strategies that appear to be promising. One major class of these designs takes advantage of the temporal sequencing of the intervention components, the measurements, or both. For example, the components of multicomponent interventions are often introduced sequentially over the duration of a multi-week program. It may be possible to collect measures of each of the putative mediators and the outcome variable at the point of completion of each program component. Mediational analyses can then be used to probe the effect of each component on the outcome. Additional information about mediation may also be gleaned from analyses using measures of the mediators and outcome collected at the posttest and follow-up measurement waves. However, this strategy is often comprised by the popularity of wait list control designs in many preventive trials which contaminate the control group following the delayed intervention. Finally, designs in which a small subsample of individuals is *randomly* selected for intensive study from each of the conditions in the randomized trial can potentially yield strong information about the processes of change. Although the full range of design and analysis issues have not been outlined for this class of interventive designs, Stone, Kessler, and Haythornthwaite (1991) and West and Hepworth (1991) present discussions of many of these issues in intensive studies of daily experience.

In this article we have presented a number of design and analysis options, many of which have not been widely used in prevention research. Some of these will turn out to be of widely useful, having applications in prevention research beyond those envisioned here. Others may become useful only after some further adaptation or only in limited areas of application. The promise of this class of techniques that examine the role of individual components in prevention research is considerable. These techniques improve the construct validity of our interventions and may enhance the contribution of large scale prevention trials to our understanding of basic psychosocial development. These techniques also identify key program components and the processes necessary to produce favorable program outcomes, increasing our ability to successfully export good programs to new sites. Addressing such worthy basic science and applied science goals is likely to be a new and important focus of the next generation of prevention research.

ACKNOWLEDGMENTS: The first author was partially supported by NIMH Grant P50MH39246 during the writing of this article. The research described in the section on mediational analysis was supported by National Cancer Institute Grant R03-CA46736. We thank Edward Seidman and four anonymous reviewers for their helpful suggestions for revision.

REFERENCES

Aiken, L. S., & West, S. G. (1991). *Multiple regression: Testing and interpreting interactions.* Newbury Park, CA: Sage.

Aiken, L. S., & West, S. G. (April 1993). Outcome evaluation of community based programs to increase mammography screening. In L. S. Aiken and S. G. West (Chairs), Development, Implementation, and Evaluation of Interventions to Increase Mammography Screening: A Symposium. Western Psychological Association, Phoenix, AZ.

Aiken, L. S., West, S. G., Sechrest, L., & Reno, R. R. (1990). Graduate training in statistics, methodology, and measurement in psychology: A survey of PhD programs in North America. *American Psychologist, 43*, 721–734.

Aiken, L. S., West, S. G., Woodward, C. K., Reno, R. R., & Reynolds, K. R. (1994). Increasing screening mammography in asymptomatic women: Evaluation of a second generation, theory-based program. *Health Psychology, 13*(6), 526–538.

Anderson, V. L., & McLean, R. A. (1984). *Applied factorial and fractional designs.* New York: Marcel Dekker.

Atkinson, A. C. (1985). An introduction to the optimum design of experiments. In A. C. Atkinson and S. E. Fienberg (Eds.), *A celebration of statistics: The ISI centenary volume.* New York: Springer-Verlag, pp. 465–473.

Baron, R. M., & Kenny, D. A. (1986). The moderator-mediator variable distinction in social psychological research: Conceptual, strategic and statistical considerations. *Journal of Personality and Social Psychology, 51*, 1173–1182.

Bentler, P. M., & Bonett, D. G. (1980). Significance tests and goodness of fit in the analysis of covariance structures. *Psychological Bulletin, 88*, 588–606.

Borenstein, M., & Cohen, J. (1988). *Statistical power analysis: A computer program.* Hillsdale, NJ: Erlbaum.

Box, G. E. P., & Draper, N. R. (1987). *Empirical model-building and response surfaces.* New York: Wiley.

Box, G. E. P., Hunter, W. G., & Hunter, J. S. (1978). *Statistics for experimenters: An introduction to design, data analysis, and model building.* New York: Wiley.

Bryk, A. S., & Raudenbush, S. W. (1992). *Hierarchical linear models: Applications and data analysis methods.* Newbury Park, CA: Sage.

Caplan, R. D., Vinokur, A. D., Price, R. H., & Van Ryn, M. (1989). Job seeking, reemployment and mental health. *Journal of Applied Psychology, 74*, 759–769.

Cohen, J. (1988). *Statistical power analysis for the behavioral sciences* (2nd ed.). Hillsdale, NJ: Erlbaum.

Coie, J. D., Watt, N., West, S. G., Hawkins, D., Asarnow, J., Markman, H., Ramey, S., Shure, M., & Long, B. (1993). The science of prevention: A conceptual framework and some directions for a national research program. *American Psychologist, 48*, 1013–1022.

Cook, T. D., & Campbell, D. T. (1979). *Quasi-experimentation: Design and analysis issues for field settings*. Boston: Houghton-Mifflin.

Cooper, W. H., & Richardson, A. J. (1986). Unfair comparisons. *Journal of Applied Psychology, 71*, 179–184.

Duncan, O. D. (1975). *Introduction to structural equation models*. New York: Academic.

Durlak, J., Wells, A., Cotten, J., & Lampmann, C. (June 1993). A review of primary prevention programs for children and adolescents. In J. Durlak (Chair), Evaluating Primary Prevention: Programs, Outcomes, and Issues. Symposium presented at the Fourth Biennial Conference on Community Research and Action, Williamsburg, VA.

Fienberg, S. E., Singer, B., & Tanur, J. M. (1985). Large-scale social experimentation in the United States. In A. C. Atkinson and S. E. Fienberg (Eds.), *A celebration of statistics: The ISI centenary volume*, New York: Springer-Verlag, pp. 287–326.

Flay, B. R. (1985). Psychosocial approaches to smoking prevention: A review of findings. *Health Psychology, 4*, 449–488.

Greenwald, A. G. (1976). Within-subject designs: To use or not to use? *Psychological Bulletin, 83*, 314–320.

Hansen, W. B., Johnson, C. A., Flay, B. R., Graham, J. W., & Sobel, J. (1988). Affective and social influences approaches to the prevention of multiple substance abuse among seventh grade students: Results from Project SMART. *Preventive Medicine, 17*, 135–154.

Harackiewicz, J. M., Sansone, C., Blair, L. W., Epstein, J. A., & Manderlink, G. (1987). Attributional processes in behavior change and maintenance: Smoking cessation and continued abstinence. *Journal of Consulting and Clinical Psychology, 55*, 372–378.

Hawkins, J. D., Catalano, R. F., & Miller, J. Y. (1992). Risk and protective factors for alcohol and other drug problems in adolescence and early adulthood: Implications for substance abuse prevention. *Psychological Bulletin, 112*, 64–105.

Higginbotham, H. N., West, S. G., & Forsyth, D. R. (1988). *Psychotherapy and behavior change: Social, cultural, and methodological perspectives*. New York: Pergamon.

James, L. R., & Brett, J. M. (1984). Mediators, moderators, and tests for mediation. *Journal of Applied Psychology, 69*, 307–321.

Judd, C. M., & Kenny, D. A. (1981a). *Estimating the effects of social interventions*. New York: Cambridge University Press.

Judd, C. M., & Kenny, D. A. (1981b). Process analysis: Estimating mediation in treatment evaluations. *Evaluation Review, 5*, 602–619.

Kazdin, A. E. (1980). *Research design in clinical psychology*. New York: Harper & Row.

Kazdin, A. E. (1986). The evaluation of psychotherapy: Research design and methodology. In S. L. Garfield and A. E. Bergin (Eds.), *Handbook of psychotherapy and behavior change* (3rd ed.), New York: Wiley, pp. 23–68.

Kenny, D. A. (1979). *Correlation and causality*. New York: Wiley.

Kreft, I. (August 1992). Hierarchical Linear Models: Potential Applications in Psychological Research. Invited Address at the meeting of the American Psychological Association, Washington, D.C.

Lipsey, M. W. (1992). Theory as method: Small theories of treatments. In L. B. Sechrest and A. G. Scott (Eds.), *New directions for program evaluation* (No. 57). San Francisco: Jossey-Bass, pp. 5–38.

Maccoby, N., & Farquhar, J. W., (1975). Communication for health: Unselling heart disease. *Journal of Communication, 25*, 114–126.

MacKinnon, D. P., & Dwyer, J. H. (1993). Estimating mediating effects in prevention studies. *Evaluation Review, 17*, 144–158.

MacKinnon, D. P., Johnson, C. A., Pentz, M. A., Dwyer, J. H., Hansen, W. B., Flay, B. R., & Wang, E. (1991). Mediating mechanisms in a school-based drug prevention program: First year effects of the Midwestern Prevention Project. *Health Psychology, 10*, 164–172.

Mason, R. L., Gunst, R. F., & Hess, J. L. (1987). *Statistical design and analysis of experiments: With applications to engineering and science.* New York: Wiley.

Mead, R. (1988). *The design of experiments: Statistical principles for practical application.* Cambridge: Cambridge University Press.

Myers, R. H., Khuri, A. I., & Carter, W. H., Jr. (1989). Response surface methodology: 1966–1988. *Technometrics, 31*, 137–157.

Pentz, M. A., Dwyer, J. H., MacKinnon, D. P., Flay, B. R., Hansen, W. B., Wang, E. Y. I., & Johnson, C. A. (1989). A multi-community trial for primary prevention of adolescent drug abuse: Effects on drug use prevalence. *Journal of the American Medical Association, 261*, 3259–3266.

Perri, M. G., McAllister, D. A., Gange, J. J., Jordan, R. C., McAdoo, W. G., & Nezu, A. M. (1988). Effects of four maintenance programs on the long-term management of obesity. *Journal of Consulting and Clinical Psychology, 56*, 529–534.

Pilz, J. (1983). *Bayesian estimation and experimental design in linear regression models.* Leipzig: Teubner-Texte.

Reynolds, K. D., West, S. G., & Aiken, L. S. (1990). Increasing the use of mammography: A pilot program. *Health Education Quarterly, 17*, 429–441.

Rossi, J. S. (1990). Statistical power of psychological research: What have we gained in 20 years? *Journal of Consulting and Clinical Psychology, 58*, 646–656.

Sandler, I. N., West, S. G., Baca, L., Pillow, D. R., Gersten, J. C., Rogosch, F., Virdin, L., Beals, J., Reynolds, K. D., Kallgren, C., Tein, J.-Y., Kriege, G., Cole, E., & Ramirez, R. (1992). Linking empirically-based theory and evaluation: The Family Bereavement Program. *American Journal of Community Psychology, 20*, 491–521.

Sechrest, L., West, S. G., Phillips, M. A., Redner, R., & Yeaton, W. (1979). Some neglected problems in evaluation research: Strength and integrity of treatments. In L. Sechrest and associates (Eds.), *Evaluation studies review annual* (Vol. 4), Beverly Hills, CA: Sage, pp. 15–35.

Sedlmeier, P., & Gigerenzer, G. (1989). Do studies of statistical power have an effect of the power of studies? *Psychological Bulletin, 105*, 309–316.

Shadish, W. R. (2002). Randomized experiments: Rationale, designs, and conditions conducive to doing them. In W. R. Shadish, T. D. Cook, & D. T. Campbell (Eds), *Experimental and quasi-experimental designs for generalized causal inference* (pp. 246–278). Boston: Houghton Mifflin.

Shaffer, D., Philips, I., & Enzer, N. B. (Eds.) (1989). Prevention of Mental Disorders, Alcohol and Other Drug Use in Children and Adolescents. U.S. Department of Health and Human Services, Office for Substance Abuse Prevention, Rockville, MD, DHHS Publication No. (ADM) 90–1646.

Shure, M. B. (1988). How to think, not what to think: A cognitive approach to prevention. In L. A. Bond and B. M. Wagner (Eds.), *Families in transition: Primary prevention programs that work* (pp. 170–199). Newbury Park, CA: Sage.

Silvey, S. D. (1980). *Optimal design.* New York: Chapman & Hall.

Steinberg, D. M., & Hunter, W. G. (1984). Experimental design: Review and comment (with discussion). *Technometrics, 26*, 71–130.

Stone, A. A., Kessler, R. C., & Haythornthwaite, J. A. (1991). Measuring daily events and experiences: Decisions for researchers. *Journal of Personality, 59*, 575–608.

Tharp, R. G., & Gallimore, R. (1979). The ecology of program research and evaluation: A model of evaluation succession. In L. Sechrest and Associates (Eds.), Evaluation studies review annual (Vol. 4). Beverly Hills, CA: Sage, pp. 39–60.

Webster-Stratton, C., Kolpacoff, M., & Hollinsworth, T. (1988). Self-administered videotape therapy for families with conduct-problem children. *Journal of Consulting and Clinical Psychology, 56*, 558–566.

Weissberg, R. P., Caplan, M. Z., & Sivo, P. J. (1989). A new conceptual framework for establishing school-based social competence promotion programs. In L. A. Bond and B. E. Compas (Eds.), *Primary prevention and promotion in the schools*, Newbury Park, CA: Sage, pp. 255–296.

West, S. G., & Hepworth, J. T. (1991). Statistical issues in the study of temporal data: Daily experiences. *Journal of Personality, 59*, 609–662.

West, S. G., Newsom, J. T., & Fenaughty, A. M. (1992). Publication trends in JPSP: Stability and change in the topics, methods, and theories across two decades. *Personality and Social Psychology Bulletin, 18*, 473–484.

Whalen, C. K., Henker, B., Swanson, J. M., Granger, D., Kliewer, W., & Spencer, J. (1987). Natural social behaviors in hyperactive children: Dose effects of methylphenidate. *Journal of Consulting and Clinical Psychology, 55*, 187–193.

Wolchik, S. A., West, S. G., Westover, S., Sandler, I. N., Martin, A., Lustig, J., Tein, J.-Y., & Fisher, J. (1993). The children of divorce intervention project: Outcome evaluation of an empirically based parenting program. *American Journal of Community Psychology, 21*, 293–331.

Woodward, J. A., Bonett, D. G., & Brecht, M.-L. (1990). *Introduction to linear models and experimental design*. San Diego, CA: Harcourt Brace Jovanovich.

2

From Field Experiments to Program Implementation: Assessing the Potential Outcomes of an Experimental Intervention Program for Unemployed Persons

Amiram D. Vinokur, Richard H. Price, and Robert D. Caplan

Demonstrated a procedure suggested by Bloom (1984) to provide estimates for the effects of an intervention on its actual participants compared to global effects on study participants in the intervention group, whether or not they showed up. Analyses were based on data collected in a field experiment that tested a preventive intervention for unemployed persons (Caplan, Vinokur, Price, & van Ryn, 1989). Effect size estimates were two to three times larger for the actual participant group than for the entire experimental group on employment outcomes (e.g., earnings) and mental health (anxiety and depression). Further analyses produced results showing that compared to participants, the nonparticipants achieved significantly higher levels of reemployment at posttests and did not differ significantly from participants on all other outcomes. The results suggest that persons who most needed the intervention and benefited from it were drawn into it through self-selection processes.

Originally published in the *American Journal of Community Psychology, 19*(4) (1991): 543–562.

Ecological Research to Promote Social Change: Methodological Advances from Community Psychology, edited by Tracey A. Revenson et al. Kluwer Academic/Plenum Publishers, New York, 2002.

In field experiments evaluating preventive interventions, nonparticipation of persons who decline to participate at the outset, or later, by not showing up to the experimental treatment, constitutes a serious threat to the validity of the findings. However, in social intervention programs nonparticipation is a commonplace reality. Since nonparticipation is a pervasive reality in virtually every type of social intervention program, field experiments that are used to test the intervention for effectiveness should be designed and evaluated with this reality in mind.

Thus, the analyses of randomized field experiments need to be concerned with three research questions, two of which derive from the fact of nonparticipation. First, there is the fundamental question of the overall global effect of the treatment program. Second, there is the question of the effect of the treatment on those who actually participated in the intervention. An intervention program may have an overall low impact due to high no-show and dropout rates, but its treatment may have very strong effects on those who participate. Third, there is the question of what the intervention program might achieve if fully implemented with its target group, that is, if improved recruitment strategies can produce full participation.

It is important to realize that these are each distinct research questions. Furthermore, the answer to these questions may have both theoretical and practical implications for redesigning and implementing tested interventions. For example, if statistically significant global effects were detected for the program, but only weak effects on the participants, the weak effects on the participants would suggest the need to redesign and strengthen the intervention itself. If, however, the effects of the treatment on the actual participants are shown to be strong, then redesigning recruitment and retention strategies would be indicated. And finally, if full participation is insured by newly designed recruitment and retention methods, the effects of the new intervention cannot be extrapolated on the basis of the results of the earlier test that involved partial participation. The reason is that the effects of the intervention on participants with the earlier recruitment methods and incentives may not be the same as those on the type of individuals who chose not to participate then, but now are successfully recruited. Thus, a valid answer to the third question mentioned above can only be obtained through the testing of the new intervention with full participation.

Standard statistical procedures are available for providing a valid answer to the question of the overall effect of the intervention program by comparing the full experimental condition to the control condition. This comparison unequivocally preserves randomization (Cook & Campbell, 1979) and represents a true experimental design. In contrast, answering the latter two questions is limited to the application of specialized methods that depend on the specific conditions of the field experiment.

The purpose of this paper is to explicate the nature of the problems that nonparticipation poses for answering the second and third research questions, for utilizing the findings of field experiments, and for the implementation of the tested intervention in new settings. Furthermore, using data from a field experiment conducted in our program of prevention research (Caplan, Vinokur, Price, & van Ryn, 1989), we demonstrate how to approach and resolve some of these problems. In particular, we analyze experimental data that include a large percentage of nonparticipants to derive estimates of the intervention's actual effects on those who actually did participate. Finally, we conduct analyses that examine the need for increasing resources to reduce nonparticipation, encouraging a larger proportion of those eligible to take advantage of the program.

The problem posed by nonparticipation of a large proportion of eligible subjects in the experimental test of a social intervention program is twofold. First, nonparticipation seriously threatens the internal validity of the experimental findings. Second, even if the internal validity of the findings is protected, high rates of nonparticipation may drastically restrict the external validity (i.e., the generalizability of the findings). The threat to external validity is a major concern when the levels of participation or the types of persons participating in the experiment are substantially different from what could be achieved when the program is later routinely implemented. In other words, it is not known, and cannot be easily estimated, whether nonparticipants are the type of individuals who would be able to benefit from the intervention as did the original participants. Since the overall effectiveness of an implemented program is dependent on who actually participates, the experimental findings that serve as the basis for the implementation need to be examined with respect to this issue.

The question of how to target the intervention based on who might benefit most can be addressed by comparing the achieved outcomes of the experimental group participants with those of the nonparticipants. If the outcomes of participating individuals are superior to nonparticipants, an argument can be made for the need to increase resources in the implementation phase to reach higher levels of participation. However, if nonparticipants' outcomes are on the same level, or superior to what has been achieved with participants, then it can be argued that the implementation should not aspire to increase rate of participation. Instead, the emphasis should be on using the same methods of recruitment to obtain more participants by having more programs in more locations, but not on intensifying efforts to convince people to participate in order to achieve higher rates of participation in each location.

In the remaining sections we discuss two ways for providing estimates of the experimental effects on the participants in addition to those based on the standard technique of comparing the fully randomized experimental and control conditions irrespective of participation. After demonstrating the application of one of these estimation methods we conduct analyses that address the question of who may benefit more form the intervention.

One way to provide an estimate of intervention effects on participants is based on the construction of a statistical model to predict those who chose to participate and those who declined to participate. Such a predictive model can be constructed and tested using data collected during a pretest from *all* the subjects randomized into the experimental condition. That is, using a multiple regression analysis on the pretest data of the experimental condition, the best predictors of participation can be identified with their respective weights. The model can then be applied to identify the subset of subjects within the control group who would be active participants had they been invited to take part in the intervention (i.e., had they been randomized into the experimental group). More specifically, the multiple regression weights developed from the experimental condition data could be applied to the control condition data to predict the persons most likely to participate in the same proportion as the proportion of participants in the experimental condition. Once this most likely subset of the control group of "would-be participants" is identified, it can be compared with the subgroup of participants in the experimental condition. In the same vein, Heckman (1979) proposed modeling attrition and entering the attrition indicator, assignment to treatment, and their interaction as predictors in a multiple regression equation. The interaction term in this equation represents the net effect of being exposed to the treatment, that is, participation in the intervention program.

The validity of the estimate provided by this method depends on the effectiveness of the modeling; that is, on finding variables that account for a substantial percentage of the variance in participation. In addition, it depends on the extent to which nonparticipants in the experimental group have been treated in the same manner as the control group subjects. If, for example, the control group subjects received an alternative treatment that is hypothesized to produce some effects, this method of estimation cannot be used with any confidence.

Another way to provide a comparison between experimental participants and control group would-be participants is by estimating the latter's contribution of mean score to the total *mean* of the control group using the method suggested by Bloom (1984). Estimating the contribution of the mean of this subgroup to the total mean precludes the need to identify the specific subset of would-be participants in the control group. This method is based on the logic and execution of the randomization procedure, in that the control group is likely to contain the same proportion of persons (with same personal characteristics) who would, if invited to the intervention, be participants as obtained in the experimental group. It is also based on meeting the condition that due to their nonparticipation, the nonparticipants in the experimental group are treated in fundamentally the same way as the control subjects. If the above conditions hold, according to this method, the mean of the control group's would-be participants can be estimated by subtracting the estimated mean of the would-be nonparticipants from the total mean of the control group. This latter estimate of would-be nonparticipants is based on the *known* mean of the nonparticipants in the experimental group. In other words, the known mean of the actual nonparticipants in the experimental group is substituted for the unknown mean of the would-be nonparticipants in the control group. In this subtraction, the appropriate weights need to be assigned to the various means based on known proportion of such subjects in the experimental group. Specifically, if the proportion of participants in the experimental condition is designed by P, we can represent the total mean of the control group as:

Mean of Control Group = P * Mean of Would-be Participants
$+(1 - P)$* Mean of Would-be Nonparticipants

We can then extract the mean of the control group would-be participants from the above formula, and substitute the known mean of the experimental nonparticipants for the unknown mean of the control group would-be nonparticipants. The resulting formula is

Mean of Control Would-be Participants
$=[P$* Mean of Total Control Group
$- (1 - P)$ * Mean of Experimental Nonparticipants$]/P$

Finally, to obtain the effect of the experimental intervention on the participants we subtract the estimated mean of the control group would-be participants from the mean of the experimental group actual participants. (For more details see Bloom, 1984, pp. 228–229.)

The validity of this second estimation method depends only on the two conditions, which are also essential for the validity of the former method, that is, (a) successfully executed randomization, and (b) the extent to which the nonparticipants have been treated in the same manner as the control group subjects. This method, however, does not require and therefore is not dependent on predictive modeling of participation. Since the statistical modeling of participation in our study did not yield an adequate predictive model, we focus our examination on the application of the second method for estimating the effects of participation as offered by Bloom (1984).

The implications of our discussion and analyses are demonstrated using the data from a study conducted by Caplan et al. (1989). In this study, theories of adherence to difficult courses of action and findings from previous survey research on coping with a major life event—job loss—were used to generate a preventive intervention that was tested in a randomized field experiment on a broad cross-section sample of the unemployed. The aim was to promote reemployment in high-quality jobs and to prevent poor mental health and loss of motivation to seek reemployment among those who continued to be unemployed.

METHOD

Since a detailed presentation of the methods is included in Caplan et al. (1989) only brief summaries are provided below.

Sample

Sites of Recruitment. Recruitment took place at four offices of state employment compensation offices in southeastern Michigan. Trained interviewers recruited 1,087 persons into the study.

Characteristics of the Sample. The sample was intended to represent a broad range of unemployed people. It was similar in some ways to the U.S. unemployed population over 16 years of age (U.S. Bureau of Labor Statistics, 1986) and to representative community survey samples of unemployed persons (e.g., Kessler, Turner, & House, 1988). Males constituted 46% of the sample compared to 60% in the community survey and 56% in the U.S. population. Blacks constituted 15% in our study compared to 20% in the community survey and 22% in the U.S. population. The average age was 35.9 years ($SD = 10.6$) and the average education was about 12.9 years ($SD = 1.9$). Similarly, the average age in the community survey was 35.0 years ($SD = 10.5$) and the average education was about 12.0 years ($SD = 2.4$), as it is in the U.S. population.

Method of Recruitment. Respondents were approached while waiting in line at state employment offices and were briefly told about two programs being offered by the University of Michigan on how to seek jobs. One program was described as a 2-week series of morning sessions (the experimental condition); the other was described as a self-guided booklet program (the control condition). Persons were asked if they were interested in participating. Their responses were used to assign them to the conditions listed in Table I.

Control, Experimental, and Refusers Groups. Among persons who said they *were* interested in participating, the interviewer asked whether they preferred the seminar or the self-administered booklet program. To ensure equal motivation to enter one or the other condition, only persons who expressed no preference were randomly assigned to the experimental and control conditions. Those who expressed a preference were sent job search materials and eliminated from the sample. The majority of these persons preferred the booklet program. In addition to the above two groups, a random sample of 190 unemployed persons who expressed no interest and declined to participate in one program or another, henceforth referred to as refusers, were nevertheless asked to fill out the self-administered questionnaires that were used for data collection to assess the various outcomes.

Dropouts and Participants. Among the 752 persons *assigned* to the experimental condition, 440 (nearly 59%) failed to show up for the intervention and are considered in the analyses as nonparticipants. This percentage varied only by about 5% over the course of recruiting 15 experimental groups in a 4-month period during which successively recruited groups were entered into the experimental and control conditions. "Participants," by contrast, were defined as having completed at least 1 of 8 sessions. The mean number of sessions attended by those who showed up was 6.2 ($SD = 2.1$).[1]

Table I. Study Design

Respondent type	Pretest Jan.–June 1986 T_1		Posttests[a] 1.5 months T_2		4 months T_3	
	n	%	n	%	n	%
Control	322	87	281	88	214	67
Experimental	606	81	412	89	414	89
Participants	308	99	282	90	285	92
Dropouts[b]	298	68	130	87	129	86
Refusers	159	84	132	83	132	83
Total[c]	1087	83	825	88	760	81

[a] Of the 1087 Ss, only 938 were sampled to be included in the posttests. A random half of the T_1 dropouts (149 Ss) were not included in the posttests.
[b] Fifty percent of the sample of dropouts from T_1 were selected for follow-up at T_2 and thereafter. At T_2, for example, 130/149 dropout respondents (as opposed to 130/298) for a rate of 87%. The percentages are computed as (number received/number of questionnaires mailed at the wave) × 100.
[c] Based on the number of eligible participants, dropouts (see Footnote *b*), and refusers.

[1] To provide a clear operational definition of nonparticipants, only those who did not show up for the intervention were considered as nonparticipants. The 73 persons who completed between 1 and 5 sessions were included in the participant group. Preliminary analyses showed that the basic findings of the study were not altered by omitting from the analyses the data of these 73 persons.

Timing of Data Collection

Approximately 2 weeks before the intervention began, a self-administered pretest (T_1) questionnaire was mailed to all the respondents. The mailed materials included a $5 bill as payment for completing the questionnaire and a prepaid return envelope. Posttests were, likewise, administered by mail along with similar payments at 4 weeks (T_2) and 4 months (T_3) after the intervention. Finally, data to monitor the intervention's process were collected at the end of training sessions 1, 7, and 8.

Response Rate

Table I presents the number of respondents and the response rates for the study. Of those experimental, control, and refusers group respondents who received a pretest questionnaire, 83% mailed it back. The response rates for those receiving the T_2 and T_3 posttest questionnaires were 88 and 81% of the preceding T_1 pretest, respectively. The reported analyses were based on the subset of persons who had complete data at all three waves. The response rate varied little from subgroup to subgroup, and as indicated in Table I, the rate for the control group was somewhat lower than those for the experimental group only at T_3. This T_3 variation, as described in the results, did not contribute to significant pretest treatment differences.

Treatment Conditions

The experimental condition consisted of eight 3-hour training sessions distributed over 2 weeks, 4 mornings per week. All persons in the experimental condition were mailed an advance $5 incentive to cover transportation costs. Experimental participants were also told that they would receive a $20 payment for completing at least 6 of the 8 sessions and a certificate of participation.

The design for the eight sessions included the application of problem-solving and decision-making processes, inoculation against setbacks, receiving social support and positive regard from the trainers, and learning and practicing job-seeking skills. The intervention sessions were delivered to groups of 16 to 20 participants by male–female pairs of trainers. The sessions covered a wide range of substantive, skill-related topics. The topics included examples and exercises in identifying and conveying one's job-related skills, using social networks to obtain job leads, contacting potential employers, preparing job application and resumes, and going through a job interview.

The control condition consisted of a booklet briefly describing job-seeking tips equivalent to 2.5 single-spaced pages of text. This booklet was mailed to persons after they were randomized into the control condition. The booklet contained useful information, but it was extremely brief, in comparison to self-help paperback books available on job-seeking.

Measures

In most cases, the major construct assessed in the study consisted of multiitem indices. Most of the resultant measures have coefficient alphas in the .70s and .80s. The major dependent variables included reemployment, job-related variables, and measures of mental health such as anxiety and depression. Other relevant measures included economic hardship and valence of work. In addition, assessments of the immediate perception of the process within the intervention provided an indication of the intervention's integrity and strength (Yeaton & Sechrest, 1981). These assessments were based on a composite measure, "Participant Psychological Engagement."

The job-related measures that were included for the reemployed respondents were indicators of the quality of the job such as monthly earning, quality of work, having a job in one's main occupation, and having a permanent (vs. temporary) job. The measures for the unemployed included motivation to seek reemployment and job-seeking confidence.

In this study, reemployment status was determined by a combination of two measures. To be classified as "reemployed" the person had to report working at least 20 hours per week *and* had to characterize the number of hours employed as "working enough." Persons working less than 20 hours per week *and* characterizing that amount "not working enough" were categorized as "not reemployed." Persons who did not clearly fall into either of these categories (14%) were omitted from analyses that include the reemployment measure. This operational definition provides an unambiguous characterization in that the person is coded as employed only when meeting both subjective and objective criteria.

RESULTS

Effectiveness of Randomization

To examine the effectiveness of randomization, the experimental and control group were compared on demographic variables, job-seeking motivation, mental health, and other dependent variables assessed at pretest. There were no significant differences on any of these variables.

Manipulation Checks, Integrity, and Strength of the Intervention

A good indication of the integrity and strength of the intervention was provided by the measures of degree of participant engagement. The high mean scores on these measures, ranging from 3.6 to 4.6 on the 5-point scales, suggested that the intervention process produced trust among the participants and that the participants actively practiced skills and dealt with potential setbacks. Furthermore, the participants found both the trainers and the group attractive and supportive. It thus appears that the intervention was perceived as psychologically and socially positive by the participants.

Comparing the Intervention Effects in the Original Experimental Design vs. Participation

Comparison of the effects of the intervention according to the original randomized assignment with the effects based on participation is provided in Table II. The left side of the table contains the means for the full intact experimental and control group, effect sizes (J. Cohen, 1977), and t tests for the difference between the means. In contrast, the right side of the table contains the data for the experimental subgroup who participated in at least one session, and *estimates* of means and percentages for the control group would-be participants. It also contains effect sizes and t tests for the mean differences. The results are presented separately for those who became reemployed and for those who remained unemployed at Time 2 and 3 posttests. As discussed above, the estimates for the control group would-be participants were produced using the procedure developed by Bloom (1984).[2]

---

[2] To compute the t test statistics for the effects of participation, Bloom suggested using an unbiased estimate of the standard error based on the standard deviations of the control group, the experimental shows, and the experimental noshows with the appropriate weights (Bloom, 1984, p. 229, Equation 6). Because this estimate relies on three parameters and their weights, its own sampling distribution has a large standard deviation; and therefore, it results in an exceedingly conservative and inefficient estimate of the standard error. Consequently, the t tests based on this estimate produce invariably smaller t statistics than those based on the entire sample, even when the degrees of freedom are adjusted to be equal. The unbiased estimate is unreasonably conservative: While the difference between the means of our participants and their counterparts is about twice as large as the difference between the mean of the experimental and control groups, the t statistics for this comparison is much smaller than that for the full groups. To overcome this problem, our calculations of the t tests are based on the standard formula for the t test statistics for difference in means between the shows in the

Effects of the Intervention on Reemployment. These intervention effects are examined by comparing the effect sizes across the left and right side of Table II. This comparison demonstrates clearly that the effects of the intervention were far more dramatic for the participants than might be inferred from the results based on the full experimental design. For example, regarding the percentage of reemployed, the effect size for the participants at T_2 and T_3 is .60 and .48, which is over three times larger than the .15 and .17 for the full experimental design groups. Among the reemployed, at the T_2 1-month posttest, there was a significantly higher level of earnings in the full experimental than the control group, $t(118) = 2.52, p < .05$. By the 4-month posttest, this difference was no longer significant. Furthermore, the percentage of persons who had found reemployment in what they characterized as their main occupation was significantly higher for the experimental group at both T_2 (82% compared to 64%), $t(145) = 2.54, p < .05$, and T_3 (87% compared to 76%), $t(290) = 2.28, p < .05$. The same results appear in the comparisons for the participants (right side of the table) with consistently larger effect size and t statistics. In addition, the comparisons for the participants display statistically significant benefits at both posttests with respect to two additional outcomes. Compared to their control counterparts, the reemployed participants enjoyed better quality of life at work, $t(88) = 2.43, p < .05$ for T_2 and $t(190) = 3.37, p < .01$ for T_3, and were more likely to obtain jobs which were characterized as permanent rather than temporary, $t(91) = 2.91, p < .01$ for T_2 and $t(187) = 2.45, p < .05$ for T_3.

Effects of the Intervention on the Unemployed. Once again, on the right side of Table II, the effects on job-seeking confidence and motivation of the unemployed group were far more pronounced in the comparisons for the participants with statistically significant effects for these variables at T_3, $t(139) = 2.89, t(140) = 2.73$, respectively, both $p > .01$. In comparison to the

---

experimental group and the would-be shows in the control group. The numerator includes Bloom's Equation 4. In the denominator, the unknown standard deviation of the would-be shows in the control group is replaced by the known standard deviation of the entire control group. Similarly, the unknown number of would-be shows in the control group is estimated as the number of cases in the control group multiplied by the proportion of shows in the experimental group. Although our method deviates from the statistical elegance of unbiased estimation, which in this case produces extremely conservative estimates, it provides a more reasonable one. In this study as well as another one conducted by our colleagues (Haney, 1991), each using about a dozen dependent variables, we found that the known variances of the three subgroups, the experimental shows, no-shows, and the controls were similar. In each case, even a conservative estimate of the denominator based on the largest of the three variances was still much smaller than the unbiased estimate as suggested by Bloom.

Table II. Means, Effect Sizes, and t Tests for Differences Between Full Experimental and Control Groups and Between Experimental Group Actual Participants and Control Group Would-be Participants in Reemployment, Quality of Reemployment, Job-Seeking Confidence, Motivation, Depression, and Anxiety

Outcome variables	Time	Full experimental and control groups				Experimental actual participants and control would-be participants			
		Experimental	Control	Effective size	$t(df)$	Actual participants	Would-be part.	Effective size	$t(df)$
All subjects									
% Reemployed[a]	T_2	33	26	0.15	1.70(527)	22	-4	0.60	4.86(319)[e]
	T_3	60	51	0.17	1.90(532)	53	29	0.48	4.12(338)[e]
Depression	T_2	1.84	1.91	-0.09	-1.12(630)	1.82	1.97	-0.20	-1.85(383)
	T_3	1.84	1.92	-0.11	-1.30(623)	1.82	2.01	-0.24	-2.19(381)[c]
Anxiety	T_2	1.87	1.88	-0.03	-0.36(630)	1.82	1.84	-0.03	-0.28(383)
	T_3	1.89	1.86	0.04	0.45(622)	1.84	1.74	0.12	1.16(380)
Reemployed subjects									
Monthly earnings ($)	T_2	1461	1084	0.48	2.52(118)[c]	1597	658	1.26	5.58(76)[e]
	T_3	1465	1372	0.10	0.75(263)	1466	1244	0.23	1.49(175)
Quality of life at work[b]	T_2	5.02	4.81	0.20	1.15(138)	5.10	4.58	0.51	2.43(88)[c]
	T_3	4.97	4.75	0.20	1.60(284)	4.94	4.41	0.51	3.37(190)[d]
% in main occupation	T_2	82	64	0.44	2.54(145)[c]	84	40	1.03	4.98(92)[e]
	T_3	87	76	0.28	2.28(290)[c]	85	60	0.67	4.42(192)[e]
% in permanent jobs	T_2	65	53	0.25	1.47(144)	66	36	0.60	2.91(91)[d]
	T_3	71	64	0.15	1.17(285)	67	49	0.37	2.45(187)[c]
Depression	T_2	1.73	1.57	0.24	1.41(146)	1.63	1.26	0.63	3.04(92)[d]
	T_3	1.67	1.78	-0.17	-1.39(289)	1.61	1.85	-0.38	2.52(191)[c]
Anxiety	T_2	1.75	1.61	0.23	1.36(146)	1.65	1.30	0.62	3.03(92)[d]
	T_3	1.71	1.72	0.03	-0.21(289)	1.65	1.66	-0.02	0.16(191)

Unemployed subjects									
Job-seeking confidence	T_2	3.91	3.77	0.17	1.67(379)	4.00	3.82	0.23	1.42(225)
	T_3	3.93	3.73	0.25	1.89(231)	3.96	3.50	0.58	2.89(139)[d]
Job-seeking motivation	T_2	4.92	4.84	0.08	0.73(374)	4.94	4.80	0.13	0.82(223)
	T_3	4.64	4.38	0.21	1.55(231)	4.59	3.90	0.53	2.73(140)[d]
Depression	T_2	1.89	2.01	−0.16	−1.52(377)	1.88	2.16	−0.38	−2.33(223)[c]
	T_3	1.93	2.02	−0.11	−0.86(233)	1.99	2.30	−0.36	−1.84(140)
Anxiety	T_2	1.93	1.97	−0.06	−0.54(377)	1.87	1.90	−0.03	−0.22(223)
	T_3	1.98	1.94	0.04	0.27(232)	1.96	1.87	0.10	0.52(139)

[a] Unemployed and reemployed were coded, respectively, 0 and 1. Tests of significance are based on t test of these codes, which produce results identical to test of differences between proportions.
[b] Quality of life at work (index based on 9 major life domains).
[c] $p < .05$.
[d] $p < .01$.
[e] $p < .001$.

would-be participants, the intervention had the effect of maintaining confidence and a sense of efficacy even in the face of setbacks.

Effects on Mental Health. The comparisons based on the full experimental design did not yield any statistically significant results with respect to mental health indicators such as depression, anxiety, anger, and self-esteem. In contrast, a number of significant differences on these variables, in particular on depression, were revealed in the analyses for the participants. Depression in particular was consistently lower for the unemployed participants at T_2, $t(223) = -2.33$, $p < .05$, and also T_3, $t(140) = -1.84$, $p < .05$, one-tail. Surprisingly, the reemployed participants displayed significantly higher level of depression and anxiety at T_2 than their counterpart controls. However, the direction of this difference was reversed at T_3, with the reemployed participants showing significantly lower levels of depression, $t(191) = -2.52$, $p < .05$.

The overall pattern of results is striking in showing greater and more pervasive effects on the actual participants than on the entire experimental group. This is not surprising since over half of the experimental group received no training at all. With respect to the employment variables presented in Table II, 3 of the 14 comparisons based on the experimental design were statistically significant whereas no more than 1 would be expected by chance. In contrast, when the comparisons for the participants are considered, 11 of the 14 comparisons were statistically significant and with larger effect sizes than those yielded by the full experimental design comparisons. Moreover, using the full experimental design comparisons, we did not find significant differences on any of a number of mental health variables. In contrast, using the comparisons for the participants and their counterpart controls, we found that the participants, reemployed and unemployed, reported significantly lower levels of depression at Time 3. Finally, the pattern of results consistently showed that the comparisons based on the full experimental design produced exceedingly conservative estimates for the effects of the intervention on the participants. The effect size estimates were lower by a factor of two to three times than those produced by the comparisons that focused on the participants and their counterparts in the control group.

Comparisons of Participants with Nonparticipants on the Achieved Outcomes: Who Needs the Intervention Most?

To examine the question of who needs the intervention most, our analyses shifted to comparisons between those who participated in the intervention and those who declined participation. The latter consisted of two subgroups: those persons from the experimental group who did not show up for the intervention and those who expressed no interest in the program at the time of recruitment and are labeled "refusers." Prior analyses found the two subgroups to be very similar, and most importantly, to differ from the experimental participants group in the same way. Consequently, the data from all the nonparticipant subgroups were combined in the ensuing analyses.

In these analyses we sought to examine the following two questions: First, can nonparticipants be identified based on their psychosocial and demographic characteristics? Second, do nonparticipants show poorer outcomes than the participants who were shown to have benefited from the intervention with respect to achieving reemployment and mental health? A positive answer to these questions would suggest the need to intensify recruiting and to identify the subgroups who should be targeted for the intensified efforts.

T tests were computed on the mean differences between the participant and nonparticipant groups. The results of the analyses that focused on reemployment outcomes are presented in Table III.

Compared to the participants, the nonparticipants were younger (34 vs. 40 years of age), $t(449) = 5.72, p < .001$, less educated, $t(447) = 2.11, p < .05$, had lower incomes in the past year, $t(411) = 2.94, p < .01$, reported greater economic hardship, $t(443) = -1.95, p < .06$, and greater confidence in their job seeking skills, $t(445) = -5.06, p < .001$.

In terms of reemployment outcomes, a higher proportion of nonparticipants than participants became reemployed at T_2, $t(379) = -4.04, p < .001$. This difference continued as a trend at T_3, $t(386) = -1.62, p < .10$. However, the nonparticipants who became reemployed at T_2 had lower monthly earnings than the participants, $t(90) = 2.15, p < .05$. Of those who remained unemployed, nonparticipants had lower confidence in their job seeking skills at T_2 than participants, $t(265) = 3.36, p < .001$. The nonparticipants also showed a trend of having lesser motivation for job seeking at T_2, $t(267) = 1.93, p < .10$.

Contrary to expectations, these results suggest that compared to the participants, the nonparticipants were in fact better off at both posttest periods with respect to becoming reemployed. Additional comparisons between these groups on the mental health outcomes failed to produce significant differences. Since nonparticipants are not at greater risk of unemployment or poor mental health than participants, any additional efforts to achieve higher rates of participation by persuading nonparticipants to take part in the intervention may not be justified on the ground of achieving equality of outcomes. Achieving equality can best be served by providing the intervention in more locations to those who select themselves to take part in it.

Table III. Means, Standard Deviations, and t Tests for Differences, Between Experimental Participants and Nonparticipants in Demographics, Quality of Reemployment, Job-Seeking Confidence, and Motivation[a]

Outcome variables	Time	Experimental participants M	SD	Experimental nonparticipants M	SD	$t(df)$
All subjects						
Age (in years)	T_1	40.33	10.67	34.62	10.39	5.72(449)[e]
Sex (M = 1, F = 2)	T_1	1.53	0.50	1.56	0.50	−0.56(447)
Education	T_1	13.18	1.88	12.81	1.84	2.11(451)[c]
Income	T_1	6.13	2.80	5.27	3.12	2.94(411)[d]
Economic hardship	T_1	2.70	1.14	2.92	1.21	−1.95(443)
Work valence	T_1	3.99	0.75	3.95	0.71	0.57(448)
Job-seeking motivation	T_1	4.89	0.96	4.81	1.04	0.79(436)
Job-seeking confidence	T_1	3.42	0.87	3.83	0.84	−5.06(445)[e]
Quality of past work	T_1	4.37	0.87	4.36	1.00	0.01(443)
% reemployed[b]	T_2	19	0.39	37	0.48	−4.04(379)[e]
	T_3	56	0.50	64	0.48	−1.62(386)
Reemployed subjects						
Monthly earnings ($)	T_2	1676	724	1307	733	2.15(90)[c]
	T_3	1501	778	1411	817	0.81(209)
Unemployed subjects						
Job-seeking motivation	T_2	4.05	0.76	3.87	0.80	1.93(267)
	T_3	4.02	0.77	3.96	0.84	0.42(149)
Job-seeking confidence	T_2	5.04	1.02	4.58	1.21	3.36(265)[e]
	T_3	4.55	1.32	4.61	1.29	−0.27(150)

[a] Nonparticipants include no-shows from the experimental group a sample of refusers (those who expressed no interest in participating in either the control or the experimental group).
[b] Unemployed and reemployed were coded respectively 0 and 1. Tests of significance are based on t test of these codes, which produce identical results to test of differences between proportions.
[c] $p < .05$.
[d] $p < .01$.
[e] $p < .001$.

Finally, there remains the question of whether the difference in the achieved reemployment outcomes between the participants and the nonparticipants can be accounted for by differences in their psychosocial and demographic characteristics that were identified at T_1. Although the answer to this question may not suggest new or different recruiting policies, it may highlight the dynamics that contribute to reemployment.

To examine this last question we repeated the above tests of differences between the participant and nonparticipant groups using analyses of covariance. In these analyses, the Time 1 demographic and psychosocial variables that are listed in Table III were entered as covariates. The results of these analyses failed to modify any of the significant differences found before or to produce other differences. Thus, the obtained differences in reemployment outcomes are not the results of the initial differences identified at pretest.

DISCUSSION

The design of field experiments to test the effectiveness of social interventions too often only focuses on the restricted goal of providing internally valid demonstrations of the benefits of the intervention. Even when successful demonstrations are achieved, the implementation of the intervention may be questioned on grounds of external validity, or generalizability. That is, the conditions of the field experiment may not represent those that will prevail for the actual implementation of the preventive program.

Two related problems often arise in field experiments that impede the direct estimation of the impact of the experimental intervention in its field implementation as an intervention program. Both problems derive from the reality of partial or selective participation in the experimental group by those who were randomly assigned to it. In a more fundamental form, partial participation appears when a certain proportion of experimentally assigned participants decline to participate, either at the outset when invited, or, later by not participating in the intervention itself.

At the earliest stage of the implementation of many social interventions, potential participants are offered the opportunity to take advantage of the program. The offer to participate usually includes information on the potential benefits of the program. In deciding whether or not to take part in a program, the candidates weigh the potential benefits of the intervention against the real and potential costs of participation. The real costs involve the time and effort of participation. Potential costs include foregone opportunities.

Depending on the circumstances, the offer to participate is often accompanied by the requirement to share some costs of participation, for example, through registration or other fees, or in contrast, an offer of reimbursement for various costs incurred such as transportation. Participation is then the end result of a complex decision process whereby the various potential and real costs and benefits are considered by the candidate.

Since participation is based on the program's candidates decisions, the wisdom or quality of these decisions determine, at least in part, the usefulness of the preventive program. The most valuable programs are those that attract participants who derive the maximum benefit from their participation while omitting those who are least likely to benefit. Traditional assessments of intervention programs focus on the extent to which participants benefited from the program by comparing them to a control group of nonparticipants. Obviously, a valid comparison requires that participation and nonparticipation be determined by a random procedure, not by candidates' choice. A more comprehensive assessment of the value of a social program must include an answer to the question of whether the program attracts the participants that (a) have the greatest need for improvement, and/or (b) are most likely to benefit from it. If the answer is negative, the value of the program can be enhanced by additional efforts to improve the recruitment of the more appropriate candidates.

When the experimental condition of a tested intervention includes a significant proportion of nonparticipants, special analyses are needed to determine the intervention's effects on those who actually participated, not just the entire experimental group. These analyses attempt to preserve the internal validity of the experimental design and at the same time provide an externally valid estimate of the treatment effects on participants. It is possible to provide such an estimate when certain conditions prevail in the study design and its execution. The most critical condition is the attempt to treat experimental subjects who did not show up, or dropped out of the experiment early, in exactly the same fashion as the control subjects who did not receive the experimental treatment, including collection of follow-up data. If care is provided to insure this requirement, then Bloom's (1984) procedure for estimating the effects of participation should be the method of choice.

However, since in all cases, an offer to participate would have been made to the nonparticipants but not to the control subjects, there is a need to consider the possibility of an interaction effect between offering of the treatment and a personalogical variable. As described in the Methods section, our procedures insured that only respondents who expressed no pre-ference for the experimental or the control condition were recruited for randomization into these conditions. Consequently, it seems implausible that an interaction between offering and personalogical variable influenced our results.

Once the effects on participants are determined, the question of who is in greater need for an intervention, and who can benefit more, participants or nonparticipants, should be addressed. The answers to these questions have implications to allocation of resources for recruitment policies when the intervention is implemented. As noted by Bloom (1984), the usefulness of his method of estimating the effects of participation extends to many circumstances where social programs, agencies, or services prohibit the provision of treatment strictly on the basis of randomization. These circumstances arise when the number of applicants for the program exceeds the number of placements available, but when the administrators of the program insist upon using certain criteria to select applicants for the program. The researcher may then randomly assigned applicants to experimental and control conditions. The agency or program can continue to use their preferred method of selecting applicants for treatment. If the agency or program agrees to restrict their selection to those that were assigned to the experimental condition then Bloom's estimation method can be used. Those who are assigned to the experimental condition but are not selected for treatment should be considered nonparticipants in the same manner as those who become nonparticipants by their own choice. These two types of subjects can be pooled in the analyses as the experimental nonparticipants subgroup.

Using data collected in a field experiment of preventive intervention for unemployed persons (Caplan et al., 1989), this paper applied a procedure suggested by Bloom (1984) to provide estimates for the effects of the intervention on actual participants. Effect size estimates were two to three times larger for the actual participant group than for the entire experimental group on employment outcomes (e.g., earnings) and mental health (anxiety and depression).

Additional analyses compared the achieved outcomes of the participants and the nonparticipants. The results demonstrate that the nonparticipants achieved significantly higher levels of reemployment at posttests and did not differ significantly on all the other outcomes including mental health. Eligible participants appear to engage in effective self-selection processes into and out of the intervention. These self-selection processes drew into the intervention the persons who needed it most. Thus, in implementing interventions with this pattern of results, resources could be better used in replicating the intervention in new sites rather than in making attempts to recruit a larger proportion of participants.

Nevertheless, the self-selection processes are not well understood insofar as they were not identified and measured in the course of our study but remain a subject for future research. The question of whether the self-selection processes *out* of the intervention were also effective in allowing the nonparticipants to maximize their own opportunities and benefits as well could not be answered using our data. An answer to this question requires a greater understanding of the role of psychosocial and demographic variables that contribute to reemployment and psychological well-being, and also requires unique research data on people who initially refuse and are then persuaded to participate.

ACKNOWLEDGMENTS

This article is based on research conducted under NIMH grants #39675 and #2P50MH38330, the latter representing the Michigan Prevention Research Center.

REFERENCES

Bloom, H. S. (1984). Accounting for no-shows in experimental evaluation designs. *Evaluation Review, 8*, 225–246.

Caplan, R. D., Vinokur, A. D., Price, R. H., & van Ryn, M. (1989). Job seeking, reemployment, and mental health: A randomized field experiment in coping with job loss. *Journal of Applied Psychology, 74*, 759–769.

Cohen, J. (1977). *Statistical power analysis for the behavioral sciences*. New York: Academic Press.

Cook, T. D., & Campbell, D. T. (1979). *Quasi-experimentation design and analysis issues for field settings*. Boston: Houghton Mifflin.

Haney, C. (1991). Enhancing social support at the workplace: Assessing the effects of the caregiver support program. *Health Education Quarterly, 18*, 4.

Heckman, J. J. (1979). Sample selection bias as a specification error. *Econometrica, 45*, 153–161.

Kessler, R. C., Turner, J. B., & House, J. S. (1988). The effects of unemployment on health in a community survey: Main, modifying, and mediating effects. *Journal of Social Issues, 44*, 69–85.

U.S. Bureau of Labor Statistics. (1986, July). Current labor statistics: Employment data. *Monthly Labor Review*. Washington, DC: U.S. Bureau of Labor Statistics.

Yeaton, W. H., & Sechrest, L. (1981). Critical dimensions in the choice and maintenance of successful treatments: Strength, integrity, and effectiveness. *Journal of Consulting and Clinical Psychology, 49*, 156–157.

3

Research on the Cost Effectiveness of Early Educational Intervention: Implications for Research and Policy

W. Steven Barnett and Colette M. Escobar

In the last decade, the "cost effectiveness" of early educational intervention has become a familiar argument for the expansion of such services to young children who are handicapped or living in poverty. Indeed, the claim is often broadened to support public provision of universal early childhood programs. At least two reasons are apparent for the popularity of the cost-effectiveness argument: (a) the commonsense appeal of early intervention as an investment in the future, and (b) the positive public response to programs that work and are fiscally responsible. One major purpose of this paper is to provide the information needed to evaluate the cost-effectiveness arguments for early educational intervention. The other major purpose is to introduce psychologists to the methods of cost-effectiveness research so that they may be better equipped to evaluate, and participate in, cost-effectiveness studies. Thus, the core of this paper is a critical review of empirical research on the cost effectiveness of early educational intervention which serves both purposes. A context is provided for the review by the first two sections of the paper which discuss the broader empirical literature on early educational intervention and define economic concepts. In a final section, we offer our conclusions regarding interpretation of the research and recommendations for further research.

Originally published in the *American Journal of Community Psychology, 17*(6)(1989): 677–704.

Ecological Research to Promote Social Change: Methodological Advances from Community Psychology, edited by Tracey A. Revenson et al. Kluwer Academic/Plenum Publishers, New York, 2002.

OVERVIEW OF EFFICACY RESEARCH

Research on the effects of early educational intervention can usefully be divided into short-term and long-term studies, where short-term is defined as less than 24 months of follow-up beyond the intervention period. There are well over 100 short-term studies of early educational intervention for children from low-income families. Only a handful of studies explore long-term effects. With so many short-term studies, one practical approach to a comprehensive review is meta-analysis. In brief, a meta-analysis is conducted by obtaining all studies or a representative sample of studies on a topic, converting the findings of each study to a common metric, coding variables for the characteristics of studies that might have affected the results (e.g., age of children, type of treatment, type of outcome, design, statistical method), and then using statistical analyses to summarize study findings and to explore relationships between findings and study characteristics (Glass, 1976).

Recently, two meta-analyses were conducted on early educational intervention (McKey et al., 1985; White & Casto, 1985). The most basic finding of these meta-analyses is that a variety of types of programs in a wide range of settings have produced meaningful short-term improvements in cognitive, academic, and language abilities. Relatively few studies have examined other types of outcomes such as self-concept, motivation, social competence, and family and peer relationships so that whether effects are generally produced in these domains is less clear. Although more specific conclusions about the relationship of program characteristics such as intensity, duration, and parent involvement have been drawn from the meta-analyses, it is our judgment that the underlying data and procedures used in these meta-analyses cannot support those conclusions. In particular, the simple analyses performed seem to run a high risk of confounding the effects of program characteristics with each other and with sample characteristics, and some of the operational measures of program characteristics are misleading at best. Limitations of the meta-analyses have been discussed at length elsewhere (Dunst & Snyder, 1986; Gamble & Zigler, 1989; Schweinhart & Weikart, 1986; Strain & Smith, 1986).

The much smaller number of long-term studies can be found in reviews by the Consortium for Longitudinal Studies (1983); Ramey, Bryant, and Suarez (1985); and Berrueta-Clement, Schweinhart, Barnett, Epstein, and Weikart (1984); and in reports by Copple, Cline, and Smith (1987); and Lally, Mangione, and Honig (1987). The Consortium's review is actually an extremely detailed meta-analysis that includes seven of the best known long-term preschool education studies. As with most longitudinal field studies, design issues and attrition make interpretation of the findings difficult.

In general, a variety of preschool education programs for disadvantaged children appear to have produced persistent effects on school success, although the precise effects vary from study to study. Some studies have found effects on non-school outcomes such as delinquency and employment. These persistent effects have been the basis for research on the cost effectiveness of early educational intervention. In the remainder of this paper, our concern is with studies to which economic analysis has been applied. Readers interested in the more general literature on long-term effects should consult the sources cited above.

INTRODUCTION TO ECONOMIC ANALYSIS

Although we have followed the ordinary language convention and referred to the cost effectiveness of early educational intervention, the convention in economics is to use the term "economic efficiency." Roughly speaking, an educational program is economically efficient if the value of its benefits exceeds its costs. One program is more efficient than another if its benefits net of costs are greater. The tools most commonly used to determine if a program is economically efficient or to determine which of several programs is the most efficient are cost–benefit analysis (CBA) and cost-effectiveness analysis (CEA). In CBA, all program outcomes—costs and effects—are translated into dollars. If a program is economically efficient, the value of benefits minus costs will be positive. In CEA, the value of costs is estimated in dollars, but one or more program effects are not translated into dollars. Obviously, it is more difficult to judge the efficiency of a program based upon a CEA. Typically, CEA is most useful for comparing alternative programs that have the same, or very similar, objectives.

The essential rationale for any type of economic analysis is that good decisions about programs require information about effects *and* costs. Some early intervention programs may cost society more than they give back. The most effective early intervention program may be much more costly than a slightly less effective program, offering relatively minor increases in effects for a much higher cost. On the other hand, the least expensive early intervention program may be completely ineffective. These are, of course, efficiency considerations. A secondary rationale for economic analysis is that it provides information about the *equity* of the distribution of program costs and effects. Thus, economic analysis can provide information about who gains and loses from a program, as well as whether the net benefits to society as a whole are positive.

Economic analysis has much in common with the ecological approach to developmental research (e.g., Bronfenbrenner, 1979, 1986), which has been adopted in recent early intervention studies (e.g., Berrueta-Clement et al., 1984; Ramey, MacPhee, & Yeates, 1982). Economic analysis requires the researcher to specify in detail: (a) the alternative "treatments" being studied, (b) the ecology within which the alternatives exist, and (c) relevant environmental interactions. Moreover, the issues of economic efficiency and equity are dealt with from the perspective of society as a whole. Whether or not a program is efficient cannot be determined if one knows only how that program affects the target population. To be complete, an economic analysis must estimate the direct and indirect effects (including costs) of a program on the rest of society.

Like other approaches to research, economic analysis can be methodologically complex and its strengths and weaknesses have been extensively debated. A complete discussion of economic analysis, its advantages and disadvantages, and its rigorous application is beyond the scope of this paper. However, the detailed presentation of the benefit–cost analysis of the Perry Preschool Project (Barnett, 1985a) in the next section serves as an introduction to the application of economic analysis to early intervention studies as well as to convey the study's important findings. The Perry study is focused on because it provides the broadest evidence and most extensive economic analysis to date. For further information, the application of economic analysis to early intervention has been discussed elsewhere (Barnett, 1986, 1988; Barnett & Escobar, 1987), and well-written introductions to the economic analysis of educational and social programs are available (Levin, 1983; Thompson, 1980).

ECONOMIC ANALYSIS OF THE
PERRY PRESCHOOL PROGRAM

The Perry Preschool Project is a longitudinal study of the effects of an early childhood program that was begun with 3- and 4-year-olds in the early 1960s. Its findings through age 19 were reported by Berrueta-Clement et al. (1984). The 123 subjects of the study were children with low IQs from low-income African-American families. Many of the children had IQs that would classify them as mentally retarded, and half of the control group eventually received special education. Thus, the subjects can be considered to come from a disadvantaged population that has many mildly handicapped members, and the study has some relevance to early intervention with handicapped as well as disadvantaged children. As the study has been reported elsewhere, we report only what is needed for our purposes. Readers desiring more detailed information about the program, research design, and findings should consult the reports by Weikart, Kamii, and

Radin (1967), Weikart, Bond, and MacNeil (1978), and Berrueta-Clement et al. (1984).

The Perry Preschool program ran from October to June and consisted of a $2\frac{1}{2}$ hour per day classroom program which met 5 days per week and $1\frac{1}{2}$ hour weekly home visits by the teachers. Children attended the program at ages 3 and 4, except for a small group of children the first year who attented only at age 4. Public school teachers with early childhood and special education training staffed the program. The staffing ratio was 5 to 6 children per teacher. Teachers taught in the morning and conducted home visits in the afternoon. A cognitive-developmental curriculum was used as described by Weikart et al. (1967). All study subjects entered public kindergarten at age 5.

Measurement of Program Effects

The Perry Preschool study employed an experimental design to study immediate and long-term effects. Subjects were assigned in a manner approximating random assignment either to an experimental group that entered the program or to a control group that did not enter the program (Weikart et al., 1978). Analyses indicate that no biases were introduced by incidental initial differences between the groups or subsequent attrition (Berrueta-Clement et al., 1984). Thus, comparison of the two groups can be considered to yield unbiased estimates of the effects of the intervention. A broad range of measures of child development and success has been obtained periodically since the first year of preschool.

The Perry Preschool study found a series of effects stretching from preschool to early adulthood. Some of the most important effects are displayed in Table I. As can be seen, the intervention's effects were pervasive as well as persistent. The intervention's first measured effects were IQ gains for the experimental group at ages 3 and 4. The IQ difference between experimental and control groups began to decline after school entry and ceased to be statistically significant by second grade. Despite the decline in IQ, the experimental group performed better on achievement tests and on teacher ratings throughout the school years and was less likely to be placed in special education (Schweinhart & Weikart, 1980). By the time they were young adults, it was clear that the experimental group was also experiencing nonacademic as well as academic advantages. They were not only more likely to be pursuing higher education but they had higher employment rates and higher incomes, less involvement in crime and delinquency, and a lower incidence of teenage pregnancy (Berrueta-Clement et al., 1984).

Table I. Representative Findings of the Perry Preschool Project

Variable	Experimental	Control	p^a	n
Early childhood				
Postprogram IQ	96	83	<.01	123
Late childhood				
School years in special education	16%	28%	.04	112
Ever classified mentally retarded	15%	35%	.01	112
Adolescence/early adulthood				
Age 15 mean achievement test score	122.2	94.5	<.01	95
High school graduation	67%	49%	.03	121
Postsecondary education	38%	21%	.03	121
Arrested or detained	31%	51%	.02	121
Employed at age 19	50%	32%	.03	121
Receiving welfare at age 19	18%	32%	.04	121
Some savings	62%	48%	.09	120
Median earnings at age 19[b]	$3,860	$1,490	.06	121
Teen-age pregnancies (per 100 women)	68	117	.08	49

[a] Two-tailed p-values.
[b] 1988 dollars.

The Monetary Value of Costs and Benefits

The heart of the economic analysis is an estimation of the program's economic value based on the resources used and estimated program effects. A complete cost estimate was produced based on program records. Annual cost was about $6,900 per child (all figures are reported in 1988 dollars). This cost was calculated based upon the *opportunity cost* of the resources used rather than the *accounting cost*. Opportunity cost is a key concept in economic analysis and refers to the value of a resource in its best alternative use (its true cost to society) rather than what was paid for the resource. In this case, the only significant instance of a difference between opportunity cost and accounting cost was for facilities. The Perry Preschool program operated in a church basement free of charge its first year. A cost was estimated for facilities in that year as well as for the years in which public school buildings were used.

The dollar value of benefits was estimated for effects on child care, elementary and secondary education, postsecondary education, earnings and employment, crime and delinquency, and welfare. The estimated value of benefits was in each case based on observed program effects, although in some cases it was necessary to predict continued benefits beyond age 19.

Just as every day care program can be considered an educational environment, every center-based preschool education program provides some day care. For the Perry program, this was a relatively minor benefit, a few hours each morning, but for other intervention programs it could be more important. The value of each hour of care was estimated based upon what families like those in the program typically paid for comparable care, less than $1.40 an hour. The estimated value of day care to parents was $416 per year.

The economic value of intervention's effects on elementary and secondary education was estimated based on cost-savings that were mostly the result of reduced special education placement. Educational costs were about $9,900 lower per child for the experimental group, despite the experimental group's lower dropout rate and higher educational attainment.

The cost estimates for postsecondary education demonstrated that it is possible to have "negative benefits." Costs of public higher education were about $1,626 per child higher for experimental subjects who were more likely to graduate from high school and enter postsecondary education.

Employment and earnings of the experimental group were found to be higher. Median earnings were roughly $2,400 higher per person through age 19. Obviously, some participants had barely begun their adult careers, and others had postponed work in order to continue their education. The benefit from increased compensation (wages plus fringe benefits) over the balance of the lifetime was estimated to be more than $100,000 per child.

Both self-report data and police and court records on criminal activity, arrest, and imprisonment indicated that crime and delinquency were reduced as a result of the preschool program. Costs to victims and costs to the police, court, and prison systems were estimated for each arrest of a study subject. The estimated cost of crime and delinquency was about $2,600 lower per child through age 20 for the experimental group. Projecting costs beyond age 20 produced an estimate of over $7,400 per child in additional cost reductions over the subjects' lifetimes.

The intervention's effect on welfare was estimated from the subjects' reports of welfare payments at age 19. The estimated effect on annual welfare payments at age 19 was $1,140 per child. The effect of the program on welfare payments beyond age 19 was projected to be about $44,000. As less is known about long-term patterns of welfare assistance than about other patterns over the life-cycle such as earnings, the lifetime welfare cost reductions are the most problematic estimates in the benefit–cost analysis. However, the estimated cost savings to society are only a small fraction of the reduction in welfare payments. Welfare is primarily a shift of resources from one person to another, which has no net effect on society as a whole. Only the administrative cost of welfare is a cost to society as a whole, and that amounts to roughly 10% of the payments.

Aggregation and Interpretation

A summary of the Perry Preschool program's costs and benefits is presented in Table II. Benefit estimates before and after age 19 are presented separately so that the importance of each can be assessed. Notice that the figures in Table II are significantly lower than those cited in the text. The estimates in the text are undiscounted, whereas those in the table are discounted using a discount rate of 5% per year above inflation. Discounting is performed because even inflation-adjusted dollar values from different years are not equivalent in value: Money has an opportunity cost over time. A dollar today can be invested to yield more than a dollar (even without inflation) next year. The discount rate is an estimate of the annual opportunity cost and is used to convert all dollars to their *present value*, which is their value at the beginning of the project, in a procedure that is the inverse of calculating compound interest. Calculation of discounted present value (or use of another approach that makes dollars comparable over time) is critical in economic analysis of long-term investments in order to avoid overstating the value of future benefits relative to program costs.

Table II. Present Value of Costs and Benefits From 2 Years
of the Perry School Program[a]

	Costs and benefits (1988 dollars)[b]		
	To society	To participants	To taxpayers
Preschool program	−12,570	0	−12,570
Custodial child care	773	773	0
School cost savings	5,500	0	5,500
Crime reduction	1,260	0	1,260
Earnings increase	621	466	155
Welfare reduction	50	−499	549
Subtotal to age 19	−4,366	740	−5,106
College costs[c]	−673	0	−673
Crime reduction	1,500	0	1,500
Earnings increase	15,588	12,590	2,998
Welfare reduction	1,075	−10,747	11,822
Subtotal from age 19 on	17,490	1,843	15,647
Total net benefits	13,124	2,583	10,541

[a] Source: Barnett, 1985b.
[b] Discounted at a 5% real rate.
[c] All attended state institutions and most of the cost was borne by the public. Costs to the students could not be estimated, except for "forgone earnings," which are accounted for in the "earnings increase" category.

The bottom line in Table II indicates that the estimated net present value (discounted benefits minus discounted costs) of the Perry Preschool program was positive. Thus, the Perry Preschool program was found to be a sound economic investment for society. It is the kind of investment that requires a long time horizon, however. The investment in 2 years of the program was not completely "paid off" until some years after the participants left school and became adults, although the conclusion that the program was a sound investment requires only about a quarter of the estimated benefits beyond age 19.

Given the difference in costs, it would be valuable to know if 1 year of the program produced essentially the same benefits as 2 years. Unfortunately, the Perry Preschool study cannot really answer this question. Although there was no statistically significant difference in effects between the 1-year and 2-year subjects, the 1-year sample was so small ($n=13$) that the study had little power to detect differences due to the number of years. Information on this issue will have to be obtained from other studies.

Distributional Consequences

Having determined that society as a whole gained, further analysis was directed to the issue of the distribution of costs and benefits from the Perry Preschool program. More specifically, the analysis investigated the distribution to two conceptually distinct groups: taxpayers who paid for the program and participants who attended the program (and their families). The results can be seen in Table II. Most of the present value of the benefits accrued to the taxpayers, and taxpayers' benefits more than justified the program's cost. The participants and their families received relatively small monetary benefits because the primary source of these was increased earnings, and these were largely offset by decreased welfare payments. Welfare is much more important in the distributional analysis than it is in the analysis of efficiency. Participants no longer qualify for welfare and lose the payment. Taxpayers gain the amount of the payment plus administrative costs.

Two significant policy implications arise from the distributional analysis. First, in the Perry Preschool program, it appears everybody was a winner. Both participants and taxpayers come out ahead. Such a program should be very popular politically. Second, the distribution of benefits offers a strong rationale for public funding. There is no economic incentive for families like those in the Perry Preschool study to buy preschool services on their own, because their economic benefits are much less than the cost. The economic incentive for early intervention lies with the taxpayers who receive more than enough economic benefits to make it an attractive investment.

Sensitivity to Assumptions

Every economic analysis requires assumptions about which there is some uncertainty. Extensive analyses were conducted to investigate the effects of departures from key assumptions on the study's conclusions (see Barnett, 1985b). One of the most crucial assumptions in this or any other CBA is the discount rate. The discount rate chosen has a large impact on the results of studies with long-term horizons, and the "correct" discount rate is a matter of endless debate. Thus, net present value was calculated using a wide range of discount rates. Our judgment is that 7% is at the high end of reasonable real (with inflation removed) rates. Others argue that this is too high (e.g., Gramlich, 1981). The net present value of 2 years of the program was positive at real discount rates up to 8%. Obviously, the net present value of 1 year assuming the same benefits except for child care would be positive even at much higher discount rates. Extensive analyses were conducted varying the assumptions used to project benefits beyond age 19. Even major changes that cut earnings estimates in half and eliminate completely other benefits in adulthood did not alter the conclusion that the program was a sound investment. The results of the sensitivity analyses increase the confidence that can be placed in the study's conclusion.

Limitations

Perhaps the most serious limitation of the Perry Preschool CBA was that cost was more completely estimated than benefits. This tends to be true of CBAs of early intervention because the economic value of many benefits is difficult to assess. In the Perry Preschool study, the economic value of some important benefits such as a safe, healthy, and enriched learning environment for young children, early IQ gains, school success, satisfaction with school, and a 40% lower rate of teen-age pregnancy could not be estimated. Other benefits were incompletely estimated. The estimated benefits from reduced crime did not include: the value of increased feelings of safety; reduced pain and suffering by victims; or, decreased expenditures on locks, guards, and other security measures. When weighing a program's value, it is useful to bear in mind those indicators of increased well-being for which monetary values could not be estimated. For the Perry Preschool program, these were hardly trivial.

OTHER ECONOMIC ANALYSES OF EARLY EDUCATIONAL INTERVENTION

Although the economic analysis of the Perry Preschool Project is the most comprehensive of its kind, a number of other studies have explored the economics of early educational intervention. All the economic analyses we could identify from previous reviews and a search of indexes of the literature are listed and described in Tables III and IV. The most interesting of these studies were selected for detailed review. These are also the methodologically strongest studies. The remaining studies and their methodological strengths and weaknesses are discussed more briefly. A well-known study not included in this review is Skeels (1966) Iowa orphanage preschool study follow-up. Although pathbreaking at the time, the economic methodology lacks precision by today's standards, and the study addresses the issue of institutional deprivation as much as preschool intervention.

STUDIES SELECTED

The National Day Care Study (NDCS)

Ruopp, Travers, Glantz, and Coelen (1979) conducted a CEA that examined the relationships between characteristics of child care programs and quality, efficacy, and cost. Direct observation was used to measure the activities of children and teachers in classrooms in order to assess program quality—the link between program characteristics and efficacy. Effects on children were measured by observation of the children's experiences and two standardized tests used to predict school readiness: the Preschool Inventory (PI; Caldwell & Freund, 1980) and the revised Peabody Picture Vocabulary Test (PPVT-R; Dunn & Dunn, 1981). Children in the study were primarily 3- and 4-year-olds. Most were economically disadvantaged, and about 65% were black. The research design consisted of a natural study of 64 centers in Atlanta, Detroit, and Seattle; a quasi-experimental study of a subsample of 49 centers in those cities; and, an experiment with 29 classrooms in Atlanta in which program characteristics were systematically varied and children were randomly assigned to classrooms. Two supporting studies were conducted: A national profile of day care supply was obtained through a survey of 3,100 centers, and an analysis of care for infants and toddlers was performed on a sample of 54 centers.

The major finding of the NDCS was that across all parts of the study manipulable program characteristics significantly affected the quality of

Table III. Characteristics of Studies of Disadvantaged Samples

Study	Sample size	Ages	Research design	Statistical analyses	Completeness of cost analysis
Barbrack & Horton (1976)	29 27 27	4–5	Nonequiv. group	t test	No details given
Barnett (1985b) Weber et al. (1978)	121	3–4	Experimental	Multivariate with pretest and demographic covariate	All program costs; parents' time
Begley & Liston (1975)	200	0–5	1-group pre-post	Mean gains with no statistical tests	Budgeted program costs
Burkett (1982)	166	4–5	Nonequiv. group	ANCOVA with pretest as covariates	Budgeted program costs
Love et al. (1976)	228 237	3–4 3–4	Experimental Nonequiv. group	Multivariate with pretest and demographic covariates	All program costs
Ruopp et al. (1979)	230 1,370 1,600 735	3–5 3–5 3–5 0–3	Experimental Nonequiv. group Natural Natural	Multivariate with pretest and demographic covariates	All program costs; volunteers and donations
Seitz et al. (1985)	36	0–3	Time-lag control matched pairs	t test, chi-square	No details given
Weiss (1981)	114	3–5	Experimental by classroom	ANCOVA with pretest as covariates	No details given

Table IV. Characteristics of Studies of Handicapped Samples

Study	Sample size	Ages	Research design	Statistical analyses	Completeness of cost analysis
Barnett et al. (1988)	39	3–5	Experimental	Multivariate with pretest and demographic covariate	All program costs;parent and volunteer time
Casto and Tolfa (1981)	60 60	0–3 3–5	1-group pre-post	Correlated t test	Program costs except capital and administration
Hutinger (1981)	34	0–3	1-group pre-post	MANOVA reported	Program costs except capital and administration
Liberman et al. (1979)	97	0–21	1-group pre-post	Wilcoxin T & t test	Budgeted program costs
Macy and Carter (1980)	819	>3	1-group posttest only	None	Staff salaries
Rule et al. (1987)	24	2–5	Nonequiv. group	ANCOVA on matched pairs pretest as covariate	Program costs except for capital
Snider et al. (1974)	10	?	1-group posttest only	None	No details given
Stile and Thompson (1982)	8 10	0–3 3–5	1-group pre-post	None	No details given
Stock et al. (1976)	130	0–6	1-group pre-post	t test, actual posttest vs. posttest estimated from pretest	Costs of direct service staff
Taylor et al. (1984)	50	2–4	Nonequiv. group	ANOVA on matched pairs	All program costs; parents' costs; volunteers & donations
Walker (1981)	15	0–5	1-group pre-post	None	Program costs except capital and administration
Weiss and Jurs (1984)	72	2–5	1-group pre-post	t test, actual posttest vs. posttest estimate from pretest	All program costs

care and scores on the PI and PPVT-R. Moreover, the program characteristics with the greatest effects were the least costly to improve. For
preschoolers, smaller group size was consistently related to better quality
and greater gains on the PI and PPVT-R. Teacher–child ratio was not
related to quality or test score gains (with group size held constant), within
the relevant range for the study (1:5 to 1:10). The finding that group size
but not ratio has important effects is curious, and it may reflect aspects of
organization and process that are not necessarily related to group size.
For example, programs that have 2 care-givers with 10 children may be
less likely to have each child consistently assigned to one care-giver than
programs that have 1 care-giver with 5 children. Teacher training in early
childhood education was associated with higher quality care and somewhat greater gains on the PI, but had relatively little impact on cost.
Unfortunately, the costs of the training per se were not included, a significant omission, so that this last finding should be viewed with caution.
It should be noted that training was not necessarily expensive as much of
the variation in the NDCS was accounted for by a short-term program provided by one city. However, much more needs to be known about the
effects and costs of training than is learned from the NDCS.

The study produced several additional findings that depend solely on
the nonexperimental portions of the study. First, center philosophy was
associated with the extent of test score gains by children. Larger gains on
the PI and PPVT-R were observed in centers where children often engaged
in reflective and innovative behavior and in centers with an emphasis on
cognitive development or school readiness. Second, group size and staff
education in teaching young children had especially strong associations
with program quality and test scores in centers serving the most economically disadvantaged children. Third, group size *and* teacher–child ratio
were strongly associated with program quality for infants and toddlers.

Ruopp et al. (1979) demonstrated that cost-effectiveness analysis, at its
best, is not a simple comparison of the effects per dollar spent for two
programs. Program characteristics hypothesized to have significant impacts
on program effects or cost were analyzed through experimental variation
and multivariate statistical analyses that "controlled" for variations in other
program characteristics and child characteristics. The large sample size and
use of multiple approaches that did not rely solely on naturally occurring
variation instill confidence in the internal and external validity of the findings. Attrition was moderate and correlations between attrition and program characteristics were near zero (Travers, Goodson, Singer, & Connell,
1980).

Nevertheless, there are important limitations to the NDCS's generalizability. Most children were economically disadvantaged, and identifiably

handicapped children were excluded from the study. Only center-based programs were studied. The experimental and quasi-experimental evidence applies only to 3- to 5-year-olds. Measures of effects on children were short-term and limited to the PI and PPVT-R. Long-term effects and effects on developmental domains other than cognition and language were not measured. Other studies indicate that short-term effects do not always persist (Consortium for Longitudinal Studies, 1983) and that programs can differ in their impacts across domains (Schweinhart, Weikart, & Larner, 1986).

INREAL (IN-class REActive Language)

Weiss (1981) demonstrated the usefulness of cost-benefit analysis even when benefits can be measured only very incompletely. The subjects were 3- to 5-year-old "language handicapped and bilingual" children attending preschool or kindergarten programs (Weiss, 1981, p. 40). The design matched seven pairs of classrooms on age, sex, bilingual status, socioeconomic background of children, and class meeting time. One classroom from each pair was randomly assigned to the INREAL treatment group. One third of the children from each classroom were randomly selected for pre- and posttesting. The treatment consisted of the placement of an INREAL specialist in each classroom for one school year. INREAL specialists provided language therapy through ordinary classroom activities and tried to avoid singling out children with language difficulties. Specialists served one preschool program in the morning and one or two kindergartens in the afternoon. INREAL specialists received preservice and in-service training.

Language abilities were assessed immediately before and after the school year using an individually administered language screening test (Weiss, 1981, p. 42). The experimental group significantly outperformed the control group on the posttest, with statistical adjustment for pretest differences. In addition, a 3-year follow-up was conducted to assess subsequent special education placement and retention in grade. Sample attrition over the 3 years was a substantial 34%, but did not differ between experimental and control groups. The experimental group experienced less grade retention and fewer and less restrictive special education placements. To examine the economic efficiency of the program, Weiss estimated INREAL's cost and the cost savings from the improved educational placements in the 3-year follow-up period. The estimated cost savings of $2,213 (1988 dollars) per child substantially exceeded INREAL's estimated cost of $356 per child.

Despite the generally high quality of the study, several problems in the economic analysis were found. No information was given regarding the estimation of INREAL's cost. The estimated cost of $356 per child appears sufficient to include only the salaries of direct service staff, implying that actual cost was perhaps 30 to 50% higher. In addition, cost savings occurred over several years but were not adjusted for inflation or discounted. Those adjustments would lower the benefit estimates relative to cost by about 20%. In the case of INREAL, more appropriate estimates of discounted real costs and benefits would probably sustain the conclusion that the program is economically efficient. Furthermore, it is reasonable to suppose that cost savings continued beyond the 3-year follow-up period. Thus, in this case, the failure to discount and adjust for inflation did not lead to the wrong conclusion, but this good fortune cannot be counted on generally.

The INREAL study (Weiss, 1981) indicated that even a modest addition to early childhood education could have meaningful long-term consequences for later schooling. That finding is not evidence of the efficiency of preschool education per se, because all of the children in the study attended a preschool program. The results do suggest that "ordinary" preschool programs could be made more efficient through the addition of programs like INREAL. The population to which the results apply appears to be economically disadvantaged and bilingual 3- to 5-year-olds. The posttest scores of the control group were high enough to cast doubt on their classification as handicapped (Weiss, 1981, p. 43).

Yale Family Support Project

Seitz, Rosenbaum, and Apfel (1985) reported the results of a 10-year follow-up of economically disadvantaged families who participated in the Yale Family Support Project. The intervention focused on parents and provided social services, pediatric care, an educational day care program, and developmental examinations. The intervention program began during the mother's pregnancy and continued until the child was 30 months old. Twenty families expecting their first child were recruited from records of a hospital in a disadvantaged area. Twenty-five families were contacted in order to obtain 20 who would participate. One child was stillborn and another was biologically impaired and so was excluded from the study. One family quit the study during the intervention period. This left a sample of 17 families and 18 children, as one family's second child was included in the intervention. Seitz et al. (1985) have discussed the implications of sample recruitment for generalization.

A comparison group was added to the study after the intervention period was completed, by replicating the procedures used to select the experimental group with birth records from the same hospital 2 years later. Candidate children for the comparison group were matched with children in the experimental group on gender, family income, number of parents in the home, and mother's ethnicity. As with the experimental group, only biologically intact infants were eligible. Twenty-eight families were drawn for the sample in order to obtain 18 families for the comparison group. As children were 30 months old at the time contact was attempted, some had moved and could not be found. Three families declined to participate.

The strategy of replicating sample selection procedures with a later cohort seems better than most alternatives for obtaining a comparison group after a study has begun, but there were several potential threats to validity. The groups had different historical experiences and different rates of loss from the initial sample pool. The experimental group consisted of 17 of 23 eligible families, the comparison group 18 of 28. However, the only empirical evidence of a difference between groups is that the comparison group was economically better off than the experimental when the children were 30 months old. Seitz et al. (1985) speculated that families in the initial sample pool who could not be located may have been the most seriously disadvantaged. An alternative explanation is that the intervention may have led the experimental group to undertake activities like school or training that temporarily reduced employment and income. On balance, we are inclined to believe that the groups were sufficiently similar initially that later differences may be reasonably attributed to the program.

Seitz et al. (1985) estimated program effects 10 years later using a sample of 14 pairs of families for whom there were complete data. They found increased employment and educational attainment and fewer births for mothers in the experimental group. Children in the experimental group had better school attendance and required fewer special education services. No analysis of attrition was reported. Although a complete benefit–cost analysis was not attempted, estimates were reported for program cost and the economic value of some effects. Cost was approximately $26,000 per family (in 1988 dollars) over the program's 3 years. Benefits were estimated for increased employment and decreased special education services. Follow-up year benefits from increased employment were estimated to be about $2,600 per family. Follow-up year benefits from decreased special education accrued only to boys and were estimated to be about $1,400 per boy.

Several issues regarding the economic analysis should be noted. First, it appears that special education cost savings were underestimated by the omission of nonstaff costs. Second, welfare payments were not measured directly, but were assumed based on unemployment. Third, although estimates were adjusted for inflation, none were discounted. Failure to discount seriously affected the comparison of costs to benefits. At a real discount rate of 5%, discounted benefits are one half of the undiscounted figures. Fourth, it was assumed that estimated benefits for the single follow-up year accurately represented the benefits that could be expected every year. That seems unlikely. Special education costs and welfare assistance systematically change over a lifetime. On the other hand, Seitz et al. estimated the value of only two benefits. Other benefits were observed, and some benefits found in other studies were not measured. A full accounting of benefits would have increased the program's estimated economic value. A broader investigation of the economic efficiency of this intervention program would be desirable in future studies.

Home Language Stimulation Study

Barnett, Escobar, and Ravsten (1988) conducted a cost-effectiveness analysis to investigate the economic efficiency of alternative treatments for preschool children with language delays. Forty children were randomly assigned to four groups: a center-based only group, a home-based (parent-delivered) only group, a group that participated in both programs, and a control group that participated in neither program.

The center-based program was conducted in a university-based communication disorders clinic. Sessions were held $2\frac{1}{2}$ hours per day, 4 days per week for 13 weeks (1 semester). Therapy was provided by a certified speech clinician assisted by 11 student aides. All aides were enrolled in a clinic class and had previous course work in language development and phonetics. The center-based program was guided by a pragmatics approach with an emphasis on replicating the natural environment and on the social interaction of language (Ravsten, Behrman, & Nielson, 1986).

In the first 3 weeks of the home-based intervention program parents attended four $2\frac{1}{2}$-hour training sessions. They attended five additional sessions over the remaining 10 weeks. Make-up sessions ensured that all parents completed all the training sessions. The sessions, conducted by a second speech clinician, were designed to enable parents to provide a more stimulating home environment and to incorporate simple therapy techniques into ordinary activities in the home. Pragmatics again provided the guiding philosophy. Parents were given assignments to implement with their children twice each day for 15 minutes. Individual program development and additional "homework" assignments were developed based upon a log of parent–child interaction recorded by each parent. Semimonthly follow-up meetings were held with each parent to address individual needs of the child, review progress, and evaluate goals.

Ten children participated in the combined treatment group, receiving both center-based and home-based interventions. These children participated in each treatment in exactly the same manner as those receiving only one type of intervention program. Nine children (one child was lost prior to pretesting) received no intervention program during the 13 weeks and agreed not to seek services outside of the clinic during that time. In return, they were guaranteed entry to both the center- and home-based programs in the following semester.

The results of the study indicated that the home-based program produced statistically significant improvements in language development as measured by the Preschool Language Scale-Revised (PLS-R; Zimmerman, Steiner, & Pond, 1979) and the Arizona Articulation Proficiency Scale (AAPS; Fudala, 1974). The center-based program demonstrated no significant effects over the controls. The combination of center- and home-based programs was not significantly different in effects from the home-based program alone. Children who received the home-based program had a 4.8-month higher gain than the children in the center-based program, as measured by the PLS-R, and passed approximately 7% more items correctly on the AAPS. A thorough cost analysis was conducted to estimate the value of all resources used by each intervention, including donated resources such as the time and other costs (i.e., opportunity costs) to parents of attending training sessions. The cost of the home-based treatment, including the value of parents' time and expenses, was substantially less than the cost of the center-based treatment. Thus, the home-based intervention was judged to be most economically efficient.

Several limitations of the study are noted. First, the duration of intervention was extremely short. Second, only immediate effects were measured, and measures were limited to the clinic's standard test battery. Third, the center-based program was a language clinic and not a typical preschool program. Fourth, it deals only with children who have mild language handicaps and who do not live in poverty. The parents were all middle class and well educated. The home-based program might not be as successful with other types of children or parents. Nevertheless, the study indicates that there are circumstances when the most expensive early intervention is not necessarily the best.

Home Start

The National Home Start Evaluation (Love, Nauta, Coelen, Hewlett, & Ruopp, 1976) included a cost-effectiveness analysis of that home-based early education program. Low-income, English-speaking families with at least one child between the ages of 3 and 5 were randomly assigned to an experimental group of 240 families that entered a Home Start program or a control group that did not enter a Home Start program until the following year. A third group of 240 Head Start families was used to compare Home Start and Head Start. The Head Start comparison group was naturally occurring, and initial data indicated that Head Start families were economically better off than Home Start families.

Home Start was associated with significant increases in children's school readiness and parents' community involvement at both 7 and 12 months. School readiness was measured by a combination of tests and observation that included the Preschool Inventory and Denver Developmental Screening Test (DDST; Frankenburg, Dodds, Fandal, Kazuk, & Cohrs, 1975). Community involvement was measured by a parent interview. The control group that entered Home Start 1 year later, essentially caught up with the experimental group by the end of a year. Love et al. concluded that there were no practical differences in effects between 1 and 2 years of Home Start. This conclusion was supported whether children entered at age 3 or age 4. Confidence in this conclusion is tempered by attrition of 57% over the 2 years, despite assurances that "serious bias" was not introduced (Love et al., 1976, p. 42).

Few differences were found in outcomes between the Home Start and Head Start groups. As Home Start was less expensive than Head Start, Love et al. concluded that Home Start was at least as cost effective as Head Start. Their conclusion may seem overcautious as the estimated cost of Home Start was 25% below that of Head Start. However, it may not be. In view of the initial differences between Head Start and Home Start samples, and the differences in goals between the two programs, their caution in drawing conclusions about the relative cost effectiveness of Head Start and Home Start seems warranted.

There were three notable omissions in the economic analysis. First, costs and effects were not discounted. Thus, the analysis does not account for the extra year of immediate benefits or the cost of waiting a year for benefits to begin. Second, as recognized by Love et al., there were no estimates of the value of the child care provided by Head Start. Third, there were no estimates of the cost of time required of parents by Home Start and Head Start. Home Start probably required more parent time, and the value of that time was a cost of the program. Although the home visits themselves required only 3 hours per month, parents may have implemented program-related activities with their children at other times. The last two omissions tend to bias the results in favor of Home Start.

The Home Start study was strongest in comparing 1 and 2 years of Home Start. In a comfortably large sample, with an approximation to random assignment, no meaningful difference in effects was found, and 2 years were undeniably twice as expensive as one. The comparison of Home Start to Head Start was much weaker. Head Start and Home Start were complex programs with multiple goals that included providing training, employment, income, and a career ladder for low-income parents. The two programs seem likely to have differed in achieving these other goals. Also, Head Start was a potential day care provider, Home Start was not.

STUDIES NOT SELECTED

Fourteen other studies employed research designs, statistical analyses, or economic methods that, in our opinion, severely limited the potential for valid conclusions. In some cases, they presented conclusions that did not appear to be warranted by the data. These studies are discussed in less detail than the seven studies reviewed earlier. Basic descriptions of the studies are presented in Tables III and IV.

Four studies used nonequivalent comparison group designs. Two had samples composed of economically disadvantaged children (Barbrack & Horton, 1970; Burkett, 1982), and two had samples composed of children with handicapping conditions (Rule et al., 1987; Taylor, White, & Pezzino, 1984). Preexisting differences between the groups resulting from self-selection and program admission criteria posed potential threats to internal validity in all four studies. Interpretation of the results was further limited by small samples. The statistical analyses employed were less than optimal in that they did not attempt to increase precision or reduce bias due to preexisting differences through the use of covariates. Three studies concluded that treatments were equally effective based on the lack of statistically significant differences (Barbrack & Horton, 1970; Burkett, 1982; Rule et al., 1987), but presented no power calculations. One study (Taylor et al., 1984) concluded that treatments differed in efficiency based on differences in effectiveness that were not statistically significant and differences in estimated cost per child as small as 2% ($230).

Finally, only Taylor et al. (1984) described the analysis of costs in detail. Thus, it is difficult to assess the completeness of the cost estimates. We suspect that only Taylor et al. provided complete estimates, whereas the others omitted some elements of cost. For example, it appears the Barbrack and Horton (1970) included only salaries of direct service personnel.

The eight studies that employed pretest–posttest designs with no comparison group and the two studies that employed only a posttest with no comparison group were of highly questionable validity (Begley & Liston, 1975; Casto & Tolfa, 1981; Hutinger, 1981; Liberman, Barnes, Ho, Cuellar, & Little, 1979; Macy & Carter, 1980; Snider, Sullivan, & Manning, 1974; Stile & Thompson, 1982; Stock et al., 1976; Walker, 1981; Weiss & Jurs, 1984). All of these studies measured outcome variables that tend to increase over time without intervention. For example, Begley and Liston (1975) and Liberman et al. (1979) measured family income. Moreover, initially low values on the outcome variables seem likely to have been selection criteria for the samples, producing regression to the mean and related statistical problems. As can be seen from Tables III and IV, these eight studies might have benefited from the use of a wider range of analyses to address issues of selection bias, measurement error, regression to the mean, and repeated measurement (Kenny, 1975; Reichardt, 1979), some of which have been developed relatively recently (Barnow, Cain, & Goldberger, 1980; Heckman & Robb, 1985).

Most of the studies employing one-group designs gave few details regarding cost estimation. The available information indicated that these studies tended to underestimate costs by excluding resources other than direct service staff, such as administrative and support staff, facilities and other capital, and costs borne outside the program budget. None estimated costs to parents, although some interventions required substantial parent time. An exception to the tendency to underestimate program costs was the study by Weiss and Jurs (1984). They described in detail the procedures used to estimate costs, accounted for all public sector costs (including general school district administration, transportation, equipment, and facilities), and adhered to accepted practices for estimating capital costs (Levin, 1983).

DISCUSSION

Viewing all of the evidence on the efficacy of early educational intervention's effectiveness and economic efficiency together, it seems clear that a wide variety of programs "work." (The variety is even greater if we add interventions like the nurse home visitor program studied by Olds, Henderson, Tatelbaum, & Chamberlin, 1986.) There is a great deal to be learned about how programs work, the consequences of differences in the characteristics of programs and the families and communities they serve, and about the economics of programs. A substantial body of evidence of meaningful immediate impacts of early educational intervention on disadvantaged, limited English proficiency, and handicapped children exists. Relatively few studies measure long-term impacts and only one comprehensive long-term economic analysis has been conducted, but the results strongly support the view that early educational interventions for young children in poverty can be sound public investments. The small number of longitudinal studies and methodologically adequate economic studies of highly diverse programs in diverse circumstances presents difficulties for making precise generalizations.

In our view, it is time for research on the economics of early educational intervention for disadvantaged children to move on from "Are early childhood programs economically efficient?" to "How can programs produce the greatest benefits at the lowest cost?" The NDCS (Ruopp et al., 1979) and the INREAL study (Weiss, 1981) were important steps in that direction. The NDCS investigated the links between program characteristics and program costs and child outcomes. Among its most important implications is that an increased emphasis on group size might result in better program outcomes without much increase in cost. Policy making would benefit from research on *why* this might be, however. The INREAL study found that the addition of a language specialist to ordinary early childhood classrooms was highly beneficial to disadvantaged children's success in the early elementary years and more than offset its costs by reducing elementary education costs. These two studies provide excellent models for future research.

Economic research is less well developed with respect to early educational intervention for nonpoor children. Despite a lack of research on the economics of early educational intervention for children with handicaps, policy has moved ahead. Federal law (PL 99-457) now provides strong incentives for states to provide educational programs for handicapped children ages 3 to 5. As with programs for disadvantaged children, the most useful focus for research at this time may be on program inprovement. With respect to early childhood programs for ordinary middle-class children, the situation is quite different. Although some efficacy studies with middle-class children have found some positive effects (e.g., Larsen & Robinson, 1989; Pierson, Walker, & Tivnan, 1984) they have not found the kinds of long-term effects that yield economic benefits in studies with disadvantaged children. This is hardly surprising since middle-class children do not as frequently encounter the serious difficulties experienced by disadvantaged children. If there are economic benefits from early childhood programs for middle-class children, they may be quite different from those for disadvantaged children because the middle-class child's relationship with the social environment is so different.

It should be recognized that economic analysis is an essentially ecological approach to research. From an economic perspective, early intervention studies should investigate the full range of children's development and experience, with an emphasis on real-life outcomes such as educational attainment, delinquency, and teen-age pregnancy, and including potential immediate benefits to health and nutrition. The possibility that health, nutrition, and education may interact has been recognized in research in less economically developed countries and may be relevant to poor children in the United States as well (McKay, Sinisterra, McKay, Gomez, & Lloreda, 1978; Selowsky, 1981).

The economic perspective also emphasizes the extension of research beyond children to families, schools, communities, and the larger society. These larger systems in which children live are directly and indirectly affected by intervention programs and are conditioning factors for program effectiveness. In the economic analysis of the Perry Preschool program, most of the economic benefits derive from long-term effects on elements of the encompassing social systems. It follows that the program's effects depend not only on the program and the children but on the characteristics of the social environment in which they are worked out. Another study with interesting ecological implications is the Yale study, which indicates that a program can provide benefits to both parents and children and suggests that educational improvements for children might follow from improved educational attainment and employment of parents. These studies' findings recommend increased attention to comprehensive interventions that deal with families and to the elementary school experiences of children who receive early intervention.

An example of the ways in which environments can condition program effects is provided by school policies regarding grade retention and special education. Findings of positive effects of early education on either grade retention or special education placement are common (e.g., Consortium for Longitudinal Studies, 1983; Horacek, Ramey, Campbell, Hoffman, & Fletcher, 1987). Across studies, the magnitude of effects on grade retention and special education varies considerably, and there may tend to be an inverse relationship between effects on retention and on special education placement. These findings can be explained by variation in school policies and the ability of schools to substitute between retention and special education placement in dealing with "difficult" students. In a school system without either special education or grade retention, the benefits of preschool education might be considerably less than predicted by existing studies. However, without improved success in educating students, we would expect schools to develop some other way of dealing with difficult students that has its own costs and in which the effects of early educational intervention would be manifested.

For those interested in pursuing economic analysis of early educational intervention, this review finds that the quality of studies could be improved. A lack of familiarity with economic methods seems to have contributed to problems. Specifically, researchers should attend to complete estimation of costs and adjusting for differences in the value of resources over time (e.g., calculating present value). However, the underlying efficacy studies are a source of problems as well. These studies tended to have weak designs, inadequate samples, high attrition, and unimaginative statistical analyses. Increased use of true experiments or approximations to them, larger samples, and greater efforts to hold down attrition would seem prudent. Unfortunately, these decisions are rarely the researcher's alone, and improvements are almost always expensive. Widespread improvements in research methods (apart from statistical technique) may not be possible unless funding agencies can be convinced that they are worth the cost.

Even researchers uninterested in economic analysis per se may find key concepts in economics useful. In particular, the concept of opportunity cost may contribute to a better understanding of the responses of clients to social and educational programs and, thereby, to improvements in the design of these programs. In early intervention, the high dropout rates of programs directed at parents and the difficulty of maintaining substantive parent involvement in programs directed at children are well known. Yet, how often have program sponsors considered how high the costs of participation might be for parents. Just as there is no such thing as a free lunch, there is no such thing as free time. Recent estimates suggest that the costs of parent time from even child-directed interventions is far from trivial (Barnett & Escobar, 1988). If parents do not participate, one reason may be that they feel their time is better spent in other activities. As Barnett et al. (1988) found, it is possible to design highly effective interventions that depend on parents but are sensitive to their opportunity costs. On the other hand, a proposal that parents with children in Head Start be required to contribute time to the program exemplifies the lack of attention to parents' opportunity costs that sometimes occurs in program planning (Borden & O'Beirne, 1989).

Recently, researchers have brought attention to divergences between advocates' claims and empirical findings regarding early educational intervention (Woodhead, 1988; Zigler, 1987). The economic studies reviewed in this paper have figured prominently in advocacy efforts and have been among the most abused. We add our voices to the others who have protested over-generalization of the findings. The programs with evidence of long-term economic benefits are high-quality and high-cost relative to existing Head Start, state preschool education, and child care programs. The consequences of lower quality in public programs for long-term economic benefits are not easily predicted and are as yet uninvestigated. Also, it seems to us that, descriptions of study results in terms like "returning $7 for every dollar invested" may encourage people to believe that research provides a degree of certainty and precision about policies and practice that is unrealistic. It is our view that the information now possessed by the field and the general public is currently out of balance in this regard. It may be difficult to achieve balance without damaging efforts to increase public funding for early childhood programs, however.

In conclusion, we would be disappointed if our review and cautions about the limitations of economic research on early educational intervention were interpreted as dampening enthusiasm for increased public support of early childhood programs for children in low-income families or for children with handicapping conditions. Even with its limitations, the evidence that quality early educational intervention is a sound public investment is far stronger than the evidence that other publicly financed activities such as development and production of the B-2 bomber and other weapons systems, the savings and loan bail out, or the proposed cut in the capital gains tax are economically sensible policies. Moreover, in an era when tensions between equity and efficiency are expected from educational and social programs, a program that promises to reduce inequality and repay the costs to taxpayers should find almost universal support. Our primary concerns are that research findings be used to support programs with a high probability of successful outcomes and that public policies recognize the limits of our knowledge by permitting flexibility in program design and allocating adequate funds for sound research and evaluation so that the efficacy and economic efficiency of programs can be assessed and improved.

ACKNOWLEDGEMENTS

We thank the anonymous referees and the Social Policy Editor for many fine suggestions. Work on this paper was partly supported by funds from the U.S. Department of Education (Contract #300-85-0173) to the Early Intervention Research Institute at Utah State University.

REFERENCES

Barbrack, C. R., & Horton, D. M. (1970). Educational intervention in the home and paraprofessional career development: A second generation mother study with an emphasis on costs and benefits. *DARCEE Papers and Reports* (George Peabody College), *4*(4).

Barnett, W. S. (1985a). Benefit-cost analysis of the Perry Preschool program and its policy implications. *Educational Evaluation and Policy Analysis, 7*(4), 333–342.

Barnett, W. S. (1985b). The Perry Preschool program and its long-term effects: A benefit-cost analysis. *High/Scope Early Childhood Policy Papers* (No. 2), Ypsilanti, MI: High/Scope.

Barnett, W. S. (1986). Methodological issues in economic evaluation of early intervention programs. *Early Childhood Research Quarterly, 1*(3), 249–268.

Barnett, W. S. (1988). Economic analysis as a tool for early intervention research. *Journal of the Division for Early Childhood, 12*(4), 376–383.

Barnett, W. S., & Escobar, C. M. (1987). The economics of early educational intervention: A review. *Review of Educational Research, 57*(4), 387–414.

Barnett, W. S., & Escobar, C. M. (1988). *Determinants of the costs of early intervention* (EIEI Final Report). Logan: Utah State University, Developmental Center for Handicapped Persons, Early Intervention Effectiveness Institute.

Barnett, W. S., Escobar, C. M., & Ravsten, M. (1988). Parent and clinic early intervention for children with language handicaps: A cost-effectiveness analysis. *Journal of the Division for Early Childhood, 12*(4), 290–298.

Barnow, B. S., Cain, G. G., & Goldberger, A. S. (1980). Issues in the analysis of selectivity bias. In E. W. Stromsdorfer & G. Farkas (Eds.), *Evaluation studies review annual* (Vol. 5). Beverly Hills: Sage.

Begley, C., & Liston, J. S. (1975). *Early childhood development programs in Texas: An analysis of benefits and costs.* Austin: Texas State Department of Community Affairs, Office of Child Development.

Berrueta-Clement, J. R., Schweinhart, L. J., Barnett, W. S., Epstein, A. S., & Weikart, D. P. (1984). *Changed lives: The effects of the Perry Preschool program on youths through age 19.* Ypsilanti, MI: High/Scope.

Borden, E., & O'Beirne, K. W. (1989). False start? The fleeting gains at Head Start. *Policy Review, 47*, 48–51.

Bronfenbrenner, U. (1979). *The ecology of human development: Experiments by nature and design.* Cambridge: MA: Harvard University Press.

Bronfenbrenner, U. (1986). Ecology of the family as a context for human development: Research perspectives. *Developmental Psychology, 22*, 723–742.

Burkett, C. S. (1982). Effects of frequency of home visits on achievement of preschool students in a home-based early childhood education program. *Journal of Educational Research, 76*(1), 41–44.

Caldwell, B. M., & Freund, J. H. (1980). *The preschool inventory.* Little Rock: University of Arkansas at Little Rock, Center for Child Development and Education.

Casto, G., & Tolfa, D. (1981). Multi-agency project for preschoolers. In T. Black & P. Hutinger (Eds.), *Cost-effective delivery strategies in rural areas: Programs for young handicapped children.* (Vol. 1, pp. 11–17). (HCEEP Rural Network Monograph.) Macomb: Western Illinois University Press.

Consortium for Longitudinal Studies. (1983). *As the twig is bent ... lasting effects of preschool programs.* Hillsdale, NJ: Erlbaum.

Copple, C. E., Cline, M. G., & Smith, A. N. (1987). *Path to the future: Long-term effects of Head Start in the Philadelphia school district.* Washington, DC: U.S. Department of Health and Human Services.

Dunn, L. M., & Dunn, L. M. (1981). *Manual to the Peabody picture vocabulary test—revised.* Minneapolis, MN: American Guidance Service.

Dunst, C. J., & Snyder, S. W. (1986). A critique of the Utah State University early intervention meta-analysis research. *Exceptional Children, 53*, 269–276.

Frankenburg, W. K., Dodds, J., Fandal, A., Kazuk, E., & Cohrs, M. (1975). *Denver developmental screening test.* Denver: University of Colorado Medical Center.

Fudala, J. B. (1974). *Arizona articulation proficiency scale.* Los Angeles: Western Psychological Services.

Gamble, T. J., & Zigler, E. F. (1989). The Head Start Synthesis Project: A critique. *Journal of Applied Developmental Psychology, 10*(2), 267–274.

Glass, G. V. (1976). Primary, secondary, and meta-analysis of research. *Educational Researcher, 5*, 3–8.

Gramlich, E. (1976). *Benefit-cost analysis of government programs.* Englewood Cliffs, NJ: Prentice-Hall.

Heckman, J., & Robb, R. (1985). Alternative methods for evaluating the impact of interventions. In J. Heckman & B. Singer (Eds.), *Longitudinal analysis of labor market data*. New York: Cambridge University Press.

Horacek, H. J., Ramey, C. T., Campbell, F. A., Hoffman, K. P., & Fletcher, R. H. (1987). Predicting school failure and assessing early intervention with high-risk children. *Journal of American Academy of Child and Adolescent Psychiatry, 26*, 758–763.

Hutinger, P. (1981). The Macomb 0–3 regional project. In T. Black & P. Hutinger (Eds.), *Cost-effective delivery strategies in rural areas: Programs for young handicapped children* (Vol. 1, pp. 19–27). (HCEEP Rural Network Monograph). Macomb: Western Illinois University Press.

Kenny, D. A. (1975). A quasi-experimental approach to assessing treatment effects in nonequivalent control group designs. *Psychological Bulletin, 82*, 345–362.

Lally, R., Mangione, P., & Honig, A. (1987). *Long-range impact of an early intervention with low-income children and their families*. San Francisco: Far West Laboratory, Center for Child and Family Studies.

Larsen, J., & Robinson, C. (1989). Latter effects of preschool on low-risk. *Early Childhood Research Quarterly, 4*(1), 133–144.

Levin, H. (1983). *Cost-effectiveness: A primer*. Beverly Hills: Sage.

Liberman, A., Barnes, M. M., Ho, S. E., Cuellar, I., & Little, T. (1979). The economic impact of child development services on families of retarded children. *Mental Retardation, 17*(3), 158–159.

Love, J., Nauta, M., Coelen, C., Hewlett, K., & Ruopp, R. (1976). *National home start evaluation final report: Findings and implications*. Cambridge, MA: Abt Associates.

Macy, D. J., & Carter, J. L. (1980). *Triple T infant consortium follow-up study*. Dallas: Macy Research Associates.

McKay, H., Sinisterra, L., McKay, A., Gomez, H., & Lloreda, P. (1978). Improving cognitive ability in chronically deprived children. *Science, 200*, 270–278.

McKey, R. H., Condelli, L., Ganson, H., Barrett, B., McConkey, C., & Plantz, M. (1985). *The impact of Head Start on children, families, and communities* (Final report of Head Start Evaluation, Synthesis, and Utilization Project). Washington, DC: CSR.

Olds, D., Henderson, C., Tatelbaum, R., & Chamberlin, R. (1986). Improving the delivery of prenatal care and outcomes of pregnancy: A randomized trial of nurse home visitation. *Pediatrics, 77*, 16–28.

Pierson, D., Walker, D. K., & Tivnan, T. (1984). A school-based program from infancy to kindergarten for children and their parents. *Personnel and Guidance Journal, 62*(8), 448–455.

Ramey, C. T., Bryant, D., & Suarez, T. (1985). Preschool compensatory education and the modifiability of intelligence: A critical review. In D. Detterman (Ed.), *Current topics in human intelligence* (pp. 247–296). Norwood, NJ: Ablex.

Ramey, C. T., MacPhee, D., & Yeates, K. O. (1982). Preventing developmental retardation: A general systems model. In L. A. Bond & J. M. Joffe (Eds.), *Facilitating infant and early childhood development* (pp. 345–401). Hanover, NH: University Press of New England.

Ravsten, M. T., Behrman, J., & Nielson, S. (1986). *Training parents as facilitators of language and speech development*. Logan: Utah State University, Early Intervention Research Institute.

Reichardt, C. S. (1979). The statistical analysis of data from nonequivalent group designs. In T. D. Cook & D. T. Campbell (Eds.), *Quasi-experimentation: Design and analysis issues for field settings* (pp. 147–205). Chicago: Rand McNally College Publishing.

Rule, S., Stowitschek, J., Innocenti, M., Striefel, S., Killoran, J., Swezey, K., & Boswell, C. (1987). The social integration program: An analysis of the effects of mainstreaming handicapped children into day care centers. *Education and Treatment of Children, 10*, 175–192.

Ruopp, R., Travers, J., Glantz, F., & Coelen, C. (1979). *Children at the center: Summary findings and policy implications of the National Day Care Study*. Cambridge, MA: Abt Associates.

Schweinhart, L. J., & Weikart, D. P. (1980). *Young children grow up: The effects of the Perry Preschool program on youths through age 15*. Ypsilanti, MI: High/Scope.

Schweinhart, L. J., & Weikart, D. P. (1986, January). What do we know so far? A review of the Head Start Synthesis Project. *Young Children*, pp. 49–55.

Schweinhart, L. J., Weikart, D. P., & Larner, M. B. (1986). Consequences of three preschool curriculum models through age 15. *Early Childhood Research Quarterly, 1*, 15–46.

Seitz, V., Rosenbaum, L. K., & Apfel, N. H. (1985). Effects of family support intervention: A ten-year follow-up. *Child Development, 56*, 376–391.

Selowsky, M. (1981). Nutrition, health, and education: The economic significance of complementarities at early age. *Journal of Development Economics, 9*, 331–346.

Skeels, H. M. (1966). Adult status of children with contrasting early life experiences. *Monographs of the Society for Research in Child Development, 31*(3, Serial No. 105).

Snider, J. N., Sullivan, W. G., & Manning, D. (1974). Industrial engineering participation in a special education program. *Tennessee Engineer, 1*, 21–23.

Stile, S. W., & Thompson, J. (1982, April). *Intervention efficiency, subsequent placements, and cost-effectiveness of two preschool programs for handicapped children*. Paper presented at the 60th International Conference of the Council for Exceptional Children, Houston, TX.

Stock, J. R., Wnek, L. L., Newsborg, J. A., Schenck, E. A., Gabel, J. R., Spurgeon, M. S., & Ray, H. W. (1976). *Evaluation of the handicapped children's early education program*. Columbus, OH: Battelle Memorial Institute.

Strain, P. S., & Smith, B. J. (1986). A counter-interpretation of early intervention effects: A response to Casto and Mastropieri. *Exceptional Children, 53*, 260–265.

Taylor, C., White, K. R., & Pezzino, J. (1984). Cost-effectiveness analysis of full-day versus half-day intervention programs for handicapped preschoolers. *Journal of the Division for Early Childhood, 9*(1), 76–85.

Thompson, M. A. (1980). *Benefit-cost analysis for program evaluation*. Beverly Hills: Sage.

Travers, J., Goodson, B., Singer, J., & Connell, D. (1980). *Research results of the National Day Care Study*. Cambridge, MA: Abt Associates.

Walker, K. (1981). Project sunrise. In T. Black & P. Hutinger (Eds.), *Cost-effective delivery strategies in rural areas: Programs for young handicapped children* (Vol. 1, pp. 28–35). (HCEEP Rural Network Monograph.) Macomb: Western Illinois University Press.

Weber, C. U., Foster, P. W., & Weikart, D. P. (1978). *An Economic Analysis of the Ypsilanti Perry Preschool Project*. Ypsilanti, MI: High/Scopp.

Weikart, D. P., Bond, J. T., & McNeil, J. T. (1978). *The Ypsilanti Perry Preschool Project: Preschool years and longitudinal results through fourth grade*. Ypsilanti, MI: High/Scope.

Weikart, D. P., Kamii, C. K., & Radin, N. L. (1967). Perry Preschool Project progress report. In D. P. Weikart (Ed.), *Preschool intervention: A preliminary report of the Perry Preschool Project* (pp. 1–61). Ann Arbor, MI: Campus.

Weiss, R. S. (1981). INREAL intervention for language handicapped and bilingual children. *Journal of the Division for Early Childhood, 4*, 40–51.

Weiss, S., & Jurs, S. (1984, October). *Cost-effectiveness of early childhood education for handicapped children*. Paper presented at the annual meeting of the Atlantic Economic Society, Montreal.

White, K., & Casto, G. (1985). An integrative review of early intervention efficacy studies with at-risk children: Implications for the handicapped. *Analysis and Intervention in Developmental Disabilities, 5*, 7–31.

Woodhead, M. (1988). When psychology informs public policy: The case of early childhood intervention. *American Psychologist, 43*, 443–454.

Zigler, E. (1987). Formal schooling for four-year-olds? No. *American Psychologist, 42*, 254–260.

Zimmerman, I. L., Steiner, V. G., & Pond, R. E. (1979). *Preschool language scale—revised edition*. Columbus, OH: Merrill.

II

Ecological Assessment

Marybeth Shinn

Researchers in laboratory settings take great care to manipulate or control every aspect of the experimental situation, so that they may ignore the effects of all of the variables that may influence participants' behavior, with the exception of those that are the focus of the study. Researchers who step outside the laboratory door, however, do not have the luxury of ignoring situational influences. With the aid of statistical tools, they must devote far more energy to assessing the contexts of human behavior in order to model transactions between people and settings. The second section of this volume offers five excellent examples of how this endeavor is accomplished.

There are three primary reasons to undertake the difficult task of ecological assessment. First, prevention and intervention researchers may wish to manipulate settings, just as laboratory researchers manipulate experimental conditions, in order to influence behavior. For example, Felner, Ginter, and Primavera (1982) restructured a high school and the roles of teachers in order to reduce flux and to increase clarity and support for students, resulting in increased grade point averages, attendance, and self-concept. To understand the influences of settings, researchers must be able to identify and assess those ecological characteristics with the most functional significance.

Second, investigators who are not in a position to manipulate settings may nevertheless want to understand the influences of these settings on behavior. Failure to attend to the influences of social settings can lead to critical errors of inference, particularly when, as is generally the case, people are not randomly distributed across settings. For example, Wilson (1987) has pointed out that African Americans, regardless of their socioeconomic

Marybeth Shinn • Department of Psychology, New York University, New York, New York 10003.

level, are far more likely to live in neighborhoods of concentrated poverty than are white Americans of comparable education, occupation, and personal wealth. And neighborhood poverty has adverse associations with variables such as childhood IQ, teen birth rates, and school dropout, rates even after controlling for family characteristics (e.g., Brooks-Gunn, Duncan, Klebanov, & Sealand, 1993). Thus, if neighborhood characteristics are ignored, their influences can be mistakenly attributed to race. As a consequence, racist stereotypes are perpetuated, and possible targets for intervention are ignored.

Finally, social contexts may moderate or condition more proximal influences on behavior. For example, Gonzales, Cauce, Friedman, and Mason (1996) found that the parenting styles that were associated with good grades for African-American adolescents depended on the levels of risk in the neighborhoods in which they lived. Lower levels of restrictive control were optimal in low-risk, but not in high-risk neighborhoods. Ignoring the moderating influences of community context here could lead to overgeneralization of conclusions about optimal parenting styles, and to counterproductive interventions.

As these examples show, the ability to assess important aspects of social ecologies is critical to understanding the influences of settings on human behavior (and the influences of people on settings), avoiding errors of inference, designing effective preventive interventions, and understanding ecological limits on generalizations that social scientists might otherwise draw. The science of ecological assessment is still in its infancy, but the five chapters in this section provide creative examples of the art.

The first two chapters, by Coulton, Korbin, and Su (1996), and Perkins and Taylor (1996)—both drawn from a special issue of the *American Journal of Community Psychology* on ecological assessment (Shinn, 1996)—offer several strategies for assessing neighborhoods. The papers take different approaches, because they are driven by different theoretical questions. Coulton, Korbin, and Su are concerned with characteristics of neighborhoods associated with the risk for abuse and neglect of children. They interviewed parents and other caregivers of young children and found that reports of both neighborhood characteristics, such as residential stability and the availability of specific facilities for children were associated with a lower risk for abuse and neglect. The associations of some neighborhood characteristics with outcomes depended on the racial makeup of the area. For example, block associations were more common and more important to children's welfare in African-American than in European-American neighborhoods. Perkins and Taylor used three different approaches to assess neighborhood characteristics that were associated with fear of crime (measured a year later). These included residents' perceptions, gathered via interviews, ratings conducted by trained observers, and content analysis of newspaper articles about crime and disorder.

Both papers address the important question of how individual perceptions can be combined to inform readers about an ecological unit, rather than simply about the individual who is reporting on the unit. Coulton, Korbin, and Su examined the extent to which residents of the same neighborhood agreed with each other in their perceptions, and offer the intriguing suggestion that in some cases, degree of consensus among respondents may be more important than the average response. Perkins and Taylor used random regression or hierarchical linear modeling (cf. Bryk & Raudenbush, 1992) to distinguish variation among neighborhoods from individual-level variation within neighborhoods, and to relate neighborhood characteristics to residents' fear of crime.

The next paper by Tausig (1987) examined the structure of mental health services in one county in order to understand problems in linkages among agencies that might lead to poor services for clients. He interviewed directors of 45 agencies serving a single county about their agencies' patterns of interactions with other agencies. Then he applied the tools of network analysis to identify missing links between agencies that might have been expected to interact based on their missions, unstructured patterns of relationships among clusters of similar agencies, and conflicted relationships. Each type of "crack" in the service system suggested a way in which agencies might fail to make appropriate referrals of clients to one another. He showed that useful results can be gained from ecological assessment strategies within a single community, and that not all ecological assessment strategies are as laborious as some of the other approaches illustrated here.

The last two papers, like the first two, examine variation among multiple settings of a particular type. In Rizzo and Corsaro's paper (1995), the settings are three early childhood programs. In Luke, Rappaport, and Seidman's study (1991), there are 13 mutual-help groups for people with serious problems in living. Rizzo and Corsaro used ethnographic and interpretive methods to show how children's patterns of interaction and friendship were congruent with the social-ecological conditions within each setting. Despite the differences across settings, the authors argued that friendships served similar functions in all three programs, including social integration and meeting the settings' specific emotional and task demands. For example, in a first-grade classroom, friendships facilitated schoolwork, whereas in a university preschool they protected ongoing peer activities and space. Luke, Rappaport, and Seidman also used observational methods to study social interactions, but took a much more quantitative approach. The authors cluster-analyzed the mutual-help groups into four types, based on the frequencies with which different types of interactions (e.g., small talk) took place. Cluster membership was associated with other characteristics of the groups, such as their size and the average level of psychological functioning of group members, and also predicted psychological improvement among newcomers to the groups.

Collectively, the five papers in this section demonstrate a variety of techniques for ecological assessment. They demonstrate close linkages between theoretical constructs and measurement strategies, careful attention to statistical reliability and validity, and sophisticated examples of both qualitative and quantitative analyses. The papers also suggest some continuing challenges for the field of ecological assessment. The practical challenges of finding efficient methods for collecting data in enough settings to be able to undertake appropriate analyses, and of understanding convergence and divergence among methods, are themselves daunting. More conceptual tasks include identifying the characteristics of settings that bear the greatest significance for individual behavior, defining the physical and conceptual boundaries of settings such as neighborhoods (see also Livert & Hughes, 2002), and discerning the relationship between culture and other aspects of social ecology. A final set of challenges shares both conceptual and statistical aspects. It includes determining how to use data collected from individuals to characterize settings, balancing the goals of finding common patterns and uncovering diversity among settings, and determining when to use multiple separate dimensions (cf. Perkins & Taylor, 1996) and when to develop typologies (cf. Luke, Rappaport, & Seidman, 1991) to characterize settings. This collection of papers provides an excellent start, but there is far more work to be done.

REFERENCES

Brooks-Gunn, J., Duncan, G. J., Klebanov, P. K., & Sealand, N. (1993). Do neighborhoods influence child and adolescent development? *American Journal of Sociology, 99*, 353–395.

Bryk, A. S., & Raudenbush, S. W. (1992). *Hierarchical linear models: Applications and data analysis methods.* Newbury Park, CA:Sage.

Coulton, C. J., Korbin, J. E., & Su, M. (1996). Measuring neighborhood context for young children in an urban area. *American Journal of Community Psychology, 24*, 5–32.

Felner, R. D., Ginter, G., & Primavera, J. (1982). Primary prevention during school transitions: Social support and environmental structure. *American Journal of Community Psychology, 10*, 277–290. Reprinted in T. A. Revenson, A. R. D'Augelli, D. L. Hughes, D. Livert, S. E. French, E. Seidman, M. Shinn, & H. Yoshikawa (Eds.) (2002). *A quarter century of community psychology: Readings from the* American Journal of Community Psychology (pp. 147–161). New York: Kluwer Academic/Plenum Publishers.

Gonzales, N. A., Cauce, A. M., Friedman, R. J., & Mason, C. A. (1996). Family, peer, and neighborhood influences on academic achievement among African-American adolescents: One-year prospective effects. *American Journal of Community Psychology, 24*, 365–387. Reprinted in T. A. Revenson, A. R. D'Augelli, D. L. Hughes, D. Livert, S. E. French,

E. Seidman, M. Shinn, & H. Yoshikawa (Eds.) (2002). *A quarter century of community psychology: Readings from the* American Journal of Community Psychology (pp. 541–562). New York: Kluwer Academic/Plenum Publishers.

Livert, D., & Hughes, D. L. (2002). The ecological paradigm: Persons in settings. In T. A. Revenson, A. R. D'Augelli, D. L. Hughes, D. Livert, S. E. French, E. Seidman, M. Shinn, & H. Yoshikawa (Eds.) *A quarter century of community psychology: Readings from the* American Journal of Community Psychology (pp. 51–63). New York: Kluwer Academic/Plenum Publishers.

Luke, D. A., Rappaport, J., & Seidman, E. (1991). Setting phenotypes in a mutual-help organization: Expanding behavior setting theory. *American Journal of Community Psychology, 19*, 147–167.

Perkins, D. D., & Taylor, R. B. (1996). Ecological assessments of community disorder: Their relationship to fear of crime and theoretical implications. *American Journal of Community Psychology, 24*, 63–108.

Rizzo, T. A., & Corsaro, W. A. (1995). Social support processes in early childhood friendship: A comparative study of ecological congruences in enacted support. *American Journal of Community Psychology, 23*, 389–418.

Shinn, M. (Ed.) (1996). Ecological assessment. [Special Issue] *American Journal of Community Psychology, 24*(1).

Tausig, M. (1987). Detecting "cracks" in mental health service systems: Application of network analytic techniques. *American Journal of Community Psychology, 15*, 337–351.

Wilson, W. J. (1987). *The truly disadvantaged: The inner city, the underclass, and public policy.* Chicago: University of Chicago Press.

4

Measuring Neighborhood Context for Young Children in an Urban Area

Claudia J. Coulton, Jill E. Korbin, and Marilyn Su

Awareness of worsening conditions in urban areas has led to a growing interest in how neighborhood context affects children. Although the ecological perspective within child development has acknowledged the relevance of community factors, methods of measuring the neighborhood context for children have been quite limited. An approach to measuring neighborhood environments was tested using the average perceptions of caregivers of young children sampled from high- and low-risk block groups. Individual- and aggregate-level reliabilities and discriminant validity were acceptable for dimensions of neighborhood quality and change, participation in block organizations, disorder and incivilities, service usage and quality, and retaliation against adults. However, for measures of neighborhood interaction and the tendency of adults to intervene with children, there was virtually no agreement among respondents within block groups, resulting in poor aggregate reliability. A model of variability may be a more promising way of characterizing neighborhoods along these dimensions.

Communities have long been recognized as potentially important contexts for child development (e.g., Bronfenbrenner, Moen, & Garbarino, 1984;

Originally published in the *American Journal of Community Psychology, 24*(1) (1996): 5–32.

Ecological Research to Promote Social Change: Methodological Advances from Community Psychology, edited by Tracey A Revenson et al. Kluwer Academic/Plenum Publishers, New York, 2002.

Cicchetti & Lynch, 1993). Recent interest in measuring these contexts has been spawned by concern about neighborhood decline. Dramatic industrial restructuring and continuing patterns of racial segregation have given rise in the last two decades to a growing geographic concentration of poverty and isolation of poor families from mainstream influences (Jargowsky & Bane, 1991; Kasarda, 1993). Many inner-city neighborhoods have experienced social transformations in which single-parent families live amidst the highest rates of violence, drug trafficking, and housing deterioration. Their children experience increasing rates of delinquency, school failure, and developmental problems (Wilson, 1987). Concurrently, scientific interest in documenting the effects of urban communities on children and families is being renewed but has been hampered by limited methodologies for measuring aspects of neighborhood contexts that are relevant to parents and their young children.

This paper explores a method of measuring neighborhood environments using the average perceptions of caregivers of young children who reside in proximity to one another. The method is distinctive in several ways. First, questions posed to residents about their neighborhoods were chosen because they reflect salient themes from our previous ethnographic research comparing neighborhoods classified as high-, medium-, and low-risk for children (Korbin & Coulton, 1994). Second, the block group rather than the census tract is used as the unit of analysis, overcoming concerns about much existing neighborhood research that census tracts may be too large to be relevant to young children. Third, the reliability of these measures of neighborhood contexts are assessed using a generalizability theory model at the aggregate level.

BACKGROUND

The impact of neighborhood conditions on children and families is experiencing a resurgence of interest. However, the importance of an ecological perspective has been a long-standing paradigm in child development theory and research (e.g., Belsky, 1980; Bronfenbrenner, 1979, 1988; Cicchetti & Lynch, 1993; Garbarino, 1977) and in environmental and community psychology (Holahan & Wandersman, 1987; Taylor, 1988). Developmentalists using an ecological perspective have viewed both the objective and perceived aspects of neighborhoods as part of the exosystem affecting child development (Bronfenbrenner, 1988). Environmental and community psychologists have identified physical and social aspects of neighborhoods that are important determinants of individual behavior (Holahan & Wandersman, 1987; Taylor, 1988).

Research on Neighborhoods and Children

Efforts to model the effects of neighborhoods on parents and children have been constrained by the lack of suitable measures of neighborhood environments that are pertinent to parents and young children. Most existing survey research that has included neighborhood measures has relied on census indicators of socioeconomic status (SES) of neighborhood residents as a proxy for neighborhood conditions and processes. However, when socioeconomic composition is the only measure of neighborhood contexts, the demonstrated effects on children are relatively weak and not uniform across population subgroups (Clark, 1992; Crane, 1991; Jencks & Mayer, 1990). Nevertheless, the findings that living near affluent neighbors produces higher IQ among low birth weight infants and lower rates of teen births and dropping out of school for some groups, even after family factors are controlled, is suggestive of the potential importance of neighborhood quality for childhood outcomes (Brooks-Gunn, Duncan, Klebanov, & Sealand, 1993; Duncan, 1993).

Unfortunately, the socioeconomic composition measures used in these studies do not reveal the multitude of differences associated with affluent compared to poor neighborhoods that affect children. Socioeconomic status may be a proxy for a wide range of factors including the prevalence of role models, social influences on parenting style, institutional strength and resources, and a variety of other conditions. It is clear that more refined and complete measures of factors in the neighborhood that affect families and children are needed.

A more direct depiction of social processes within neighborhoods appears in research on community social organization (Bursik & Webb, 1982; Figueira-McDonough, 1991; Freudenburg, 1986; Sampson, 1992) even though these studies do not typically focus on young children. Most closely related to the work in this paper is Sampson's (1991) analysis which used interviews with random samples of residents to develop community level measures of density of acquaintanceships, social cohesion, and stability. Each measure reflected the mean of response ratings from the interviews. Using a similar method to this analysis, Sampson found these aggregate measures to be reliable for British polling districts as the unit of analysis and to predict deviant behavior among youth.

Alternatively, qualitative research has provided a rich description of a few neighborhoods and the processes that affect parents and children, but these techniques have not been suitable for larger scale research. Ethnographic portraits, although revealing many aspects of neighborhood life that are important to children, have been difficult to generalize (Anderson, 1990, 1994; Jarrett, 1994; Keiser, 1969; Liebow, 1966; Stack, 1974; Whyte, 1955).

However, qualitative studies have shown that parenting strategies differ depending upon the danger and other risks to children in neighborhoods (Furstenberg, 1993). Also, qualitative studies comparing neighborhoods with similar economic conditions but different rates of child maltreatment have suggested the importance of social resources in reducing risk for children (Garbarino & Crouter, 1978; Garbarino & Kostelny, 1992; Garbarino & Sherman, 1980).

Coleman (1987) used the term "social capital" to refer to the community resources that support child development. His contention is that structural changes in employment, households, and neighborhoods have eroded the effectiveness of community norms, adult-sponsored youth activities, and informal relations among adults and children. He noted that in some communities these functions are being replaced by other mechanisms, often more formal institutions. Yet, in poor communities with sparse resources for private or public investment, such conversion to formal mechanisms has been limited. It is, in part, this elusive concept of social capital that this study seeks to measure.

Defining Neighborhood and Community

The term *community* is a social rather than a geographic unit, but the concept of neighborhood implies local communities that are bounded spatially. Neighborhood boundaries are often difficult to draw because there is little consensus about what constitutes a neighborhood. Social scientists hold varying perspectives on the degree to which the term implies homogeneity, social interaction, and place identity on the part of the residents (White, 1987). Most definitions of neighborhood imply a degree of social cohesion that results from shared institutions and space, but it is also widely accepted that neighborhoods differ in their levels of community social organization and integration (Lyon, 1987). Further, it seems that neighborhoods that are the least cohesive and organized may be the poorest environments for rearing children (Coulton, Korbin, Chow, & Su, 1995; Garbarino, Dubrow, Kostelny, & Pardo, 1992; Sampson, 1992).

Despite the definition ambiguities of neighborhoods or other meaningful localities, research on community context for families and children typically requires geographic boundaries. These boundaries may be established on the basis of phenomenological, interactional, or statistical information.

At the phenomenological level, each resident has a sense of the boundaries that are personally meaningful. These vary, even for the same individual, depending upon the context (Galster, 1992). Although for some purposes it is useful to use the consensus of residents as the basis for drawing geographic boundaries for neighborhoods, our previous research has revealed some places where there is considerable agreement among neighbors on the boundaries they draw for their neighborhoods, while in other locales neighborhood boundaries seem virtually idiosyncratic. Consensus seems to be greater in areas with higher levels of community identity and attachment (Korbin & Coulton, 1994). Thus, the lack of consensus seems to prohibit measurement of neighborhood contexts in just those areas where there would be greatest concern about negative effects.

A second approach to generating neighborhood boundaries is to use the patterns of social interaction of residents. This involves a process of "mapping locally based social interaction onto a spatial grid" (Entwisle, 1991). Friendship patterns and daily activities have both been used as methods of tying interaction patterns to spatial locations. Although this approach fits research where interactional patterns are the primary focus, neighborhoods as a context for families and children have many aspects in addition to social interaction.

Standardized statistical definitions of neighborhood areas represent a third approach. To date census tracts and zip codes have been most widely used in research on neighborhood effects on children and youth. However, concerns have been raised about the degree to which these units resemble the space that is meaningful to residents (Tienda, 1991). Block groups (i.e., areas defined by a group of city blocks) have also served as proxies for neighborhoods (Taylor, Gottfredson, & Brower, 1984) and, because their size is fairly consistent with "walking distance," may represent the most immediate influence on families with young children.

Aggregation to Higher Level Units

In this analysis, we aggregate the responses of individuals for the purpose of determining the properties of a higher level unit: their neighborhoods. This is not the only approach to measuring neighborhood characteristics. Some properties of aggregates can be measured independently of the individuals contained within them. For example, the housing density or distance from the center of the city are features of neighborhoods that do not depend upon aggregating individuals and are conceptually independent from the neighborhood residents.

When aggregation of individuals is used to capture a feature of a neighborhood, two possible perspectives apply. One is that the residents are a set of observers reporting on a fact, perhaps imperfectly, but there is a referent that is independent from the observers. For instance, if residents

were asked whether certain signs of deterioration exist in their neighborhood it can be assumed that they are a knowledgeable set of observers of
these facts (Romney, Weller, & Batchelder, 1986).

Other social properties of a neighborhood, however, have a different
status. They are actually compositional in nature. In other words, their
conceptualization reflects the properties or characteristics of the individual
residents combined. The degree to which each resident is actively involved
in organizations when aggregated becomes a property of the neighborhood,
namely, resident participation level, for example.

When residents are treated as observers of an external reality, combining
their responses is a straightforward method of obtaining a more reliable
measure than could be provided by using a single observer. However,
if the purpose of aggregation is to represent a concept that derives from the
composition of individuals, greater consideration needs to be given to
the meaning of this indicator when it becomes a property of an aggregate
rather than an individual. Using aggregations of individuals to represent
neighborhood properties implies that the composition itself represents
a theoretically meaningful concept. In other words, the composition is a
proxy for a property of the neighborhood that is not directly observed but
can be approximated by combining individual perceptions, self-reported
behaviors, or personal characteristics.

METHOD

The purpose of this study was to develop and test a survey measure
that would represent aspects of the neighborhood context that are salient
to the well-being of young children in that neighborhood. Two hypotheses
are tested in this analysis. The first is that multiple aspects of the neighborhood can be measured reliably by aggregating resident responses to survey
questions. The second hypothesis is that these measures can differentiate
high- and low-risk neighborhoods for children.

The perceptions of caregivers of young children living in proximity to
one another were used to characterize the neighborhood. Rather than
treating the individual caregiver as the primary unit of analysis, through,
the caregivers' responses were aggregated to characterize their neighborhoods. This approach does not deny that the pathway through which neighborhoods may affect children is their parents' perceptions of those
neighborhoods. However, the purpose of this study was not to test that
proposition but to determine whether selected aspects of neighborhood
contexts could be measured reliably using responses from multiple resident
caregivers.

Design and Sampling

The block group was chosen as the unit to represent neighborhoods because our previous ethnographic work suggested that geographic areas smaller than census tracts may be needed to identify neighborhood characteristics relevant to young children. Block groups are defined by the United States Census Bureau and consist of several contiguous blocks. In urban locations they usually represent an area that is fairly small, in which residents get around by walking. Face-to-face interaction and direct knowledge of the area is, therefore, possible. They are considerably smaller than census tracts, and census tracts vary in the number of block groups contained within them. Block groups are generally fairly homogeneous, and in this study there was little within-block group variability in housing stock, economic status of households or race, and ethnic group.

As one of the purposes of this study was to test whether the measures could discriminate between neighborhoods that were better or worse contexts for children, we chose block groups that represented known extremes of risk and had been studied in our previous epidemiological and ethnographic research (Coulton et al., 1995; Korbin & Coulton, 1994). Child maltreatment report rates were used as an indicator of adverse conditions for children. Maltreatment rates were calculated using all child maltreatment reports to the County Department of Family and Children's Services. All cases determined by the department to be "substantiated" and "indicated" neglect and/or abuse in 1991 were included in the calculation of rates. The addresses of the children on whom the reports were made were geocoded so that rates could be calculated for specific geographic areas. Because we were interested in the effect of residential locations on rates of child maltreatment, incidents were excluded that reportedly occurred in schools and day care centers. In a few cases (9.4%), the same child had several reports of maltreatment during the year. In the calculation of rates, these cases were counted only once because we were interested in the proportion of children who experienced maltreatment rather than the number of reports that were made. The rates were calculated by counting the total number of children living in each tract who experienced one or more confirmed instances of maltreatment, and dividing by the population of the tract, ages 0 through 17.

Child abuse and neglect reports are often thought to underestimate the incidence and prevalence of maltreatment and to be biased against poor and minority families (Newberger, Reed, Daniel, Hyde, & Kotelchuck, 1977; O'Toole, Turbett, & Nalpeka, 1983). Official reports are often considered an imperfect source of data because of problems in record-keeping, variability in definitions, and misidentification of cases. Further, official reports reflect child consequences serious enough to come to the attention of an agency rather than reflecting all behaviors that pose dangers to children (Straus, Gelles, & Steinmetz, 1980). However, child abuse and neglect reports are an indicator of the distribution of recognition of, and response to, child maltreatment and have usefully been applied in past research (Garbarino & Sherman, 1980; National Center for Child Abuse & Neglect [NCCAN], 1988; Pelton, 1981; Zuravin, 1989). Studies show that the percentage of all maltreatment reported to Child Protective Services has remained steady over the years (NCCAN, 1988).

Sixteen block groups were selected from four census tracts that were in the top (high rate) or bottom (low rate) quartile of child maltreatment report rates in our previous study (Coulton et al., 1995; Korbin & Coulton, 1994). Eight block groups from high-risk census tracts and eight from low-risk census tracts were selected randomly. Half of the block groups in each risk category were composed predominantly of African American families, and the other half of predominantly European American families. Ten households were selected randomly from each block group for an anticipated sample size of 160.

Data Collection

Maps of block group boundaries were computer generated, and all housing units in each block group were listed by the interviewers through direct observation and mapping. Interviewers began the sample selection process with a housing unit randomly selected from this block group mapping, and solicited interviews from every second housing unit. If nobody was home, interviewers were required to make at least two "call backs" on different days and at different times of the day to try to reach a household member for screening.

At each sampled household, interviewers asked a series of screening questions to determine if there was at least one child under 6 years of age living in the household along with a parent, guardian, or other caregiver who provided at least half of the child's care in the home. The inclusion of other significant caregivers allowed a grandparent or other relative who provided much of the child's everyday care at home to be interviewed. Paid child-care providers or caregivers who did not live in the home were not eligible for the interview.

A total of 156 caregivers were actually interviewed after obtaining informed consent. Table I reports the numbers of households contacted and the reasons for nonparticipation. Interviewers never found anyone at home for approximately 16% of sampled housing units. Only about 27%

Table I. Stages of Sample Selection

	Low-risk block groups ($n = 8$)	High-risk block groups ($n = 8$)	Total ($n = 16$)
Housing units sampled	635	278	922
Unavailable in 4 visits	117	29	146
Total households contacted	518	258	776
No children <6 years	411	157	568
Unwilling to be interviewed	28	24	52
Households interviewed	79	77	156

of households, where a member was contacted, qualified for the study through having a child in the specified age range. Of the 208 eligible participants, 16% were unwilling to participate in the interview process. As Table I suggests, it was more difficult to obtain interviews in the low-risk neighborhoods because of a higher frequency of individuals who were not available after three contacts (the initial contact and two return attempts) on different days of the week and different times of the day. This supports our past research that individuals in low-risk neighborhoods are more likely to have jobs and other activities that take them out of the home. Refusals to participate were not substantially different between the block group types, but low-risk block groups had more households without young children.

The demographic characteristics of the sample are presented in Table II. The respondents were predominately female in their 30s. Those in high-risk neighborhoods were more likely to be unmarried and have lower income and educational attainment. Relatively high proportions of respondents in all neighborhoods reported having worked at least part time during the previous year. There was considerable variation in length of residence in the neighborhood but on the average it was longer in African American neighborhoods.

Development of Questionnaire Items

Since the purpose of the study was to measure aspects of neighborhood contexts that were salient to caregivers of young children, the general areas covered by the interview schedule were derived from our previous ethnographic work that compared 13 neighborhoods with high, medium, and low rates of reported child maltreatment and other adverse outcomes for children (Korbin & Coulton, 1994). The ethnographies included physical mapping of each area and of the institutions and areas of economic and

Table II. Demographic Characteristics of Sample by Risk Status and Ethnicity of Block Group

Variable	High-risk European American (n = 38)	High-risk African American (n = 39)	Low-risk European American (n = 40)	Low-risk African American (n = 39)
No. of children in household, M (SD)	3.0 (1.7)	3.1 (2)	1.8 (0.8)	2.6 (1.2)
Respondent's age, M (SD)	31.4 (9.0)	34.0 (12.2)	32.8 (5.9)	33.0 (12.6)
Years of residence in the neighborhood, M (SD)	7.9 (9.6)	17.1 (13.2)	6.7 (6.2)	13.7 (11.4)
% Married	42	26	95	41
% Employed	47	64	68	67
% With at least a high school education	63	79	98	90
% Household income ≤ $20,000	62	55	2	21
% Household income > $40,000	6	8	68	31
% Female	84	85	80	90
% White	76	0	100	0

residential activity; in-depth interviews with selected residents; observations of activity in public places; and interviews with neighborhood service providers, church officials, business people, and leaders.

The in-depth interviews with residents and observations in the ethnographies suggested several aspects of the neighborhood contexts that seemed pertinent to parents and children. These themes generally were consistent with community social organization theory and with the research discussed in the background section of this article. However, by drawing on the ethnographic descriptions of neighborhoods, the questionnaire items were able to make concrete some of the more abstract theoretical concepts. It should be noted that although the focus of this study is the neighborhood contexts for young children, the ethnographies suggested that the resources generally available to families were important as well.

The questionnaire items initially were generated to represent the following thematic areas: availability of resources and services; participation in neighborhood activities; social interactions with neighbors; willingness to intervene with children and expectations regarding reactions to intervention; neighborhood quality; neighborhood stability; direction of neighborhood change; neighborhood disorder and fear of violence; and neighborhood identity. Items were pretested to determine their clarity and feasibility.

Scale Construction

The items representing each conceptual area were examined individually and as a group. For some conceptual areas, it was anticipated that the items might form several distinct dimensions. Exploratory factor analysis, employing principal components and a varimax rotation, was used to determine the number of dimensions. Where more than one factor was found, the items were grouped into scales accordingly.

Item analysis examined the correlation between each scale item and all other items. A few items were found to be insufficiently related to the rest of the scale and were dropped. For each respondent, a score was calculated on each of the scales. The scale score was calculated by adding the score on the individual items and dividing by the number of nonmissing items for that individual. Missing values were rare and seemed to justify this method of mean substitution at the individual level. All scales were then standardized to a 10-point scale.

The resulting scales were consistent with the themes derived from the ethnography. However, several of the thematic areas were multidimensional and required several scales. The questionnaire items associated with each scale appear in the Appendix along with a shortened name, in upper case letters, to identify the scale.

For the theme availability of resources and services, three scales were developed. *Facility Availability* measured the existence of neighborhood institutions and services; *Facility Usage* represented the degree to which neighborhood facilities were used by residents; *Facility Quality* reflected resident judgments of the facilities in their neighborhood.

For the theme of participation in neighborhood activities, only two types of involvement were successfully captured by scales: *Church Activities* and *Block Club Activities*. The neighborhood social interaction theme was reflected in the *Interaction* scale that asked about acquaintanceships, activities, and mutual aid among neighbors.

The expectations surrounding intervention with neighborhood children proved to be a multidimensional area, with five factors. The scale labeled *Intervene* contained general statements about whether or not neighbors would intervene with other people's children. *Retaliate* reflected the degree to which caregivers perceived a risk of verbal or physical retaliation for such intervention. Three other scales queried residents about which behaviors and situations (pertaining to a 5- or 6-year-old child) would stimulate or provoke neighbors' intervention. The scale labeled *Stop Delinquency* referred to serious behaviors that were dangerous or law breaking. *Stop Misbehavior* pertained to mischievous acts. *Assist* referred to situations in which children might be hurt or need assistance.

The theme of the quality of the neighborhoods included a number of caregiver judgments on the positive and negative aspects of their neighborhood and whether or not they would like to continue living in their neighborhood. The scale is labeled *Neighborhood Quality*.

The amount of instability in neighborhoods is reflected by *Mobility*, which included questions about the turnover of neighborhood residents. The direction of neighborhood change was represented by a question asking residents whether their neighborhoods were changing for better or worse or staying about the same. This item is labeled *Positive Change*.

Disorder included items to tap perceptions of deleterious conditions in neighborhoods. It included conditions such as litter, boarded buildings, unkempt yards or homes, and loitering and disorderly behavior. Some of these items were adapted from a questionnaire used to evaluate the Dorchester Cares project (Earls, McGuire, & Shay, 1994). *Victimization* questions asked residents their degree of worry about becoming victims of crime and violence. Some of these items were adapted from a questionnaire used to evaluate the Dorchester Cares project (Earls et al., 1994). *Identity* of neighborhood was based on whether respondents had a name for their neighborhood.

Reliability at the Individual Level

Since these scales were newly created, it was necessary to first examine their reliability as a measure of individual perceptions. Coefficient alpha was calculated for each scale to determine the internal consistency of each scale. We used scales with an internal consistency reliability of .45 or greater in subsequent analyses, because the primary purpose of this analysis was to examine aggregate reliability at the neighborhood level.

Reliability at the Aggregate Level

To determine whether the above scales were useful indicators of neighborhoods as contexts for children, the next step was to determine the reliability of each scale at the aggregate or block group level. In other words, it was necessary to test whether the mean of a sample of individual observations could be used to characterize the neighborhood in which the individuals reside. As mentioned previously, block groups were used as proxies for neighborhoods.

A generalizability theory model was used to estimate aggregate reliability (O'Brien, 1990). The model had one facet, the block groups, with individual caregivers nested within the block groups. The generalizability coefficient was calculated by comparing the variance attributable to block groups with the variance due to individuals and random error within block groups. The variance due to block groups is conceptually similar to the true score variance in classical test theory.

As demonstrated by O'Brien (1990, p. 482), the reliability of an aggregate measure using the average scores of individuals within block groups can be estimated by:

$$E\hat{\rho}^2 = \frac{\sigma^2(a)}{[\sigma^2(a) + \sigma^2(r{:}a, e)/n_r]}$$

where $E\hat{\rho}^2$ is the generalizability coefficient, a is the aggregate or block group, r is the respondent nested within a block group, e is error, and n is the number of respondents within block groups.

The generalizability coefficient can be estimated by manipulating the mean squares from a one-way analysis of variance where block groups are the factor and individuals are nested within block groups. Both the aggregates and individuals are tested as random, not fixed. The output from a standard, random effects, analysis of variance was used to calculate the reliability coefficients according to the following formula (O'Brien, 1990, p. 484):

$$E\hat{\rho}^2 = \frac{[MS(a) - MS(r{:}a)]}{MS(a)}$$

where $MS(a)$ is the mean squares for block groups and $MS(r{:}a)$ is the mean squares for residents nested within block groups.

A scale is most reliable at the aggregate level when the variance between block groups is high and there is little variation among individuals within block groups. When there is little consensus among the individuals within block groups, the aggregate reliability is low. Thus, aggregate reliability can be low even when the scale performs well when applied to individual residents (i.e., has an acceptable coefficient alpha). Indeed, it is possible for individual variation within block groups to exceed variation among block groups to such a degree that a negative generalizability coefficient is obtained.

A cautionary note is in order because the study estimated aggregate level reliability using only 16 neighborhoods. The stability of generalizability coefficients is dependent upon the sample size of aggregate units (Johnson & Bell, 1985). The relatively small n in this analysis means that these results may be somewhat unstable.

RESULTS

Reliability

Table III presents the reliability of the scales. The generalizability coefficients for the aggregate reliability of the scales are in the third column of Table III. It can be seen that individual reliability is a necessary but not sufficient condition for aggregate reliability. In fact, several scales that are reliable for assessing individual perceptions do not seem to be reliable for describing the neighborhood contexts.

The most reliable neighborhood measures are achieved for Disorder, Mobility, Identity, Neighborhood Quality, and Retaliate. The relatively high generalizability coefficients of these measures imply that all respondents within the block group are observing these conditions and making similar judgments about their level or desirability. Facility Availability, Facility Usage, and Facility Quality, Block Club Activity, and Victimization are measured with modest aggregate reliability. Residents are somewhat heterogeneous in their responses to these scales, resulting in greater measurement error at the neighborhood level.

Table III. Reliability Coefficients for Individual- and Aggregate-Level Measures

Scale	Individual level: Cronbach's alpha ($n = 156$)	Aggregate level: generalizability coefficient ($n = 16$)
Facility availability		
Existence of institutions and services	.58	0.55
Facility Usage		
Usage of facilities in the past 2 months	.65	0.52
Facility Quality		
Perceived quality	.89	0.56
Church Activities		
Participation in church activities	.68	0.38
Block Club Activities		
Participation in block club meeting and neighborhood watch	.55	0.55
Interaction		
Neighborhood interaction	.82	−0.46
Intervene		
Tendency to intervene with children	.46	0.17
Retaliate		
Expected response to intervention	.90	0.71
Stop Delinquency		
Response to delinquent acts	.89	0.32
Stop Misbehavior		
Response to misbehavior	.72	−1.33
Assist		
Intervene to prevent harm	.72	0.02
Neighborhood Quality		
Satisfaction with neighborhood	.81	0.76
Mobility		
Renters and residential mobility	.52	0.83
Positive Change		
Neighborhood changed in the past couple of years	N/A	0.52
Disorder		
Conditions that occur in neighborhood	.95	0.84
Victimization		
Worry about victimization in neighborhood	.94	0.43
Identity		
Have a name for the neighborhood	N/A	0.74

Neighborhood interaction and most of the dimensions of intervening with children cannot be measured reliably by using the average of neighborhood residents' answers to this set of questions. In fact, for some of these scales, the disagreement among residents of the same block group is so extreme relative to the total variation in the sample that the coefficient is near zero or negative. The responses to these items, while internally consistent with the individual, were relatively idiosyncratic and showed little consensus among neighbors.

Validity

The sampling design we used allowed for the exploration of the discriminant validity of the scales that displayed at least modest aggregate reliability. We anticipated that if these aggregate measures were valid indicators of neighborhood contexts for young children, they should show a pattern of significant differences between high- and low-risk areas. We also expected that there would be few differences between African American and European American neighborhoods that were similar on level of risk.

The ability of these aggregate measures to discriminate between high- and low-risk areas was examined in a two-way analysis of variance using risk status and predominant racial/ethnic group as factors. The aggregate scores for the 16 neighborhoods were the units of analysis. Only the 11 scales that exhibited aggregate level reliability coefficients of greater than .4 were included in this analysis.

Multivariate analyses yielded Wilks's lambdas 13.5 ($p < .001$) for risk, 4.4 ($p < .001$) for race/ethnicity, and 3.2 ($p < .001$) for the race/ethnicity by risk interaction. Univariate F tests for the two-factor, fixed-effects model are presented in Table IV, along with the means and standard deviations of these scales by type of block group.

Most of the scales that achieved a reasonable level of aggregate reliability also discriminated between the high- and low-risk neighborhoods. High-risk neighborhoods had lower scores on facility availability but the facilities were used more often. Respondents in high-risk areas were more likely to expect retaliation when they intervened with children and to rate their neighborhood quality as poor. Scores on scales measuring residential mobility, disorder, and threat of victimization were higher in high-risk areas, and residents of high-risk areas were less likely to have an identity for their neighborhood.

However, two scales showed no significant differences between neighborhoods at high- and low-risk levels but were significantly different by the predominant racial/ethnic group in the neighborhood. These were the measures of facility quality and positive neighborhood change. Facility quality was generally seen as poorer in African American neighborhoods regardless of risk. Also, the residents of African American neighborhoods were less optimistic about the direction of change in their neighborhood than residents of primarily European American neighborhoods.

Table IV. Means (Standard Deviations) and F Values by Risk and Race of Block Group

Scale	High-risk European American ($n = 38$)	High-risk African American ($n = 39$)	Low-risk European American ($n = 40$)	Low-risk African American ($n = 39$)	F (1,152) Risk	Race	Risk*Race
Facility availability							
Existence of institutions and services	8.7 (1.3)	8.6 (1.4)	8.9 (1.0)	9.6 (0.5)	14.0[c]	2.3	5.0[a]
Facility Usage							
Usage of facilities in the past 2 months	6.8 (1.4)	6.6 (1.8)	6.2 (1.3)	5.1 (1.8)	19.1[c]	6.1[a]	3.6
Facility Quality							
Perceived quality	8.1 (1.2)	7.5 (1.3)	7.9 (0.9)	7.0 (1.5)	3.7	14.4[c]	0.4
Block Club Activities							
Participation in block club meeting and neighborhood watch	2.7 (2.4)	2.6 (3.0)	2.0 (2.4)	3.9 (3.3)	0.5	4.1[a]	4.5[a]
Retaliate							
Expected response to intervention	5.9 (2.5)	5.8 (2.4)	3.3 (1.6)	4.6 (2.2)	29.0[c]	2.8	3.9
Neighborhood Quality							
Satisfaction with neighborhood	5.8 (1.7)	5.6 (1.7)	7.7 (1.1)	6.9 (1.5)	46.0[c]	4.1[a]	1.6
Mobility							
Renters and residential mobility	6.1 (2.4)	5.7 (2.5)	3.0 (1.7)	2.7 (1.8)	78.4[c]	0.8	0.0
Positive Change							
Neighborhood changes in the past couple of years	5.9 (2.0)	5.5 (2.6)	6.8 (1.4)	5.1 (2.2)	0.7	9.5[b]	3.5
Disorder							
Conditions that occur in neighborhood	5.1 (2.4)	5.5 (2.4)	2.0 (0.9)	3.5 (2.0)	64.0[c]	9.7[b]	3.0
Victimization							
Worry about victimization in neighborhood	5.7 (2.7)	6.2 (2.3)	3.8 (2.0)	4.9 (2.2)	17.5[c]	4.3[a]	0.7
Identity							
Have a name for the neighborhood	3.4 (4.0)	4.7 (4.5)	9.3 (2.4)	5.8 (4.6)	31.6[c]	2.9	14.4[c]

[a] $p < .05$.
[b] $p < .01$.
[c] $p < .001$.

For the measure of block group activity there was no significant effect for risk, but there was a significant effect for race/ethnicity and for interaction. Block group activity was higher in African American neighborhoods regardless of risk status than in European American neighborhoods. Also, block group activity differed between high- and low-risk African American neighborhoods but did not differ between the low and high-risk European American neighborhoods. In other words, block groups were associated most clearly with reducing risk to children within African American neighborhoods.

In addition to a main effect for risk, there was a significant interaction effect between race and risk on facility availability and neighborhood identity. Specifically, high-risk areas all had poorer facility availability regardless of race. However, in low-risk areas, African American neighborhoods perceived the highest levels of facility availability. With respect to neighborhood identity, the interaction effect was disordinal. In the high-risk neighborhoods, African American neighborhoods had the highest rating on neighborhood identity. In the low-risk neighborhoods, it was the opposite with European American neighborhoods rating neighborhood identity highest.

DISCUSSION

The aspects of neighborhood context for children measured in this study were selected because they emerged as themes from ethnographies that contrasted high- and low-risk neighborhoods for children. While also consistent with theories of community social organization and social capital, these measures reflect the vision of people in the neighborhood as well. Thus, they are likely to represent real aspects of neighborhood life that are seen as relevant by the residents. However, to characterize the context of numerous neighborhoods, a reliable and valid method of aggregating the survey responses of samples of residents was needed. Testing such a method was the purpose of this study.

Based on a generalizability model, we conclude that it is possible to measure many aspects of neighborhood context by aggregating the scale scores of a sample of residents. Promising levels of reliability were found for facility availability, usage, and quality, block club activity, expected retaliation for intervention with children, neighborhood quality, mobility, positive change, disorder, victimization, and identity.

There is also beginning evidence of validity, in that most of the scales showed significant differences in the expected direction when neighborhoods with high and low rates of child maltreatment were compared. However, because facility availability, block club, supervision, and identity also showed significant race/ethnicity by risk interaction effects, there is a possibility that these scales may represent a case of differential validity. For example, block clubs may be important indicators of a positive context in African American neighborhoods but are not particularly important in European American neighborhoods.

For those scales, such as positive change and facility quality, that show no main effects or interaction effects for risk but only main effects for race/ethnicity, care must be taken in drawing conclusions. A possible inference is that these aspects of neighborhood context may exhibit cultural variation but not be particularly important neighborhood-level determinants of child well-being. In other words, this variation among neighborhoods is interesting but neutral with respect to childhood risk. On the other hand, the differences in neighborhoods by race/ethnicity may reflect shared perceptions that are important contextual factors to which this risk classification system is insensitive. For example, the fact that both high- and low-risk African American neighborhoods are seen as having poorer service quality may be a result of less investment in these areas. Resourceful African American parents may overcome these limitations by traveling outside their neighborhoods to use higher quality services. But this extra effort may come at a cost that has not been evaluated in this study.

It also is useful to examine the thematic areas that resulted in the lowest levels of aggregate reliability. Extremely low generalizability coefficients were found for all of the scales measuring intervention with children and the scale for social interaction in the neighborhood. These are all areas in which individuals' reported perceptions of the neighborhood could be greatly affected by their own expectations. Although all of the questions asked them to focus on what people in their neighborhood did, their personal experiences in this regard may have been influenced by their personal behavior. For instance, when asked the degree to which people in the neighborhood visit in each others' homes, the respondents' knowledge of this may be determined by their own visitation patterns.

An additional possibility is that some of the measures with poor aggregate reliability may represent phenomena that are meaningful attributes of individuals but cannot be applied to a higher level of aggregation such as a neighborhood. Simply taking an average of residents in such cases does not capture any systematic differences among neighborhoods leading to a low generalizability coefficient. This effort to characterize neighborhood social interaction may have been vulnerable to this problem as well. An individual's perception of the helpfulness or friendliness of neighbors may have little to do with the context and instead be dependent upon a variety of personal predilections and preferences. Thus, efforts to characterize this aspect of neighborhood life at the aggregate level may be inappropriate.

This initial effort to measure neighborhood context by aggregating responses from samples of residents is likely to benefit from some methodological improvements. First, the individual-level reliabilities for some of the scales might be increased by rewording some items and adding more items to some scales. Improved internal consistency reliability should add marginally to the aggregate reliability of those scales where generalizability coefficients were already acceptable but modest. Nevertheless, for the scales where aggregate-level reliability was extremely low or negative, the improvement of individual-level reliability will not change this situation.

A limitation of this study is that it used a relatively small number of neighborhoods and a small number of respondents per neighborhood. The generalizability coefficients can be improved by increasing the number of respondents in each neighborhood. Furthermore, the accuracy of the estimate of reliability will be greater when there are a larger number of aggregate units in the study (Johnson & Bell, 1985). A larger number of neighborhoods representing the entire spectrum of risk will provide a more accurate estimate of the reliability of these scales.

An additional methodological issue is whether the block group is a meaningful proxy for the neighborhood context. Residents of the block groups were asked to draw the boundaries of their neighborhood as they perceived them. Few respondents selected the exact boundaries of their block group as defined by the census. However, many respondents drew larger boundaries while only a few respondents drew somewhat smaller boundaries. This suggests that the block group is relevant to residents' perceptions of neighborhood but may omit contiguous areas that are also relevant.

An additional question is whether block groups are a practical unit for sampling neighborhood residents. Most block groups had sufficient population to yield adequate samples of families with young children. However, a few block groups had many vacant lots and empty housing units and did not have sufficient numbers of families with children under 6 years of age to make it practical to increase the sample size. For some of our aggregate measures, larger samples are necessary to increase reliability. Thus, it would be useful to experiment with combining block groups that are contiguous and similar in their demographic makeup so as to yield somewhat larger sampling units as proxies for neighborhoods. A wider age range for children in households that are sampled might also remedy the problem of adequate numbers of respondents.

Additionally, it is important in future research to distinguish various types of concepts that are of interest at the neighborhood level. These concepts may lend themselves to fundamentally different forms of measurement. One important distinction is between concepts that have a concrete, external referent apart from individual residents as compared to those that only have meaning as individual perceptions. For example, facilities existing in a neighborhood can, indeed, be viewed as attributes of the neighborhood rather than the individual residents. When a sample of residents is used to measure this attribute of the neighborhood they represent a set of observers. The important question is whether they are reliable observers of this attribute of the neighborhood. In another example, such as neighborhood social interaction, quite a different relationship can be envisioned between the individual and the aggregate. If the average individuals' experiences of social interaction within their neighborhood are used to characterize the interactional context of the neighborhood, it is assumed that social interaction is an attribute of a neighborhood. This empirical work suggests, however, that a small sample of individuals' perceptions of interaction cannot be combined to represent this characteristic of the neighborhood. The way neighborhood social interaction was operationalized here, using the mean of individuals, is not a reliable measure. It may be more appropriate to think of neighborhoods as presenting opportunities for interaction as a function of their spatial qualities, their institutions, their traditions, and make these the focus of measurement in the future.

Whether an index of variability rather than central tendency may be a better way to describe neighborhoods along some dimensions is worthy of future consideration. Quantifying consensus may be particularly important for concepts such as neighbors' intervention with children. This study found that using the mean on these scales resulted in extremely poor aggregate reliability. It is possible that neighborhoods differ in the degree to which residents agree about these matters. From a social capital perspective, it is expected that some neighborhoods experience more normative consensus than others. Theory suggests that a neighborhood in which there is more consensus about how neighbors would react to children's behavior may be one that is more stable or one in which more of the parents are acquainted with one another (Coleman, 1987). The degree of consensus about intervening with children may be a better indication of neighborhood context than is the average that was used in this analysis. In other words, an index of variation within a neighborhood may be more revealing than a measure of central tendency in such instances.

This study's approach to measuring neighborhoods uses residents' responses to scale items. Some of the scales, however, tap concepts that could be measured in other ways. For example, instead of asking residents what facilities are in their neighborhoods, this could be determined by researchers using maps and directories. Mobility within a block group could be quantified by using counts from the decennial census. An indication of neighborhood violence could be obtained by using crimes reported to the police. All of these methods are reasonable and useful but they are fundamentally different than the approach tested here. This approach captures the observations and perceptions of a random sample of people who live in the area. While their perceptions will be correlated with the census counts or with reports to public agencies, there are likely to be important differences. Especially in low-income and minority neighborhoods, for example, there is known to be a severe census undercount (White, 1987). Also reporting of crimes and other concerns to public officials is selective. Finally, if facilities exist but are not seen by residents, perceptions are likely to differ from counts made by external observers. Thus, resident perceptions may be a valuable accompaniment to other methods of measurement for some concepts.

Additionally, there are some aspects of neighborhood life that can only be ascertained from querying residents. The degree to which a neighborhood has identity for those who live there or judgments on quality of the surroundings are examples of this. It is important that researchers have well-developed methods to measure these kinds of conditions so that they can move beyond the use of proxies such as SES in studies of neighborhood effects. The method of using the aggregate responses of residents to characterize neighborhood environments is promising for quantifying some of the subtle and unobservable aspects of these contexts and their influence on children and families.

Based on this effort to measure neighborhood as a context for children, we conclude that as much care must be given to the aggregate level of measurement as has traditionally been given to the measurement of individual families and children. Policies and programs to strengthen the neighborhood context for children need to be informed by tools that can fully describe that context and identify those aspects that are important. Evaluators of special initiatives to rebuild communities require reliable methods of determining whether neighborhood context for children is improving or worsening as a result of initiatives and interventions. Multiple approaches to measuring neighborhoods, including the method presented here using the aggregated responses of samples of residents, should contribute to creating more benign or supportive community environments for children and families.

APPENDIX

Questionnaire Items and Scales

FACILITY AVAILABILITY: Residents are asked if the following facilities exist in their neighborhood:

Day care center
Playground or park

Recreation center
Supermarket/Large Chain Grocery Store
Convenience Store or Corner Store
Pharmacy or Drug Store
Clinic or doctor's office where they can take their child
Laundromat
Dry Cleaners
Bank
Check Cashing Facility, not at a bank
Elementary School
Library

FACILITY USAGE: Residents are asked if they or their family have used the following neighborhood facilities in the past 2 months:

Day care center
Playground or park
Recreation center
Supermarket/Large Chain Grocery Store
Convenience Store or Corner Store
Pharmacy or Drug Store
Clinic or doctor's office where they can take their child
Laundromat
Dry Cleaners
Bank
Check Cashing Facility, not at a bank
Elementary School
Library

FACILITY QUALITY: Residents are asked how they would rate the quality of the following facilities on a scale of 1 (very bad) to 10 (excellent):

Day care center
Playground or park
Recreation center
Supermarket/Large Chain Grocery Store
Convenience Store or Corner Store
Pharmacy or Drug Store
Clinic or doctor's office where they can take their child
Laundromat
Dry Cleaners
Bank
Check Cashing Facility, not at a bank
Elementary School
Library

CHURCH ACTIVITIES: Residents are asked if they or members of their family have participated in the following activities in the past 2 months:

Church or Religious service
Church (or other Religious) club or activity (outside of religious services)

BLOCK CLUB ACTIVITIES: Residents are asked if they or members of their family have participated in the following activities in the past 2 months:

Block club meeting
Neighborhood Watch

INTERACTION: Residents are asked to respond to the following statements on a scale of 1 (mostly false) to 10 (mostly true):

When the weather is nice, the people living in my neighborhood visit with one another outside.
The people in my neighborhood visit with one another in their homes.
The people in my neighborhood loan things to one another.
The people in my neighborhood make sure other's homes are safe when someone is away.
On Halloween, most of the children living in my neighborhood go trick-or-treating in my neighborhood.

INTERVENE: Residents are asked to respond to the following statements on a scale of 1 (mostly false) to 10 (mostly true):

Neighbors should mind their own business about their neighbors' children.
Nowadays someone will verbally correct a child's behavior if the parents are not around.
Any adult has the right to verbally correct a neighborhood child if their parents are not around.

RETALIATE: Residents are asked to respond to the following statements on a scale of 1 (mostly false) to 10 (mostly true):

Children in this neighborhood might yell or swear at someone who verbally corrects their behavior.
Teenagers in this neighborhood might yell or swear at someone who verbally corrects their behavior.
Parents in this neighborhood might yell or swear at someone who verbally corrects their children.
Children might retaliate physically against a neighbor who verbally corrects their behavior.
Teenagers might retaliate physically against a neighbor who verbally corrects their behavior.
Parents might retaliate physically against a neighbor who verbally corrects their child's behavior.
Parents should be angry if neighbors verbally correct their children.

STOP DELINQUENCY: Residents are asked how likely it is that someone in their neighborhood would intervene in the following situations with a 5- or 6-year-old child on a scale of 1 (not likely) to 10 (very likely):

A child paints or writes on a car or building.
A child has hold of a gun.
A child has hold of a knife.
A child is playing with matches.
A child is shoplifting.
A child is taking something out of a neighbor's house, garage or yard.

STOP MISBEHAVIOR: Residents are asked how likely it is that someone in their neighborhood would intervene in the following situations with a 5- or 6-year-old child on a scale of 1 (not likely) to 10 (very likely):

A child hits another child of the same age
A child picks flowers out of someone else's yard

A child throws pebbles at a dog
A child throws pebbles at another child

ASSIST: Residents are asked how likely it is that someone in their neighborhood would intervene in the following situations with a 5- or 6-year-old child on a scale of 1 (not likely) to 10 (very likely):

A child is wandering by himself/herself
A child falls off his/her bicycle and is crying
An adult is spanking a child in the street
A child is left at home alone during the day.
A child is left at home alone during the evening.

NEIGHBORHOOD QUALITY: Residents are asked to respond to the following statements on a scale of 1 (mostly false) to 10 (mostly true):

My neighborhood is a good place to live.
My neighborhood is a good place to raise children.
The people moving into the neighborhood in the past year or so are good for the neighborhood.
I would like to move out of this neighborhood.
There are some children in the neighborhood that I do not want my children to play with.
The people moving into the neighborhood in the past year or so are bad for the neighborhood.
For the most part, the police come within a reasonable amount of time when they are called.
There is too much traffic in my neighborhood.
There are enough bus stops in my neighborhood.
My neighborhood is conveniently located in the city.
If I had to move out of this neighborhood, I would be sorry to leave.

MOBILITY: Residents are asked to respond to the following statements on a scale of 1 (mostly false) to 10 (mostly true);

About half of the people in the neighborhood are renters.
People move in and out of my neighborhood a lot.

POSITIVE CHANGE: on a scale of 1 to 10, in general, would you say that your neighborhood has changed for the better, has changed for the worse, or has stayed about the same in the past couple of years with "1" being "changed for the worse" and "10" being "changed for the better?"

DISORDER: Residents are asked how frequently the following things occur in their neighborhoods on a scale of 1 (rarely) to 10 (frequently):

Litter or trash on the sidewalks and streets
Graffiti on buildings and walls
Abandoned cars
Vacant, abandoned, or boarded up buildings
Drug dealers or users hanging around
Drunks hanging around
Unemployed adults loitering
Young adults loitering
Gang activity
Houses and yards not kept up

Absentee landlords
Disorderly or misbehaving groups of young children (younger than teenagers)
Disorderly or misbehaving groups of teenagers
Disorderly or misbehaving groups of adults

VICTIMIZATION: Residents are asked how worried they are about the following items on a
scale of 1 (not worried at all) to 10 (very worried):

Having property damaged
Having property stolen
Walking alone during the day
Walking alone after dark
Letting children go outside alone during the day
Letting children go outside alone after dark
Being robbed during the day
Being robbed at night
Being raped
Being mugged or beaten up
Having a child sexually abused by a stranger
Having a child sexually abused by someone they know
Having children kidnapped
Being murdered

IDENTITY

Do you have a name for your neighborhood?

ACKNOWLEDGMENTS

This research was supported primarily by a grant from The Foundation for
Child Development, as well as support from the Cleveland Foundation.

REFERENCES

Anderson, E. (1990). *Streetwise: Race, class and change in an urban community.* Chicago:
University of Chicago Press.
Anderson, E. (1994, May). The code of the streets. *Atlantic Monthly,* pp. 81–93.
Belsky, J. (1980). Child maltreatment: An ecological integration. *American Psychologist, 35,*
320–335.
Bronfenbrenner, U. (1979). *The ecology of human development: Experiments by nature and
design.* Cambridge, MA: Harvard University Press.
Bronfenbrenner, U. (1988). Foreword. In A. Pence (Ed.), *Ecological research with children and
families: From concepts to methodology* (pp. 9–19). New York: Teachers College Press.
Bronfenbrenner, U., Moen, P., & Garbarino, J. (1984). Child, family, and community. In
R. Parke (Ed.), *Review of child development research* (pp. 283–328). Chicago: University
of Chicago Press.

Brooks-Gunn, J., Duncan, G. J., Klebanov, P. K., & Sealand, N. (1993). Do neighborhoods influence child and adolescent development? *American Journal of Sociology, 99*, 353–395.

Bursik, R. J., & Webb, J. (1982). Community change and patterns of delinquency. *American Journal of Sociology, 88*, 24–41.

Cicchetti, D., & Lynch, M. (1993). Toward an ecological/transaction model of community violence and child maltreatment: Consequences for children's development. *Psychiatry, 56*, 96–118.

Clark, R. (1992). *Neighborhood effects on dropping out of school among teenage boys.* Washington, DC: The Urban Institute.

Coleman, J. S. (1987). Families and schools. *Educational Researcher, 16*, 32–38.

Coulton, C., Korbin, J., Chow, J., & Su, M. (1995). Community level factors and child maltreatment rates. *Child Development, 66*, 1262–1276.

Crane, J. (1991). Effects of neighborhoods on dropping out of school and teenage childbearing. In C. Jencks & P. E. Peterson (Eds.), *The urban underclass* (pp. 299–320). Washington, DC: The Brookings Institution.

Duncan, G. J. (1993). *Families and neighbors as sources of disadvantage in the schooling decisions of white and black adolescents.* Ann Arbor: University of Michigan.

Earls, F., McGuire, J., & Shay, S. (1994). Evaluating a community intervention to reduce the risk of child abuse: Methodological strategies in conducting neighborhood surveys. *Child Abuse & Neglect, 18*, 473–485.

Entwisle, B. (1991). Macro-micro linkages in social demography: A commentary. In J. Huber (Ed.), *Macro-micro linkages in sociology* (pp. 280–286). Newbury Park, CA: Sage.

Figueira-McDonough, J. (1991). Community structure and delinquency: A typology. *Social Service Review, 65*, 69–91.

Freudenburg, W. R. (1986). The density of acquaintanceship: An overlooked variable in community research. *American Journal of Sociology, 92*, 27–63.

Furstenberg, F. F. (1993). How families manage risk and opportunity in dangerous neighborhoods. In W. J. Wilson (Ed.), *Sociology and the Public Agenda* (pp. 231–258). Newbury Park, CA: Sage.

Galster, G. (1992). Housing discrimination and urban poverty of African Americans. *Journal of Housing Research, 2*, 87–122.

Garbarino, J. (1977). The human ecology of child maltreatment: A conceptual model for research. *Journal of Marriage and Family, 39*, 721–735.

Garbarino, J., & Crouter, A. (1978). Defining the community context for parent-childrelations: The correlates of child maltreatment. *Child Development, 49*, 604–616.

Garbarino, J., Dubrow, N., Kostelny, K., & Pardo, C. (1992). *Children in danger: Coping with the consequences of community violence.* San Francisco: Jossey-Bass.

Garbarino, J., & Kostelny, K. (1992). Child maltreatment as a community problem. *Child Abuse and Neglect, 16*, 455–464.

Garbarino, J., & Sherman, D. (1980). High-risk neighborhoods and high-risk families: The human ecology of child maltreatment. *Child Development, 51*, 188–198.

Holahan, C. J., & Wandersman, A. (1987). The community psychology perspective in environmental psychology. In D. Stokols & I. Altman (Eds.), *Handbook of environmental psychology* (pp. 827–861). New York: Wiley.

Jargowsky, P. A., & Bane, M. (1991). Ghetto poverty in the United States, 1970–1980. In C. Jencks & P. E. Peterson (Eds.), *The urban underclass* (pp. 235–273). Washington, DC: The Brookings Institution.

Jarrett, R. L. (1994). Living poor: Family life among single parent, African American Women. *Social Problems, 41*, 30–49.

Jencks, C., & Mayer, S. E. (1990). The social consequences of growing up in a poor neighborhood. In L. E. Lynn & M. G. H. McGeary (Eds.), *Inner-city poverty in the United States* (pp. 111–186). Washington, DC: National Academy Press.

Johnson, S., & Bell, J. F. (1985). Evaluating and predicting survey efficiency using generalizability theory. *Journal of Educational Measurement, 22,* 107–119.

Kasarda, J. (1993). Inner-city concentrated poverty and neighborhood distress: 1970 to 1990. *Housing Policy Debate, 4,* 253–302.

Keiser, R. L. (1969). *The vice lords: Warriors of the street.* New York: Holt, Rinehart and Winston.

Korbin, J., & Coulton, C. (1994). *Neighborhood impact on child abuse and neglect.* Final Report of Grant No. 90-CA1494. Washington, DC: National Center on Child Abuse and Neglect, Department of Health and Human Services.

Liebow, E. (1966). *Talley's corner.* Boston: Little, Brown.

Lyon, L. (1987). *The community in urban society.* Chicago: Dorsey.

National Center for Child Abuse & Neglect (1988). *Study of national incidence and prevalence of child abuse and neglect: 1988.* Washington, DC: U.S. Department of Health and Human Services.

Newberger, E. H., Reed, R. B., Daniel, J. H., Hyde, J. N., & Kotelchuck, M. (1977). Pediatric social illness: Toward an etiologic classification. *Pediatrics, 60,* 178–185.

O'Brien, R. M. (1990). Estimating the reliability of aggregate-level variables based on individual-level characteristics. *Sociological Methods and Research, 18,* 473–504.

O'Toole, R., Turbett, P., & Nalpeka, C. (1983). Theories, professional knowledge, and diagnosis of child abuse. In D. Fenkelhor, R. Gelles, G. Hotaling, & M. Strauss (Eds.), *The dark side of families: Current family violence research.* Newbury Park, CA: Sage.

Pelton, L. (1981). *The social context of child abuse and neglect.* New York: Human Sciences.

Romney, A. K., Weller, S. C., & Batchelder, W. H. (1986). Culture as consensus: A theory of culture and informant accuracy. *American Anthropologist, 88,* 313–337.

Sampson, R. J. (1991). Linking the micro- and macro-level dimensions of community social organization. *Social Forces, 70,* 43–64.

Sampson, R. J. (1992). Family management and child development: Insights from social disorganization theory. In J. McCord (Ed.), *Advances in criminological theory* (Vol. 3, pp. 63–93). New Brunswick, NJ: Transition.

Stack, C. (1974). *All our kin: Strategies for survival in a black community.* New York: Harper and Row.

Straus, M. A., Gelles, R. J., & Steinmetz, S. K. (1980). *Behind closed doors: Violence in the American family.* Newbury Park, CA: Sage.

Taylor, R. B. (1988). *Human territorial functioning.* Cambridge, MA: Cambridge University Press.

Taylor, R. B., Gottfredson, S. D., & Brower, S. (1984). Block crime and fear: Defensible space, local social ties and territorial functioning. *Journal of Research in Crime and Delinquency, 21,* 303–331.

Tienda, M. (1991). Poor people and poor places: Deciphering neighborhood effects on poverty outcomes. In J. Huber (Ed.), *Macro-micro linkages in sociology* (pp. 244–262). Newbury Park, CA: Sage.

White, M. (1987). *American neighborhoods and residential differentiation.* New York: Russell Sage Foundation.

Whyte, W. F. (1955). *Street corner society* (3rd ed.). Chicago: University of Chicago Press.

Wilson, W. J. (1987). *The truly disadvantaged: The inner city, the underclass, and public policy.* Chicago: The University of Chicago Press.

Zuravin, S. J. (1989). The ecology of child abuse and neglect: Review of the literature and presentation of data. *Violence and Victims, 4,* 101–120.

5

Ecological Assessments of Community Disorder: Their Relationship to Fear of Crime and Theoretical Implications

Douglas D. Perkins and Ralph B. Taylor

Researchers suggest that fear of crime arises from community disorder, cues in the social and physical environment that are distinct from crime itself. Three ecological methods of measuring community disorder are presented: resident perceptions reported in surveys and on-site observations by trained raters, both aggregated to the street block level, and content analysis of crime- and disorder-related newspaper articles aggregated to the neighborhood level. Each method demonstrated adequate reliability and roughly equal ability to predict subsequent fear of crime among 412 residents of 50 blocks in 50 neighborhoods in Baltimore, MD. Pearson and partial correlations (controlling for sex, race, age, and victimization) were calculated at multiple levels of analysis: individual, individual deviation from block, and community (block/neighborhood). Hierarchical linear models provided comparable results under more stringent conditions. Results linking different measures of disorder with fear, and individual and aggregated demographics with fear inform theories about fear of crime and extend research on the impact of community social and physical disorder. Implications for ecological assessment of community social and physical environments are discussed.

Originally published in the *American Journal of Community Psychology, 24*(1) (1996): 63–107.

Ecological Research to Promote Social Change: Methodological Advances from Community Psychology, edited by Tracey A. Revenson et al. Kluwer Academic/Plenum Publishers, New York, 2002.

Community disorder is a broad and elusive concept, difficult to define or measure in a way that all would understand and agree with. It refers to social and physical conditions and events in a locale beyond the serious crimes that may be occurring there. These conditions and events may relate to any or all of the following: residents who are no longer able to maintain a satisfactory quality of community life; unregulated, uncivil, or rowdy behaviors observed on the street that may be associated with social conflict; a lack of investment in or supervision over a locale on the part of residents or external public and private institutions, or both; and a degeneration over time in neighborhood-based physical capital, reflected in diminishing quality and/or maintenance of both public and private property.

This article has three main objectives. The first is to present three different methods for measuring community-level ecological constructs. Indicators of community disorder may be drawn from several sources: residents themselves, on-site observations of conditions, or reports from the local media, for example. In the present paper, we present examples of each of these methods.

Our second purpose is to explore and compare each method's ability to predict residents' fear of crime. Theorists have argued for 20 years that community disorder strongly influences residents' concerns for personal safety. By comparing the relative impact of different indicators, we can learn whether the strength of the relationship depends on the type of data collected. Research in this area has tended to rely on the same source of data to measure both fear and disorder: resident surveys. Will we see weaker impacts using other indicators of disorder?

We pursue these first two purposes using nested, or clustered, data on individuals living on different street blocks, each located in a different neighborhood.[1] We are interested in both ecological and psychological dynamics. More specifically, with two of our three modes of data collection, we can examine both community- and individual-level effects. This is useful for descriptive purposes, but also has important theoretical ramifications. Sociological research on disorder and fear of crime has generally implied that the processes occur largely at the ecological or neighborhood level, or that the processes represent effects of different contexts on individuals in different locations. Psychologists are more likely to assume that individual differences (e.g., in the perception of disorder) are the primary determinants of fear.

---

[1] A street block is defined as both sides of a street bounded by cross streets or a cross street and a dead end. We sometimes refer to street blocks as simply "blocks." They should not be confused with (square) census blocks.

Thus, our third objective is to contrast effects at the different levels of analysis. We hope such information can be used to further sharpen our understanding of community disorder, fear of crime, and their relationship to one another. The remainder of this introduction explains the logic linking community disorder to fear of crime and then examines research linking fear with physical environment features and media sources.

THE SOCIAL RELEVANCE OF FEAR OF CRIME

Fear of crime is a serious individual- and community-level problem in urban and suburban areas, influencing how freely people move about the places where they live (Liska, Sanchirico, & Reed, 1988). It is concerned with people's emotional responses and feelings of vulnerability in the face of dangerous conditions or the possibility of victimization (Ferraro, 1994). It emerges as distinct from people's more cognitive perceptions of risk (Dubow, McCabe, & Kaplan, 1979).

Crime has been identified as an important environmental stressor (Lewis & Riger, 1986; Melnicoe, 1987; Taylor & Shumaker, 1990). Fear may be a critical factor in the related stress process. Fear has been linked with block-level shifts in anxiety and depression, suggesting that in the social ecology of the street block, changes in psychological distress are interwoven with fluctuations in safety-related concerns (Taylor & Perkins, 1994; see also Norris & Kaniasty, 1991). Fear of crime is also linked negatively with community social and psychological ties (Liska & Baccaglini, 1990; Perkins, Florin, Rich, Wandersman, & Chavis, 1990; Riger, Gordon, & LeBailly, 1981; Skogan, 1990; Steward, Perkins, & Brown, 1995; Taylor, Gottfredson, & Brower, 1984).

FEAR OF CRIME AND COMMUNITY DISORDER

On the Distribution of Fear and Victimization

Social scientists initially presumed that fear of crime and actual victimization would be closely linked (Dubow et al., 1979). This presumption foundered on two points: Fear is much more widespread than victimization and the demographic groups that are most fearful are least victimized. On the latter: Young males are victimized the most but report being the least fearful. Women and the elderly, and particularly elderly women, are especially likely to report fear (Ferraro, 1994; LaGrange & Ferraro, 1989; Lawton & Yaffe, 1980; Mulvey, Turro, Cutter, & Pash, 1995; Ortega & Myles, 1987) despite comparatively low exposure to risk (Clarke, Ekblom,

Hough, & Mayhew, 1985; Liska et al., 1988) and low victimization rates, according to official crime statistics (Balkin, 1979). The validity of crime statistics is suspect (O'Brien, 1985) and the not necessarily irrational fear felt by physically more vulnerable groups may be grounded in more serious physical, psychological, or economic consequences should victimization occur (Skogan, Cook, Antunes, & Cook, 1978). Further, if women and elderly are less often victimized by street crime, that may be due to their fear causing them to take greater precautions, such as avoiding unsafe areas at night and other behavioral adaptations (Liska et al., 1988; Norris & Kaniasty, 1992; Skogan & Maxfield, 1981). But the data still suggest that there may be more to "fear of crime" than simply fear of crime (Garofalo & Laub, 1978).

Fear May Reflect Broader Conditions in the Community

On the former point: Researchers began suggesting in the mid to late 1970s that fear of crime was more prevalent than crime because it reflected not only victimization experienced, and indirect victimization (those crime experiences heard from friends), but they proposed that it also reflected broader conditions of disorder in the community (Garofalo & Laub, 1978; Hunter, 1978; Lewis & Salem, 1985; Wilson, 1975). Those who witness this disorder may conclude that the community cannot manage these problems and that external agencies are unwilling or unable to deal with them (Hunter, 1978).

The Incivilities Theory of Neighborhood Decline

To residents and visitors alike, these conditions of disorder or "incivility," both physical and social, symbolize not only a superficial neglect of the community but also an underlying breakdown in both local norms of behavior and formal and informal social controls (Lewis & Maxfield, 1980; Lewis & Salem, 1985; Perkins, Meeks & Taylor, 1992; Skogan & Maxfield, 1981; Taylor, 1987; Taylor & Hale, 1986; Taylor & Shumaker, 1990). Social incivilities include such problems as loitering youths or homeless people, rowdy behavior, drug dealing, public drunkenness, and prostitution. Physical incivilities include such environmental stimuli as litter, vandalism, vacant or dilapidated housing, abandoned cars, and unkempt lots.

Subsequently, researchers expanded the model, adding a longitudinal perspective. They suggested that increases in social and/or physical signs of incivility might not only inspire residents' fear, but might also contribute independently to neighborhood decline. They argue that if incivilities are not dealt with promptly and effectively, residents perceive more social problems in the locale and lose confidence in their neighborhood and in law enforcement's ability to prevent or control open displays of disorder, let alone more serious crime. The theory suggests that as resident fears and avoidance behaviors increase, informal social controls weaken, incivilities proliferate, potential offenders are emboldened, criminals from adjoining areas are attracted to the locale, and the downward spiral becomes self-reinforcing (Skogan, 1990). This broader theory of disorder has, for some years, strongly influenced policy changes in community policing and community crime prevention (Greene & Taylor, 1988; Wilson & Kelling, 1982).

Resident Perceptions of Community Disorder

Regrettably, much of the research linking signs of incivility with fear has been based solely on residents' subjective perceptions of disorder, drawn from survey responses (LaGrange, Ferraro, & Supaneic, 1992; Lewis & Maxfield, 1980; Lewis & Salem, 1985; Skogan, 1990; Skogan & Maxfield, 1981). At the neighborhood level, perceptions of disorder correlate strongly with fear, and with indicators of neighborhood structure. Skogan (1990) observed a correlation of $r = .84$ between perceived disorder and neighborhood unemployment. Hope and Hough (1988) suggested that, at the neighborhood level, fear and signs of incivility may not be conceptually separable. But another interpretation is that very high fear–disorder correlations may arise in part from the two measures, when based on resident surveys, sharing method variance. We should not draw a conclusion of construct inseparability until we have examined measures of each construct drawn from different sources. A few studies have done this, using on-site observations of block and neighborhood environments recorded by trained raters.

On-Site Observations and Levels of Analysis

Studies employing measures based on on-site observations find linkages with fear that depend in part on the level of aggregation, and the community context. At the individual level, in both U.S. and British samples, Maxfield (1987) found observed measures of physical neighborhood decay related more strongly to fear than perceived vulnerability or victimization.

In a neighborhood-level model examining impacts of observed incivilities on a broad range of responses to disorder, including fear of crime, Taylor (1996) found direct effects in the expected direction; staying in more and fear of crime were more prevalent in neighborhoods with higher rated incivilities.

A very few studies have examined *both* on-site observations and resident perceptions of disorder. Taylor, Shumaker, and Gottfredson (1985) found independently rated, neighborhood-level physical and social disorder to correlate strongly with resident perceptions of disorder and fear of crime. They suggested that observed disorder might influence neighborhood fear only for neighborhoods whose future was uncertain; in extremely stable neighborhoods, and in extremely disadvantaged locales, disorder will not influence fear. In the former case, residents are buffered by their secure future; in the latter case, given other extant problems, impacts of observed incivilities become diminished through a process analogous to cognitive adaptation (Taylor & Shumaker, 1990). In Covington and Taylor's (1991) contextual reanalysis of the Taylor, Shumaker, and Gottfredson (1985) data, neighborhood-level on-site observed incivilities significantly predicted individual-level fear. But resident perceptions of incivilities, based on individual within-neighborhood deviation scores, were the strongest predictor of fear.

From the same data used in the present study, Perkins et al. (1992) found on-site observations demonstrated high interrater reliabilities and concurrent validities, significantly predicting residents' subjective assessments after controlling for block size, race, education, and home ownership. Regression analyses showed that physical incivilities were independently linked to perceptions of social and crime-related problems.

Contrary to those studies and using a similar on-site data collection instrument but in a different city, Perkins, Wandersman, Rich, and Taylor (1993) found in a block-level analysis that resident and independent ratings of block physical incivilities were not significantly correlated. But observed environmental items correlated more strongly and consistently with five different indicators of block crime over the following year than did resident perceptions of the environment. Using those same data, Perkins et al. (1990) found residential street block-level fear related modestly to certain independent observer-rated incivilities (e.g., litter) and nonsignificantly to others (e.g., graffiti, dilapidated housing). They also found that resident perceptions of physical disorder correlated significantly with fear, but not after controlling for block income, residential stability, and race.

It would be reasonable to assume that the relationship between community disorder and fear increases as the level of analysis gets smaller and "closer to home." Thus, the street block *should* be an even more relevant context for this relationship than is the neighborhood. It may be that the block-level results of Perkins et al. (1990) were not stronger and more consistent because most of the blocks in that study were well-organized with a high degree of citizen participation in crime prevention and other activities. Similar to the argument of Taylor, Shumaker, and Gottfredson (1985), the authors suggest that the formal and informal social organization of the community may help to buffer the impact of disorder on fear. What is clear, however, is that more block-level research on community disorder and fear is warranted.

In sum, recent research suggests that on-site observations of community disorder may help us understand perceptions of crime and related community problems. But these studies are limited in several ways, even if we focus on the set of studies including on-site observations and residents' perceptions of disorder. Shortcomings of the latter group include the following.

Limitations

Only two studies examine impacts of both on-site observations and resident perceptions of disorder on fear of crime. Perkins et al. (1990) used block-aggregated data only, which fails to distinguish individual and group-level effects. Covington and Taylor (1991) used cross-level (contextual) analysis, but misspecification of individual-level predictors could have biased the effects observed for the contextual incivility predictor (Hauser, 1974). Because effects may vary depending upon the level of analysis, an analytic approach allowing separation of different levels of process may help illuminate the varying dynamics. None of the previous studies allow for this. Third, none of the studies allow for correlated error structures. Since most of these studies use clustered samples, using either street blocks or neighborhoods or both as a sampling unit, errors within a sampling unit may be nonindependent. Analyses have not yet allowed for this. Finally, none of the studies has yet compared environmental measures of community-level disorder with a measure based on content-analyzed mass communication (i.e., television, radio, newspaper, or magazine reports). In the next section we turn to the research on media and fear, then conclude with a statement of an integrated model.

FEAR AND THE NEWS MEDIA

If resident perceptions of community disorder do not always match more independent and systematic ones, what else besides demography and methodology may be influencing those differences? What indirect sources of information are there about local crime and disorder? One source is of course one's neighbors, which is where theories of indirect, or "vicarious," victimization arise (Skogan & Maxfield, 1981; Taylor & Hale, 1986; Tyler, 1984). Another important source may be the news media. The degree to which public fears are influenced by the media, and precisely how they may be influenced, have been studied but remain open questions. Some presentations of crime in the media may even have a distancing effect on personal risk assessment (Gomme, 1988). Noting that it would be mal-adaptive for people to rely solely on their direct personal experience of environmental hazards, such as crime victimization, Tyler (1984) reviewed the literature on how indirect, socially transmitted information influences fear of crime. He found that people receive such information through their social networks, but that studies of naturally occurring crime-risk judgments and evaluations of media campaigns suggest that citizens do not generally accept the mass media as a source of information about personal crime risk.

That conclusion may be true for electronic media, but there is some evidence for the impact of newspapers on fear. O'Keefe and Reid-Nash (1987) found that greater attention to televised news was related to subse-quent increased fear, concern, and avoidance behaviors. They found no such effects for attention to crime news in newspapers, although greater concern was related to subsequent increased readership. But most other studies have found the relationship between fear and media coverage of crime to be significant for newspapers (Jaehnig, Weaver, & Fico, 1981; Liska & Baccaglini, 1990; Smith, 1984; Williams & Dickinson, 1993) and modest for television viewing (Sparks & Ogles, 1990).

Pawson and Banks (1991) used rape reports from the two Christ-church, NZ, daily newspapers over a 5-year period and found that surveyed fear of violence extended well beyond those groups and districts that featured prominently in the newspaper reports. Although this suggests either a non-effect or overgeneralized effect of newspaper coverage, younger women in their sample exhibited patterns of fear that indicated that were well aware of the areas with more rape news stories.

Jaehnig et al. (1981) correlated data from a survey of community residents with content analyses of newspaper crime stories. They found that the influence of newspapers on public opinion toward crime problems increases as individuals' personal knowledge of social conditions contribut-ing to crime decreases. Comparing two urban samples, they also found much higher fear of victimization in the city with a lower reported crime rate but almost twice as many news stories about violent crime. They suggest that newspaper crime stories cause an unreasonably high fear of violent crimes and an unreasonably low concern over property crimes.

Liska and Baccaglini (1990) content-analyzed daily newspaper crime stories to measure their effect on attitudes, beliefs, and fears about crime in 26 major U.S. cities based on National Crime Survey data. Homicide stories had the highest correlation with fear of crime but, interestingly, newspaper coverage of nonlocal crime appeared to make people feel safe by comparison, regardless of the local crime situation.

Three of the most important studies on the relationship between newspaper crime reporting and fear of crime were done in Great Britain. Ditton and Duffy (1983) did not focus on fear per se, but documented widespread bias toward sensationalism in the newspaper reporting of crime news in Scotland. They found that the press reported only 0.25% of the offenses reported to the police or heard by courts. Newspapers tended to concentrate on crimes involving violence, sex, and public disorder (i.e., those most likely to induce public fears).

Smith (1984) used a household survey in Birmingham, England, to measure responses to crime news and content-analyzed 7 months of crime stories in a daily newspaper. The majority of respondents reported learning of crime events through either electronic media or the local newspaper. Similar to Ditton and Duffy (1983), the newspaper content analysis revealed such distortions of police crime reports as giving more attention to "exciting" personal offenses than to nonviolent thefts and burglaries, which actually made up 84% of reported crimes. Smith (1984) also found that news stories tended to unjustifiably link crimes with ethnic minorities. She argued that such distortions may unrealistically increase fear of crime.

Indeed, Williams and Dickinson (1993) measured the amount of space and prominence given to crime in 10 British newspapers and found a positive correlation between a newspaper's crime coverage and its readers' level of fear. This effect held even after controlling for demographic factors, although they also found that tabloid newspapers, particularly those targeting a working-class readership, carried more crime reports and reported crimes more sensationally than did broadsheets. Smith (1984) concluded that fear must be studied in relation to both the urban environment and newspaper coverage of crime. By comparing impacts of newspaper coverage and other urban conditions, we can accomplish this purpose.

METHODS

Overall Design

Fifty blocks in 50 different neighborhoods throughout Baltimore City, MD, were randomly selected to participate in the 1987–1988 multimethod study. Two waves of panel survey data were collected in order to examine change in sampled individuals and neighborhoods over time and to facilitate tentative causal interpretations. Extensive data were also collected by trained, independent raters at the beginning of the study on the crime and fear-related physical environment of each block and almost 70% of the respondent households. The third source of data used in the present analyses is a 15-month archive of content-analyzed crime and disorder-related news articles from the city's major daily newspaper and a minority community newspaper. The triangulation of these diverse ecological methods helps to paint a rich portrait of the sociophysical context of each community in the study.

Sample Selection

Site Characteristics

Baltimore is a typical, large, older, Eastern U.S. city, in the midst of industrial and economic change and moderate population decline in recent decades. Its fairly high rate of serious street crime was similar to comparably sized U.S. cities during the same period. In terms of demography, Baltimore's neighborhoods, though internally homogenous, are ethnically and socioeconomically diverse. Regarding housing turnover, many of the neighborhoods are fairly stable. The relatively small scale of the neighborhoods has helped most of them organize Neighborhood Improvement Associations, many of which engage in crime prevention activities.

Neighborhood Selection[2]

A probability proportionate to size (PPS) procedure was used to systematically select the 50 neighborhoods to be included in the study. First, each of the 277 Baltimore neighborhoods (as defined by Goodman and Taylor, 1983, using ecologically validated boundaries and names) was ordered geographically in a serpentine pattern from the Northwest corner of the city to the Southeast peninsula. Then, the 1980 Census was used to construct a cumulative neighborhood household population frequency.

---

[2] Given a limitation of 412 survey respondents, the decision process for deriving the optimum number of blocks and neighborhoods to include in the sample was based on a difficult balance between statistical power at the aggregate level and an adequate sampling ratio of individuals per block. Several different approaches to drawing the neighborhood, block, and household sampling frame were considered, based on three criteria related to variability and inferential validity: Does the sampling procedure allow for capturing sufficient individual-level variability on the measures of interest (crime, fear, disorder, etc.)? Are there sufficient cases per social area unit to allow us to describe and draw conclusions about blocks or neighborhoods (i.e., does it provide for meaningful contextual variables)? Does the procedure capture sufficient variability at the aggregate (block/neighborhood) level? After weighing the various tradeoffs of (a) random selection throughout neighborhoods (i.e., ignoring blocks), (b) choosing more or fewer households per block, (c) more or fewer total neighborhoods in the sample, (d) stratifying the sample, we believe the plan chosen represents the best compromise. Regarding statistical power, an n of 50 blocks results in power values of .57 at alpha = .05 and .69 at alpha = .1 for 2-tailed, block-level analyses of a moderate effect size ($r = .3$).

Baltimore neighborhoods vary considerably in size, but the mean neighborhood population in 1980 was 2,840. Public housing projects, high-risk apartment complexes, and the central business district were excluded due to limitations on the size of the survey sample. Thus, at best our data may only be generalized to low-rise urban residential neighborhoods of moderate density.

The neighborhood sampling interval was then determined by dividing the total household population of the 250 remaining neighborhoods by 50, the number of neighborhoods sought. A random starting number was applied to the cumulative neighborhood population table to choose the first neighborhood. The interval was then added to that number in successive steps to determine Neighborhoods 2 through 50.

Block Sampling Procedure

The processes of informal social control, social cohesion, and territoriality, which are intrinsic to crime and disorder prevention, are considered most salient at the street block level (Perkins et al., 1990, 1992). Block household listings from a city address (criss-across) directory were used to conduct the random selection of one block per neighborhood with probability proportionate to size. All blocks in each of the 50 neighborhoods, excluding boundary streets and blocks with no usable household listings, were entered in a cumulative household population distribution. Unusable listings include businesses, offices, and addresses with more than 15 listings (i.e., generally, high-rise apartment buildings). Due to the tendency of Baltimore neighborhoods to be culturally homogenous and the exclusion of high-rise, predominantly commercial and boundary blocks, every block sampled appears to be reasonably representative of its surrounding neighborhood, physically and demographically. The representativeness of each block's physical characteristics was verified in person at the time of household sampling and environmental observation (below).

Household Sampling Procedure

For use with the survey and environmental measures, a field household enumeration on each selected block provided a more complete and up-to-date listing of households than the address directory permits. The field listing and systematic household selection were conducted at the same time as the environmental observation (below). This procedure entailed visual inspection of each address on the block for number of occupied units. Then, the interval selection of eight primary and four replacement households on each block with a random start was done on site.

Survey Respondent Sample

Of an initial sample frame of 601 potential respondents, no contacts were attempted for 13 addresses and 13 others were verified, in person, as vacant, thus leaving an n of 575 attempted contact households (response rate = 72%). If one looks only at those households in which someone was actually reached, however ($n = 492$), the completed interviews per household-contacted response rate is 84% (n of refusals, break-offs, and language problems = 80). Eligible respondents for this study were a randomly selected head of household. Within household replacements were not allowed. The final Time 1 survey sample ($n = 412$) comprised 270 (65.5%) females; 52.4% were African American, 46.3% white. At the time of the survey, 17% of the sample were under 30 years of age; 54.2% were between 30 and 60; and 28.8% were over 60. The mean length of residence in the current neighborhood was 14.6 years and in the respondent's current home was 12.6 years. Homeowners made up 58.5% of the sample. The mean household size is 2.9 with an average of 1 child per household. Roughly half the sample had a household income of $20,000 or more.

The Time 1 survey sample was used as the sampling frame for the follow-up survey conducted 1 year later. The panel sample ($n = 305$) had a response rate of 74%. The two samples did not differ significantly by sex, race, or fear of crime. The Time 2 sample had a higher percentage of homeowners and long-term residents and was a mean of 3.4 years older at Time 1. Weighting the Time 2 sample by home ownership (the most significant source of attrition bias) had very little effect on other differences between the samples, which suggests that those differences (less victimization and perceived block crime and disorder problems at Time 2) are probably due more to change than sample attrition.

Instruments

Block Environmental Inventory

The Block Environmental Inventory (Perkins et al., 1992) is a combination of the authors' previous separate research involving direct observational measurement of the crime and fear-related physical environment of urban residential blocks. The instrument was pilot-tested and refined throughout the training of six raters. Three teams of two raters each were sent to separate blocks in January 1987. Raters were not allowed to discuss a particular rule or rating as they conducted a block observation.

They were, however, allowed to discuss the interpretation of a rule between blocks.

The first page (Section I) of the inventory covers the number of young men and women (approximately ages 10–35), children, and adults outdoors at a given point in time and their general activities (walking, "hanging out," etc.), abandoned cars, damaged or graffiti painted public property, types and amount of open land use (vacant lots, church or school yards, parking lots, playgrounds, gardens, etc.), and whether the land is poorly maintained. Although there is undoubtedly variation in people's use of outdoor space by time of day, environmental data collection was limited to 5:00 to 8:00 p.m. on weeknights and noon to 8:00 on weekends. A more serious limitation in the present area is that they were collected in winter when people spend less time outdoors. Thus, the restriction of the variables time and weather may also restrict the influence of the independent variable "males outdoors."

For the second page (Sections II, III, and IV), the raters start over at the beginning of the block, walk down one side of the street at a time, keeping a count of the number of occupied residential units. Each non-residential (stores, schools, etc.) and mixed-use building was rated for litter in front of it, vandalism (e.g., graffiti, broken windows), and lack of exterior maintenance (peeling paint, broken fixtures) (block-level $\alpha = .76$). The eight primary survey sample households were selected (see Household Sampling Procedure, above) and rated for litter, vandalism, and lack of exterior maintenance (block-level $\alpha = .73$). (See Appendix A.)

Interrater reliability, or agreement, has been a problem for many observational measures. Table I presents means, standard deviations, and interrater reliability coefficients for the inventory. Five blocks were rated by only one rater and so were excluded from these analyses. With the exception of a few, low base-rate items, such as young males engaged in "other" outdoor activities, abandoned cars, and trash-filled empty lots, interrater agreement for block-level observations was high (mean intraclass correlation ($ICr = .78$). Interrater reliabilities were consistently high for property-level observations. The ICr for recognizing the number of abandoned buildings on a block is .92. Section III covers each nonresidential property on a block. Its mean reliability coefficient for all items is $ICr = .86$. Section IV consists of 16 items on eight sample homes per block. These may be aggregated to the block level, which renders higher reliability coefficients than at the property level. Block-level ICrs for the three disorder items range from .67 to .83 with an overall mean (including nondisorder items) of .81. See Perkins et al. (1992) for psychometric information on the entire instrument.

Table I. Disorder Items in the Block Environmental Inventory: Means and Interrater Reliability[a]

	M	SD	Intraclass r	
Section I: Block-level characteristics				
Males, 10–35, observed outdoors hanging out	0.36	1.70	.83	
Walking	0.64	1.10	.84	
Working	0.16	0.76	.91	
Other	0.05	0.25	−.02	
Total males, 10–35	1.21	2.10	.85	
Unused vacant lots as estimated % of block	0.64	1.72	.97	
Open lot lack of maintenance	0.24	0.37	.43	
Number of abandoned cars on street	0.31	0.83	.53	
Section II. All properties (per block)				
Total abandoned building	1.4	2.2	.92	
Section III. All nonresidential properties				
Total vacant nonresidential units	0.14	0.43	.86	
Litter on/in front of nonresid. property	0.39	0.92	.82	
Vandalism/graffiti on nonresid. property	0.27	0.71	.92	
Nonresidential dilapidation	0.44	1.0	.90	
			Household-level ICr	Block-level ICr
Section IV. Sample homes	M	SD		
Physical Disorder Subscale			.69	
Litter in front of house	0.44	0.29	.61	.83
Vandalism/graffiti	0.10	0.14	.47	.67
Dilapidated exterior	0.47	0.27	.53	.71

[a] See Perkins et al. (1992) for an explanation of the entire instrument. The *n* of blocks is 45. The *n* of properties in Section IV is 365.

Survey of Residents

Beginning 2 weeks after the environmental data collection, eight residents on each study block were interviewed in late winter, 1987 (Time 1), and again 1 year later (Time 2). The survey took approximately 35 minutes to complete. If the respondent could not be interviewed by telephone, an interviewer was sent door-to-door to try to conduct the survey. Of the 412 interviews completed in Time 1, 191 (46%) were by telephone and 221 were in person.

The overall survey was designed to elicit residents' perceptions of the quality of the surrounding social and physical environment, the extent of residents' social support resources—including both the format and informal network of neighbors helping neighbors, their behavioral and emotional responses to crime and victimization, and the stressful impact of persistent fear on residents' mental health status.

The present analyses use only the survey measures of demographic variables and perceptions of social and physical environmental disorder and crime problems from Time 1 and fear of crime from Time 2. Although a variety of demographic questions were asked, the ones used here are those that have been empirically linked with fear (i.e., *sex, age,* and *race*). The fourth covariate for the present analyses is criminal *victimization* in "past 12 months." A series of items prompted the type of crime attempted, whether it happened more than once, whether any attempts were success-ful, whether any attempts occurred within two blocks of home, and whether the incident was reported to the police (adapted from the National Crime Survey and Perkins et al., 1993).

Residents assessed crime and fear-related block problems on a 3-point scale (i.e., *a big problem, somewhat of a problem,* or *not a problem*) used in other community surveys (e.g., Perkins et al., 1990). The internal consis-tency of the total scale is alpha = .88. The present analyses use just two sub-scales (based on unit-weighted, z-scored items) derived by factor analysis. One is *perceived physical disorder*: "vandalism, like people breaking win-dows or spray painting buildings," "vacant housing," "people who don't keep up their property or yards," "litter or trash in the streets," and "vacant lots with trash or junk" (individual-level $\alpha = .75$; block-level $\alpha = .87$). The other subscale is *perceived social disorder*: "people who say insulting things or bother other people when they walk down the street," "groups of teenagers hanging out in the street," "people fighting or arguing," "people selling illegal drugs" (individual-level $\alpha = .80$; block-level $\alpha = .89$). We used hierarchical linear modeling (HLM) to assess how much residents on a block agreed with one another on these indices (Bryk & Raudenbush, 1992, p. 63). The way HLM handles intraclass agreement is in terms of estimated true group means as a function of how much members of each group agree with each other, how far the block mean is from the grand mean, and how large the group is. The overall reliability of the block means on perceived social disorder was .775; the overall reliability of the block means on per-ceived physical disorder was .684. These substantial reliability coefficients indicate that the observed block means are quite acceptable as indicators of the true block means on these indices.

Fear of crime is measured with a series of questions on felt and per-ceived safety of self and household members, in the neighborhood and on the block, adapted from several studies, including Greenberg, Rohe, and Williams (1982), Rosenbaum, Lewis, and Grant (1986), and Taylor et al. (1984) (see also Ferraro & LaGrange, 1987). Based on principal components analysis at the individual level, three subscales were obtained: emotional fear, worry, and comparative (geographic and temporal) risk perceptions. For the present analyses, we use the emotional component, which consists of six questions: (1) "How safe would you feel being out alone on your block during the day?" (2) The same question is then asked about how the respondent would feel "elsewhere in your neighborhood" and (3 and 4) both of those questions are again asked for "at night." The response categories for those four items were collapsed in order to be comparable to the other two dichotomous items in the emotional fear scale. (5) "Would you be afraid if a stranger stopped you at night in your neighborhood to ask for directions?" and (6) "Would you feel uneasy if you heard footsteps behind you at night in your neighborhood?" The internal consistency of the scale at the individual level and prior to collapsing is alpha = .82. Block level (intrablock agreement) reliability was an acceptable .77, indicating the observed block means adequately capture the true block means.

Baltimore Newspaper Archive

Two Baltimore newspapers were reviewed, abstracted, and coded into an archival database for the purpose of accounting for the potential fear-related influence on survey respondents of local crime and disorder news coverage between the two waves of survey data (i.e., to monitor potential "history" threats to statistical conclusion validity). The *Baltimore Sun* is the largest daily newspaper in the area. Sampling strategy is critical to validity but often overlooked in content analysis (Babbie, 1995). Thus, the semi-weekly *Baltimore Afro-American* was also used to offset any bias in favor of *Sun* coverage of predominantly white neighborhoods: 73.5% of the 321 articles selected were taken from the *Sun* and the rest were from the *Afro-American*.

Four research assistants were trained to skim and identify relevant articles in weekday issues of the *Sun* (those most likely to contain relevant articles) and all issues of the *Afro-American* from January 1, 1987, to March 31, 1988. The type of articles which were abstracted covered two general topics: Approximately 80% were reports of events expected to influence crime-related attitudes in, or in neighborhoods adjacent to, one or more study neighborhoods. These included articles reporting specific crimes, social or physical disorder problems, or the immediate community response to specific crime-related problems. Articles on "disorder" include the physical deterioration of housing or other property, racial unrest, and prison escapes or unrest. Both kinds of articles were expected to influence perceptions of personal vulnerability, attitudes toward the city's ability to reduce crime, and possibly anticrime behaviors of residents in study neighborhoods. They provided the basic sampling element, aggregated to the neighborhood level, for the present analyses. The rest of the archive included news stories about criminal justice system or community development (e.g., housing and urban planning) programs or policy changes. Articles on events occurring in unsampled neighborhoods (including all public housing projects) and surrounding counties were ignored unless they were adjacent to at least one sampled study neighborhood.

Due to the inclusion of articles on incidents either in or near study neighborhoods, there were many cases (articles) relating to more than one neighborhood of interest. For each event, we allowed for up to four possible neighborhoods that the event is in or near. (Obviously, unless an incident occurs on a neighborhood boundary as happened on two occasions, it can only be "in" one neighborhood, but it can be "near" three). With regard to data processing, all of the information was entered into a database and all but the lengthy text article title and summary fields were also exported for statistical analysis. This allowed us to summarize all the relevant and available news for each neighborhood by having the program sort through data and select if any one of the four neighborhood codes equalled the target neighborhood code. The result was a separate list of news events and issues occurring in or near each neighborhood.

One issue that arose was how to handle multiple articles on a single incident. Our purpose here was not to estimate the amount of actual crime but the amount of print media coverage of social disorder and related matters in the sample neighborhoods. Thus, a general rule we used was to discard a follow-up story to an incident if it only covered criminal justice system responses that were deemed inconsequential to community fear. We did include follow-up stories that discussed new information on an event, such as community reaction or an arrest, and both articles on the same event in each newspaper. Thus, the frequencies or means of "crimes" in the archive actually refers to different news reports of crimes, or "article-crimes," two or more of which may be on the same incident. Hence, as the British studies of crime news show, the more sensational the crime—such as a particularly brutal murder, kidnapping, or rape—the more coverage it receives and the greater it is (in effect) weighted in the present scheme. Again, we believe this is appropriate for a measure of media's expected impact on fear.

Just over 50% of the crime stories included a homicide as one of the crimes mentioned. The next most frequently mentioned crimes were, respectively, assault, robbery and weapons offenses, burglary, drug dealing, and rape. Use of a deadly weapon was reported in 70% of all crime stories. Multiple crimes occurring during the same incident were reported in 35% of the crime articles. The average number of people injured was 1.4. Excluding those articles that were unclear on the exact number, the average number of offenders was 1.6, although this may be an underestimate as accomplices were not always mentioned in a news story.

The number of articles *in* a particular neighborhood ranged from 0 ($n = 22$) to 20. The number of articles *near* a given neighborhood ranged from 0 ($n = 6$) to 54. Several examples clearly demonstrated the importance of noting crimes not only within the neighborhood's boundaries but also in adjacent neighborhoods. Many had few or even no article-crimes within them but many nearby. There were only 4 study neighborhoods in which no incidents or policy issues (i.e., no articles) were located in or near them. All are smaller neighborhoods located near the outer edges of the city.

No interrater reliability information is available for this data set. But the same coding form was used by 17 minimally trained undergraduate raters content analyzing issues of the *Salt Lake Tribune* and the *Deseret News*. Six articles were selected by only one or two of nine raters (per issue). The other 10 articles were selected by a range of 33 to 89% and a mean of 59% of the raters. If one considers *all* articles on which a decision was made (including those rejected by all raters), selection agreement would be over 95%. Furthermore, raters of the newspapers used in the following analyses received much more training and experience with the procedure. Even so, article selection reliability deserves caution in the present study and closer scrutiny in rater training and future research.

Scores for pairs of raters on the Salt Lake news data were cross-tabulated. The kappa coefficients (agreement corrected for chance) were as follows: type of crime (26 possible categories; $\kappa = .72$), policy issue (12 categories; $\kappa = .21$), use of a weapon (yes/no; $\kappa = .77$), number injured ($\kappa = .87$), number of offenders ($\kappa = 1.00$). With the main focus on crime articles, the baseline for selecting relevant policy-related articles and for assigning policy issues to all articles was low. This may be the reason that the kappa for that variable was not higher. In many cases, raters identified a policy issue where others saw none. But in the 7 cases where a pair of raters both identified a policy issue, the raters agreed on what the issue was in every case.

APPROACH TO DATA ANALYSIS

Variables

To recapitulate the variables to be used in the present analyses, disorder items have been combined within all three of the above methods into social and physical composite independent variables. From the Block Environmental Inventory, we used three measures of *observed disorder*:

The proportion (based on the number of housing units on the block) of *young men outdoors* is a possible cue for perceived social disorder. We aggregated the property-level items to the block level and combined the three *home physical disorder* (litter, vandalism, and dilapidation) into a scale. Since nonresidential property has been found to be a significant magnet for crime (Perkins et al., 1993) and disorder (Taylor et al., 1995), we combined three inventory items: (a) poorly maintained open land use, (b) the proportion of nonresidential buildings with graffiti and (c) with dilapidated exteriors into *nonresidential physical disorder*.

From the newspaper archive, we combined all stories about homicides, rapes, assaults, robberies, and burglaries into one *serious crime news* variable (neighborhood $M = 14.04$, $SD = 17.99$). Articles about other crimes were less common. We combined all stories that mentioned other non-traffic offenses (e.g., carrying a weapon, drug abuse, car theft, kidnapping, domestic disturbance, arson, prostitution, vandalism, and disorderly conduct incidents) into a *disorder crime news* variable (often referred to as "quality-of-life crimes"; neighborhood $M = 4.72$, $SD = 7.98$). The third variable of interest are stories on the physical deterioration of housing or other property, racial unrest, and prison escapes or unrest, which we labeled *disorder news* (neighborhood $M = 0.26$, $SD = 0.66$). As the standard deviations imply, all three of these variables have fairly skewed distributions, with most neighborhoods having few relevant newspaper stories and a few neighborhoods with many. All three variables were aggregated to the neighborhood level (sum of stories) and each story was weighted according to whether the event or problem took place near ($= 1$) or in ($= 2$) the target neighborhood.

We used the Time 1 resident survey, aggregated to the block level, for the demographic (sex, age, race) covariates and to combine loitering youths, harassment in the street, fights and arguments, and drug dealing into *perceived social disorder* and vandalism, vacant housing, unkempt property, litter, and trashed vacant lots into *perceived physical disorder*. We used the aggregated Time 2 survey for the criminal victimization (in the past year) covariate and the emotional subscale of *fear of crime*. Fear, the dependent variable, was thus measured 12 to 15 months after the observational and survey predictors and at the end of a year measuring victimization and crime-and-disorder-related news.

Analyses

First, we present correlations among fear, the key exogenous variables (sex, race, age, and criminal victimization), and the various measures of disorder. We also examine correlations after partialing those same exogenous variables. These correlations are analyzed at the individual level, the individual-within-block level (i.e., using pooled group variance), and the aggregate community level. For this level and for the analyses below, community is defined as the residential street block for the environmental and survey data and the neighborhood for the news data. We briefly discuss a multiple regression analysis of the data. Finally, we analyze three hierarchical linear models of the multilevel impact of disorder on fear. These analyses allow us to test a multilevel model of the impacts of community disorder on fear of crime. Before describing the multilevel model we explain how HLM operates (see Appendix B for more details).

Significance tests are two-tailed for correlation matrices and one-tailed for predictors in the HLMs. Given the number of blocks and neighborhoods in the study ($n = 50$), the degrees of freedom, and thus statistical power, are rather limited, especially for multivariate analyses. Kenny and LaVoie (1985) recommended raising the significance criterion to $p < .25$ when analyzing (more reliable) group-level data. (All of these community-level variables are based on multiple survey respondents, properties, or newspaper articles.) Instead, for just the HLM, we adopt a significance level of $p < .10$ for Level II hypothesis tests, which yields an acceptable degree of statistical power.

Relevant Features of Hierarchical Linear Modeling

HLM represents a family of models specifically devoted to analyzing hierarchical data where individuals are nested within larger units such as students in schools (Bryk & Raudenbush, 1992; Bryk & Thum, 1989). They also have been applied to changes in individuals over time (Bryk & Raudenbush, 1987; Raudenbush & Chan, 1992, 1993). Combining maximum likelihood and empirical Bayes estimation techniques they separate out between-group from within-group effects, provide estimated true scores of group means, generate empirical Bayes estimates of predictor slopes within each group, and allow cross-level interactions to be explored by permitting varying slopes for individual predictors across groups, and examining the group-level determinants of those varying slopes. HLM takes into consideration the assumption that residuals (error) within groups are correlated.

For our purposes here the following HLM advantages are pertinent. (a) We can gauge the amount of variation in fear of crime that is due to differences between communities. This is useful descriptive information. (b) We can test whether the between-community variation is significantly greater than zero. (c) After entering our community-level predictors, we can see how much of the between-community variation in fear they explain, and test whether significant between-community variation remains. (d) HLM uses precision weighting and empirical Bayes (EB) estimates of group means. Therefore data quality is taken into account across communities, and at that level we are not predicting observed means, but rather EB estimates of "true" community means.[3] (e) HLM makes assumptions about correlated within-group errors that are more appropriate to the clustered data we have than are the assumptions about error made by ordinary least squares (OLS). (f) We can simultaneously explore individual-level effects on the dependent variable. The impacts of these individual-level, or Level I, predictors are completely independent of the community level (II) impacts because we center each Level I predictor by its group mean. Thus each Level I predictor tells us about the contrast between the individual and the block mean, pooled across blocks.

In HLM it is possible to explore interactions between individual and context by allowing slopes of Level I predictors to vary across groups. We did not do this because of data limitations (see Appendix B) and because of insufficiently developed theoretical rationales.

Model to Be Tested in HLM[4]

In HLM we test the models described below to predict *fear of crime*. We enter exogenous variables at theoretically appropriate levels (individual or block) and as the data permit. In contrast to contextual analysis, exclusion of a variable at one level does not bias the coefficients or the standard errors at the other level.

---

[3] More specifically, HLM considers: size of the Level II groups (i.e., number of Level I units in each Level II unit), distance of each Level II observed mean from the estimated true grand mean, and how much respondents in each Level II unit agree with each other on the attribute in question. As a reviewer has pointed out, there are other sources of data quality variation across Level II units. But the critical point here is that many different sources of "error," including misinterpretations of questions by some respondents or varying interviewer effects, will contribute to one of the above three factors that are taken into account in HLM precision weighting.

[4] A reviewer has reminded us that HLM cannot test a multistep causal model. It seems plausible to argue that community conditions give rise to perceptions of community conditions, and that the latter influence fear. So the impact of observed, on site, disorderly conditions may be mediated by the perceptions of those conditions. HLM cannot test such a model. But as Covington and Taylor (1991) have shown, observed, on-site conditions have unmediated, direct impacts on fear, separate from the impacts of perceived conditions. So if that model was not seriously misspecified, we know that perceptions and on-site conditions each have their own independent, direct impacts on fear. It is those that we test in the HLM models here.

Victimization is entered at Level II. Blocks where more residents report victimization are likely to be blocks where street and/or property crime are higher. Controlling for block victimization helps us roughly control for the amount of crime occurring on the block. It was not possible to control for victimization at the individual level because on several blocks no respondents reported victimization.

Race. Residents on more predominantly African American blocks, all else equal, are likely to receive less aggressive police action and other services (Taylor & Covington, 1993). Skogan and Maxfield (1981) suggested that minorities are more fearful because race captures an ecological vulnerability to disorder. Race is thus entered at the block level. We are unable to enter race at the individual level because on several blocks all respondents were either white or African American. (Given the strong Level II correlations between racial composition and disorder indicators, we ran each analysis twice, once with race included, and once with it excluded. Results were closely comparable, yielding no substantive differences. We show the results here with race included.)

Age. At the individual level, residents who are older than their neighbors may feel less integrated into the block social life and may even be intimidated by being surrounded by younger residents. They may not know the teens hanging out on the block as the teens' parents probably do. At the block level, age may link with fear for two possible reasons. Skogan and Maxfield (1981) suggested older residents are more fearful because they are more physically vulnerable. On a block of predominantly elderly residents, this may translate to a collective sensing itself to be vulnerable and lacking adequate informal social controls. As a group, they may participate less in outdoor activities on the block. A dearth of adult residents viewed outside may render daily events on the block less familiar and more threatening to all residents, not just the elderly.

Gender. Sampson (1987) has argued that female-headed households in an urban locale may predominate because of joblessness and the associated lack of stable males. The problems stem not from the female-headed households per se, but rather from the associated unemployment and related male instability in the locale. His argument, originally specific to urban black communities, seems appropriate to other urban residential locations as well. Thus, gender at the block level serves as a proxy for block stability. We were unable to enter gender at Level I because on some blocks all respondents were women.

Disorder. We enter three disorder measures at the individual level. One is *physical disorder* (litter, vandalism, dilapidation) independently observed at the respondent's *home*. Disorder theory predicts that those keeping their place up less than their neighbors are less interested in their neighborhood, more alienated from neighbors, and thus more fearful. But this anticipated effect may not emerge at this level for two reasons: First, physical upkeep in many locations is the responsibility of landlords as well as residents. Second, residents are likely to be concerned about their neighbors' upkeep (the Level II effect: see below), but incivilities on one's own property may be fear-provoking only if one believes that others are directly responsible for it (e.g., gang graffiti).

The other two disorder measures at Level I are *perceived social disorder* and *perceived physical disorder* from the resident survey. Those seeing more problems than their neighbors on the same block should be more fearful than their neighbors. Those seeing the block as more problem-ridden may spend more time there or may just be more sensitive to the block context because of differential adaptation processes (Taylor & Shumaker, 1990).

The Level II predictors of community disorder will vary depending upon the specific model. In the observed disorder model we will enter mean block scores for observed *home physical disorder, nonresidential disorder*, and *number of young men outdoors*. We expect each to contribute positively to mean block fear. With regard to the last of these three measures, we do not mean to imply that all young men observed outdoors are, or should be, viewed by either residents or raters as a threat or a symbol of disorder. We are merely using it as an admittedly crude proxy for the presence of a potential source of youthful incivilities. It may also reflect relative levels of joblessness, or nearby amenities that draw foot traffic but at the same time destabilize the block setting (Taylor et al., 1995).

In the perceived disorder model we enter block means for perceived physical disorder and perceived social disorder. We expect block residents' shared views of physical and social problems to each contribute independently to their level of fear.

Finally, in the newspaper model, we enter neighborhood-level aggregates for disorder crime news and disorder news. Each neighborhood corresponds to a different block in the sample. As explained below in the multiple regression analysis, serious crime news correlated highly with disorder crime news and so was excluded from the HLM analyses. We expect that media attention to nearby quality-of-life crimes and disorder problems will each contribute independently to block fear.

SUMMARY

We have described above the specific hypotheses to be tested for Level I and Level II predictors. Level I results tell us about pooled effects of differences of individuals from their block average (on perceived social and physical disorder and one measure of observed disorder). Level II results tell us about block and neighborhood-level effects. In the first equation we include measures of observed disorder, based on block-level and aggregated property-level ratings. This model tells us whether, in addition to *psychological* processes at Level I, *ecological* processes are also at work at the block level. In the second equation we include two measures of perceived disorder, based on block mean survey responses. In the third equation we include measures of disorder crime news and noncriminal disorder-related news, based on content-analyzed newspaper articles aggregated to the neighborhood level. These last two models tell us whether, in addition to the Level I psychological processes, *social psychological* processes involving group perceptions and/or mass communications are also simultaneously at work at Level II.

RESULTS

Correlations among Fear, Demographics, Victimization, and Community Disorder

Table II presents unadjusted correlations among fear of crime, demographics, criminal victimization experienced in the year preceding the fear measure, and community disorder. These correlations represent combined between-person and between-block dynamics. Above the diagonal are partial correlations controlling for sex, race, age, and victimization. Women and African Americans were more fearful. Resident perceptions of block social and physical disorder were significantly, and about equally, related to fear. On-site observations of the respondent's own property showed only a trend with fear. It is not surprising that this trend was nonsignificant since it is disorder in the *rest of the community* rather than one's own home, that is expected to be associated with fear of street (as opposed to domestic) crime.

Table III presents individual-level correlations among the same variables as in Table II, based on pooled, within-block deviations. All variables are block-centered. Again, partial correlations, controlling for block-centered sex, race, age, and victimization, appear above the diagonal. These correlations capture solely individual-level processes. Sex was still significant, indicating that women living on blocks that were more predominantly male (based on the gender ratio of those we interviewed) were especially fearful. (An alternative explanation would be that men living on blocks with more women were less fearful.)

Table II. Individual-Level Zero-Order Correlations Among Fear of Crime, Demographics, Victimization, and Community Disorder; Partial Correlations (Above Diagonal) Controlling for Sex, Race, Age, and Victimization

	n	1	2	3	4	5	6	7	8
1. Fear of crime[a]	300	—					.14	.22[c]	.21[c]
Control variables									
2. Female	412	.27[c]	—						
3. Nonwhite	410	.15[b]	.13[b]	—					
4. Age	303	.13	.00	−.04	—				
5. Victimization[a]	305	.11	−.01	−.08	−.13	—			
Independent observation of respondent's property									
6. Physical disorder	283	.16	−.01	.28[c]	−.12	.15	—	.36[c]	.28[c]
Surveyed resident perceptions									
7. Social disorder	411	.25[c]	.05	.14[b]	−.09	.26[c]	.41[c]	—	.65[c]
8. Physical disorder	412	.25[c]	.07	.19[c]	−.02	.13	.33[c]	.67[c]	—

[a] Fear of crime and victimization were measured 1 year later than the other variables.
[b] $p < .05$, two-tailed.
[c] $p < .01$, two-tailed.

Table III. Correlations Among Individual-Level Block-Deviation Scores for Fear of Crime, Demographics, Victimization, and Community Disorder; Partial Correlations (Above Diagonal) Controlling for Sex, Race, Age, and Victimization

	n	1	2	3	4	5	6	7	8
1. Fear of crime[a]	300	—					.19[b]	.26[c]	.17[b]
Control variables									
2. Female	412	.28[c]	—						
3. Nonwhite	410	−.07	.02	—					
4. Age	303	.06	−.02	−.17[b]	—				
5. Victimization[a]	305	.09	−.00	−.08	−.11	—			
Independent observation of respondent's property									
6. Physical disorder	283	.17[b]	−.05	.09	−.09	−.15	—	.38[c]	.39[c]
Surveyed resident perceptions									
7. Social disorder	411	.27[c]	.04	−.08	−.04	.22[c]	.39[c]	—	.65[c]
8. Physical disorder	412	.20[c]	.08	−.10	.02	.10	.38[c]	.66[c]	—

[a] Fear of crime and victimization were measured 1 year later than the other variables.
[b] $p < .05$, two-tailed.
[c] $p < .01$, two-tailed.

The disorder measures also emerged significant, this time including on-site observations as well as perceived incivilities. Those who were most fearful not only perceived more disorder on the block than their neighbors; they also lived on properties with objectively more physical disorder (litter, graffiti, dilapidation) than was observed on their neighbors' homes.

Table IV contains block-level correlations among fear of crime, demographics, crime (victimization rate), and all three measures of disorder. Again, partial correlations controlling for proportion female, racial composition, mean age, and crime appear above the diagonal. These correlations capture purely block level dynamics. Fear was higher on blocks with higher proportions of women ($r = .34$, $p < .05$) or African American interviewees ($r = .45$, $p < .01$). Fear of crime was also significantly related to all of the measures of community disorder across all three methods. The largest partial correlations (controlling for sex, race, age, and victimization during the 12 months between surveys) were for the on-site observation measures, especially physical disorder around nonresidential property ($pr = .38$, $p < .01$). The number of young males outdoors ($pr = .31$, $p < .05$) and litter, graffiti, and dilapidation around homes ($pr = .32$, $p < .05$) also predicted block fear a year later.

Surveyed resident perceptions of physical disorder problems ($r = .41$, $p < .01$; $pr = .25$, $p < .05$) and social disorder problems ($r = .37$, $p < .01$; $pr = .21$, $p < .10$) also predicted block fear a year later, although the effect was reduced noticeably after controlling for demographics and victimization.

Neighborhood-level noncrime newspaper stories about social or physical disorder problems were related to fear of crime ($r = .34$, $p < .05$; $pr = .28$; $p < .05$). That result may not be completely reliable, however, due to the low frequency of such articles ($n = 9$). Disorder crime news was also related to fear ($r = .41$, $p < .01$; $pr = .24$, $p < .10$). But the correlation between fear and serious crime news was even more sharply reduced by controlling for race and the other covariates ($r = .38$, $p < .01$; $pr = .16$, ns).

Multiple Regression Analysis

A block-level hierarchical multiple regression using all three types of disorder measures was tested. Block racial and sex composition were entered first followed by the three observational measures, the two resident perception variables, and the three newspaper predictors ($R^2 = .45$, adjusted $R^2 = .31$, $p < .005$). Due to the higher degree of multicollinearity even across these very different measures of disorder (i.e., what one would

Table IV. Community-Level Correlations Among Fear of Crime, Demographics, Victimization, and Three Measures of Community Disorder; Partial Correlations (Above Diagonal) Controlling for Sex, Race, Age, and Victimization[a]

	1	2	3	4	5	6	7	8	9	10	11	12	13
1. Mean fear of crime[b]	—					.32[c]	.38[d]	.31[c]	.21	.25[c]	.16	.24	.28[c]
Control variables													
2. Proportion female	.34[c]	—											
3. Proportion nonwhite	.45[d]	.35[c]	—										
4. Mean age	.04	.17	.12	—									
5. Mean victimization[b]	.04	-.13	-.07	-.23	—								
Independent observations													
6. Home physical disorder	.45[d]	.07	.47[d]	-.14	.21	—	.39[d]	.16	.61[d]	.66[d]	.48[d]	.49[d]	.23
7. Nonresidential property physical disorder	.36[d]	-.13	.16	-.05	.12	.44[d]	—	.54[d]	.42[d]	.28[c]	.53[d]	.59[d]	.58[d]
8. Young men outdoors	.32[c]	-.16	.36[d]	-.13	-.11	.32[c]	.55[d]	—	.35[d]	.07	.38[d]	.50[d]	.41[d]
Surveyed resident perceptions													
9. Mean social disorder	.37[d]	.11	.41[d]	-.20	.23	.72[d]	.45[d]	.41[d]	—	.73[d]	.49[d]	.41[d]	.25[c]
10. Mean physical disorder	.41[d]	.12	.43[d]	-.12	.26	.76[d]	.34[c]	.20	.80[d]	—	.58[d]	.42[d]	.16
Newspaper articles													
11. Serious crime news	.38[d]	.17	.62[d]	.14	.00	.60[d]	.51[d]	.48[d]	.56[d]	.65[d]	—	.84[d]	.39[d]
12. Disorder crime news	.41[d]	.18	.48[d]	.02	.09	.61[d]	.58[d]	.53[d]	.53[d]	.55[d]	.87[d]	—	.58[d]
13. Disorder news	.34[c]	.12	.23	.12	-.11	.27	.55[d]	.40[d]	.26	.20	.44[d]	.59[d]	—

[a] All data aggregated to block level except news data (Nos. 11–13), which were aggregated to the neighborhood-level; N of blocks/neighborhoods = 50; partial correlation $df = 44$.
[b] Fear of crime and victimization were measured 1 year later than the other variables.
[c] $p < .05$, two-tailed.
[d] $p < .01$, two-tailed.

hope for in terms of construct validity), reversed valence suppression effects (positive correlations/negative betas) were found for serious crime news, resident perceptions of social incivilities, and disorder crime news.

The remaining multivariate analyses thus tested separately each of the three methods of measuring community social disorder for its ability to predict fear of crime. In a regression with only demographic and news predictors, the beta was negative for serious crime news, which correlated highly with both the proportion nonwhite and disorder crime news. We therefore excluded serious crime news from the following HLM analyses. This also makes the focus on disorder, as distinct from serious crime, more consistent across all three methods.

Hierarchical Linear Models Predicting Fear of Crime

ANOVA. An initial HLM, with no Level I or Level II predictors describes the between- and within-group variation; it is comparable to a one-way ANOVA. We are able to reject the null hypothesis that there is no between-block variation in estimated fear true scores ($\chi^2 = 93.11, p < .001$); 17% of the total variance in fear arises from between-block variation. Table V shows the variance results of the ANOVA, and subsequent models. The amount of between-block variance in fear is comparable to or somewhat larger than what has been observed in other studies. Kurtz and Taylor (1995), analyzing fear levels across 66 neighborhoods in Baltimore, found that 15% of fear was due to between-neighborhood variation. Reanalyzing surveys from residents surrounding 24 small commercial centers in Minneapolis–St. Paul, Taylor (1995) found that 4% of the variation from a neighborhood fear index, and 8% of the variation from a more specific index measuring fear while in the commercial center, arose from between-neighborhood differences. In this study we assess between-block rather than between-neighborhood differences, and this may account for a greater proportion of the outcome variance residing at Level II. Alternately, the higher proportion may be due to the smaller group sizes used here than in these other studies.

Observed Disorder. The variance results for each of three different models including both Level I (individual within-block deviations) and Level II (block-level) predictors appear in Table V. In the observed disorder model, our Level II predictors (including aggregate race, age, sex, victimization rate, both home and nonresidential exterior physical disorder and young men observed outdoors on the block) explain 37.8% of the

Table V. Hierarchical Linear Modeling Analyses of Residual and Explained Variation in Fear of Crime[a]

	Model							
	No predictors		Observed disorder		Perceived disorder		Newspaper reports	
Location of variance	Variance	% of total	Variance	% of total	Variance	% of total	Variance	% of total
			Residual variation					
Between blocks	0.148	17.0	0.092	10.6	0.085	9.8	0.082	9.4
Within blocks	0.723	83.0	0.671	77.1	0.681	78.2	0.673	77.3
Total	0.871							
χ^2	93.11	$p < .001$	68.47	$p < .01$	69.72	$p < .01$	67.79	$p < .01$

Model	% Between	% Total
	Explained between-block variation	
Observed disorder	37.8	6.4
Perceived disorder	42.3	7.2
Newspapers	44.7	7.6

[a]Due to strong Level II correlations between racial composition and disorder indicators, each model was analyzed two ways: with and without race. Results here for explained between-block variation include the race variable. The top portion of table describes between- and within-block variation. "No predictor" model is equivalent to a one-way ANOVA, and provides a descriptive breakdown on the total outcome variance. Remaining portions of the top panel describe how much unexplained variance remains at each level, after predictors have been entered. So the between-block residual variation in the observed disorder model is 0.092; this represents 10.6% of the total outcome variance. What has been explained is (0.148—0.092) or 0.056. This explained variation, as shown in the bottom panel, represents 37.8% of the between block outcome variation, and 6.4% of the total outcome variation. In other words, the bottom panel describes the explained variance as a percentage of between variance, and as a percentage of total variance. The chi-square values indicate, for each of the models, if the amount of between-block outcome variance remaining after Level II predictors have been entered, is significantly different from zero. The chi-square associated with "no predictors" tells us if the between-block variation, before predictors are entered, is significantly different from zero.

block-level outcome variation, and 6.4% of the total variation.[5] Significant unexplained block-level variation in the outcome remains ($\chi^2 = 68.47$, $p < .01$). Individual coefficients in the model appear in Table VI. Level I effects remain constant for all three models. The only significant Level I impacts are associated with perceived disorder. Residents who perceive more social and physical disorders than their neighbors report more fear 1 year later. Individual differences in age, and observed residential deterioration, make no independent contributions to individual-level differences in fear. Turning to Level II results, we first examine the *observed disorder* model. Three Level II predictors yield significant demographic impacts. Fear is higher on blocks where the average age was higher, where more women were interviewed, and where nonresidential physical disorder was more extensive. Level II predictors were z scored, allowing us to compare coefficients. The largest Level II coefficient is for the proportion of women interviewed on the block.

Perceived Disorder. When we use resident perceptions of disorder for our Level II indicators of incivility, we explain about the same amount of fear: 7.2% of total fear, and 42.3% of between-block fear. Again, the chisquare test informs us that significant, between-block variation in fear remains ($\chi^2 = 69.72$, $p < .01$). In the Level II predictors, average age and the proportion of women remain significant. Average perceived physical problems significantly influence block fear, and generate the strongest Level II coefficient. This latter result, considered in conjunction with the Level I impact of perceived physical disorder, demonstrates two channels of influence on fear. Not only are those perceiving more problems more fearful than their neighbors; in addition, on blocks where the average perceived physical problems are higher, residents are more fearful. Of course, as mentioned earlier, because of data properties, we cannot say if this independent, Level II impact would persist if we controlled for observed disorder.

Newspaper Reports. Results using news reports of so-called quality-of-life, or disorder, crimes and of noncriminal disorder problems, aggregated to the neighborhood level, yield comparable amounts of explained variance. Now our Level II predictors explain 7.6% of the total outcome variation and 44.7% of the between-group variation. Again, significant, unexplained between-group outcome variance remains ($\chi^2 = 67.79$, $p < .01$). At Level II, disorder news demonstrates a significant coefficient ($.166$, $p < .05$). Average

---

[5] Unlike OLS, HLM does not allow one to determine if the addition of specific predictors results in improved fit. This can only be done when the fixed predictors are held constant, and a random effect is added, and you compare two deviance statistics. With different models and different predictors, as is the case here, we only can gauge if the remaining, unexplained variation at Level II is significant.

Table VI. Coefficients of Level I and Level II Predictors in Three HLM Models of Disorder Predicting Fear of Crime

	Model		
Predictor	Observed disorder	Perceived disorder	Newspaper reports
Level II (Street block)			
Mean victimization	.026	.007	.031
Proportion nonwhite	.065	.075	.117[d]
Mean age	.134[e]	.136[e]	.109[d]
Proportion female	.205[e]	.179[f]	.155[e]
Home physical disorders	.066	—	—
Nonresidential property physical disorder	.163[d]	—	—
Young men outdoors	.114	—	—
Mean perceived social disorder	—	−.071	—
Mean perceived physical disorder	—	.228[e]	—
Disorder crime news[a]	—	—	.088
Disorder news[a]	—	—	.166[e]
Level I (Individual)			
Age[b]	.079	.079	.079
Home physical disorder[b]	−.009	−.009	−.009
Perceived social disorder[b]	.214[e]	.214[e]	.214[e]
Perceived physical disorder[b]	.289[e]	.289[e]	.289[e]
EB Intercept[c]	−.165	−.089	−.115

[a] News data collected for entire neighborhood within which a given block is located.
[b] Group-mean centered predictor.
[c] The EB intercept is comparable to the intercept (A) OLS multiple regression, except that it uses precision weighting and adjusts for data quality. All predictors are z-scored, so coefficients can be compared for their relative size.
[d] $p < .10$, one-tailed.
[e] $p < .05$, one-tailed.
[f] $p < .01$, one-tailed.

age and proportion female continue to have significant impacts. In this model, racial composition also has a significant impact on fear, with fear being higher on blocks where more African Americans were interviewed.

DISCUSSION

Summary and Implications

We presented three very different ecological methods for assessing community-level social and physical disorder problems: the Block Environmental Inventory based on systematic observations, aggregated subjective perceptions from a survey of residents, and a procedure for content-analysis of newspaper articles. The criterion-related validity of all three was demonstrated by their roughly equal ability to predict subsequent fear of crime, even after controlling for the influence of variables that have been linked with fear in the research literature (race, sex, age, and victimization). In each HLM model, one Level II indicator demonstrated a significant effect. The differences between the three models were minor, in part because two thirds of the Level II predictors were the same. Each explained about 6 to 8% of the total variation in estimated "true" fear scores.

These results provide some confirmation of existing theories (Skogan, 1990; Taylor, 1987; Wilson & Kelling, 1982), but also extend earlier research on the impact of community social and physical disorder (Covington & Taylor, 1991; Perkins et al., 1990, 1992, 1993; Taylor & Covington, 1993; Taylor, Shumaker, & Gottfredson, 1985). For example, as expected, women were significantly more fearful of crime in both the correlational and HLM analyses. But we found this result not only at the individual level but also at the block-centered individual level and the block level. This shows the importance of community context (e.g., being surrounded by more men than women on one's block) even for variables that seem exclusively individualistic, such as sex. The block-centered individual-level result suggests that having more men as neighbors tends to *in*duce fear, rather than *re*duce it (e.g., through a greater sense of block protection). This finding replicates Taylor et al.'s (1984) finding also using pooled within-block measures. An alternate interpretation of the block-level result is that the proportion of women may serve as a proxy for block instability and associated lack of employment opportunities (Sampson, 1987).

The effect of age on fear is less clear in these results. The fact that it was only significant as a Level II HLM predictor is an example of a multilevel result that was not found in individual or even group-level correlations. Mean block age is only a significant predictor of fear after controlling for other block and individual-level variables.

With regard to racial composition, the significant block-level correlation between fear and the proportion of nonwhite respondents on the block in the present data confirms previous studies (Taylor et al., 1984). What is interesting here is that when we control for disorder in the HLM models using observed ratings, or respondents' perceptions, racial composition does *not* have a significant impact on fear. This is because the Level II correlation between racial composition and disorder news ($r = .23$) is weaker than the correlation between racial composition and the other disorder indicators (mean $r = .42$). This weaker correlation argues against those contending that media sources tend to highlight and overemphasize physical problems occurring in predominantly African American communities.

In interpreting the HLM model for observed disorder, we see that disorder around the home and young men outdoors matter less than disorder on nonresidential property, which makes an independent contribution to block fear. The effect may arise from the physical blight itself or from the presence of nonresidential land uses, such as stores and small businesses, that are the site of the disorder. Nonresidential land use in a predominantly residential context contributes to a more deteriorated and less predictable block (Taylor et al., 1995).

The results for this model build on and clarify previous findings on the impact of observed disorder on fear of crime. Unlike Perkins et al. (1990), the present results control for block-level sex, age, and victimization and individual-level within-block deviations in perceived disorder.

Covington and Taylor (1991) accounted for those and other factors at either the individual or contextual level. But the present model extends their findings in several ways. First, Covington and Taylor (1991) used one combined, individual-level scale composed largely of perceived physical incivilities. Results here show that both social and physical perceived disorder can make independent, individual-level contributions to fear of crime. Second, results here suggest that nonresidential deterioration may contribute more to fear than residential deterioration. The prior study did not separate those two types. Third, in that study the unit of aggregation was the neighborhood. The relative impact of (individual-level) perceived disorder to (neighborhood-level) observed disorder was on the order of 3/1. In this study, using the street block as the aggregation unit and standardized predictors, we get individual coefficients of comparable size when we compare observed versus perceived deterioration.

The results of this study make several important contributions. First, we have shown that resident perceptions of disorder contribute to fear at *both the individual and aggregate levels*. Community-level effects may emerge from residents having common perceptions of the surrounding physical and social milieu and/or communicating with one another about that milieu. Further research is needed to determine the relative influence of shared information versus independent, common perceptions on community fear level. But the very high correlations found here between resident perceptions and independently observed physical disorder (see Table IV) suggest that the disorder theory of fear does not depend on perceptions being spread or exaggerated via communication among neighbors (cf., Crenson, 1983; Taylor, 1996).

Second, we found the effects of perceived disorder and observed disorder on fear to be significant 1 year later.

Third, we distinguish between social and physical disorder and found that, although both correlate with fear, *physical disorder had higher block-level and individual-level HLM coefficients than did social disorder, and this effect was triangulated using all three assessment methods.* Thus, litter, graffiti, and dilapidation may be more likely to induce feelings of vulnerability than do "groups of teenagers hanging out," perhaps because the latter are less common. Still, this effect is somewhat surprising given that the social disorder measures in the survey and news data included actual quality-of-life crime items (e.g., drug dealing, menacing, public disturbance), which should logically provoke more fear.

Fourth, in particular, we found that, although people often complain about unkempt housing exteriors, nonresidential physical disorder may contribute more to fear of crime. We do not know if the problem is the presence of nonresidential land uses per se, which can destabilize the block setting (Taylor et al., 1995), or the deterioration on the establishments.

Fifth, in comparison to Covington and Taylor (1992), these results demonstrate that the residential street block is at least as valid an ecological unit of analysis when considering disorder and fear as are neighborhoods. We observed strong block-level reliabilities for perceived disorder and fear.

Sixth, and perhaps most important, this study is the first we know of explicitly contrasting the relative impacts of three different ecological methods of assessing community disorder. We have seen that, controlling for age, race, gender, and victimization experience, all three measures perform about the same, yielding comparably sized coefficients. There are no marked differences in the proportions of Level II variance explained. Our perceived physical disorder measure yields a larger coefficient than the other indicators, but the differences are minor. The safest conclusion may be that each type of assessment yields roughly comparable measures of impact (see Choosing Methods, below).

Turning briefly to our exogenous variables, results confirm Level II but not Level I impacts of age. These results differ from prior contextual analyses (Covington & Taylor, 1991), and are relevant to the ongoing debate about the linkage between fear and age (LaGrange & Ferraro, 1989). We need more theoretical attention to the relevant processes, at the appropriate level, that might be responsible for these impacts. We failed to observe effects of block racial composition. Some prior studies using neighborhoods have observed such effects (Covington & Taylor, 1991), others have not. Prior block-level analyses have observed racial composition impacts on fear (Taylor et al., 1984). The emergence of a significant Level II race impact when we use neighborhood-level, media indicators of disorder rather than block-level indicators, suggests the following. Prior block studies may have observed race composition impacts because race and disorder correlate at the block level. In short, impacts of race at the block level may have emerged because race served as a proxy for signs of incivility. The consistent impact of gender suggests further attention. Small group studies in the residential context have not attended closely to aggregate impacts of female-headed households. Theoretical development building on the neighborhood dynamics described by Sampson (1987), and considering their application to smaller residential units, may prove profitable.

Finally, our results have something to say about fear of crime and the ongoing debate about its construct validity (Ferraro, 1994; LaGrange & Ferraro, 1989). As described above, theorists have turned to noncriminal causes of fear to explain its apparent lack of connection to criminal victimization (which, again, was not a significant predictor of fear in this study and even the correlation between serious crime news and fear was nonsignificant after controlling for block racial composition). They have focused instead on the unsettling conditions, alternately labeled sources of "urban unease," "signs of incivility," "soft crimes," or something else, which residents may encounter. Results here inform these proposals in two respects. First, they confirm that the proposed connection has underpinnings in psychological differences. Residents on the same block, although they may and do view it differently, experience the same physical and social setting. Their differences in how they perceive that setting make them more or less concerned about safety than their neighbors. Second, they confirm that the proposed connection also has ecological underpinnings. Communities with differing levels of disorder express varying fear levels.

Strengths and Limitations of These Methods and Results

The sheer combination of multiple, diverse methods for assessing a community context (i.e., data triangulation) is a major advantage. That is particularly true when it comes to contexts such as crime and disorder, whose measurement has had notorious validity problems (O'Brien, 1985). Independent observations of community disorder were related not only to fear but also to resident-surveyed perceptions of disorder and to crime and disorder news stories (see Tables II, III, and IV; see also Perkins et al., 1992), thus exhibiting good concurrent validity.

The internal consistency and interrater reliability of both the resident survey scales and the Block Environmental Inventory were tested and found to be more than adequate. The reliability of the newspaper article selection and content analysis methodology was demonstrated using the same procedure, but with other raters and newspapers. More applications and psychometric work using two or more of the methods are recommended. In particular, it would be useful to know more about survey respondents' exposure to specific environmental and media stimuli.

Choosing Methods

If the measures are about equally predictive, one might question the need to ever use more than one measure (e.g., surveyed perceptions). Other studies, using different measures with different items and different samples may obtain different results, however. Furthermore, a separate and still unresolved issue concerns the construct validity of each of these assessment procedures. The various methods may still be measuring different under-lying processes. For example, group perceptions reflect a mix of group attitudes, group communication patterns, and extant conditions. On-site observations come closer to extant conditions. Further, from a policy perspective, different foci may be relevant to different goals. Community policing initiatives have concentrated on improving extant conditions (Greene & Taylor, 1988), making on-site observations the preferred indicator. But policy-makers more concerned with distress expressed by resident groups might rather focus on the perceived disorder as their problem indicator.

Observational methods and media analyses both deserve more attention among community researchers. Their significant independent relationships with fear in the present study are noteworthy, given the advantages surveyed perceptions had. Most important, neither the Block Environmental Inventory nor the newspaper data shared method variance with the criterion as did the survey. The observational data were collected earlier than the other two methods, and more than a year before the second survey, when the criterion was measured. Only one of the three observational predictors, home physical disorder, even shares household-level sampling variance with the fear measure, again unlike the survey. The newspaper archive had the disadvantage of focusing on a larger unit of analysis altogether, the neighborhood as opposed to street block (i.e., it depends on selected residents and blocks being representative of their wider neighborhood). Most of the newspaper stories did have the advantages of being closer in time to the fear measure and being more focused on crime per se, compared to the other two methods.

Remaining Questions

Although the present results help clarify the theoretical links between community disorder and fear, several important related questions remain.

First, it is still possible that the individual-level connection between perceived disorder and fear is spurious, arising from other psychological factors. For example, people who are more worry- or anxiety-prone may be more fearful and also (inaccurately) perceive more disorder in their environment. The fact that resident perceptions of the block environment agreed closely with independent observations in this study (Perkins et al., 1992) tends to discount that explanation, however.

At the group level, although all three HLM models suggest that the conditions most troubling to residents are physical rather than social disorder, questions remain before dismissing social incivilities as a source of problems. We did find that perceived social incivilities failed to have an independent impact on fear, but they also correlated very strongly with perceived physical problems ($r = .80$). This close coupling makes the assessment of independent impacts difficult if not impossible. Take, for example, the significant impact of nonresidential disorder on fear. The sheer presence of street-corner groceries, bars, or schools inevitably attracts nonresidents to the area, disrupts informal social controls, and makes for less safe neighborhoods (Greenberg et al., 1982; Taylor et al., 1995). So although our results seem to suggest that fear of crime is in large part fear of litter, graffiti,[6] and living in a deteriorated block or neighborhood, the intertwining of social and physical disorder cautions against such a conclusion at this time.

There are many potential moderators of the impact of community disorder on fear that were not controlled for in these results. The amount of citizen participation in individual and collective crime prevention and other local organizational activity, and the nature of that participation, are likely to affect fear at both the individual and community levels (Perkins et al., 1990; Taylor & Perkins, 1994). What we know less about is precisely *how* various formal and informal communication processes operate to influence perceptions of crime and disorder within communities. For example, does information about local crimes disseminated through newspapers or community meetings increase fear directly? Or do most residents hear secondhand accounts which may be exaggerated? And how can information about crimes be presented so that it encourages awareness and a healthy and effective response but not fear and paranoia? More information is needed about residents' exposure to various forms of communication and their reactions to each form before we can answer these questions. We would

---

[6] It should be acknowledged that although we include graffiti as a form of physical disorder, it is also a crime. Indeed, respondents whose homes have been "tagged" with graffiti may be especially, and understandably, fearful of gang violence.

argue that ecological, multilevel analyses of actual communities are more likely than laboratory experiments to produce externally valid answers.

Although that is the approach we have taken here, we still cannot generalize to settings beyond urban, predominantly residential blocks of low-to-moderate density. We do not know if our results would hold for commercial blocks or public or high-rise housing, where patterns of communication and the use, territorial functioning, and even the definition of public space may differ dramatically.

Those types of land use also have a worse reputation for crime than do lower density, private residential blocks. Yet an important caveat to the present results is the apparently high degree of serious, violent crimes that happened to occur during the study in study neighborhoods, according to the newspaper archive. Probably the biggest crime story of the year was a series of unexplained murders of women in the Northwest section of the city. Police maintained that the crimes were unrelated, but the brutality of the attacks (most of them involving rapes and strangulation or multiple stabbings), as well as their timing (leading right up to the Time 2 survey) and accompanying warnings in the press for women not to walk alone at night and to avoid dimly lit areas suggest that female survey respondents in those neighborhoods may well have been affected by the news coverage.

There were also several, singular incidents that received considerable attention from both the media and the community. The one receiving perhaps the most attention was the murder of an 11-year-old girl and subsequent community crime prevention efforts in one of the study neighborhoods. Other major crime news incidents occurring in just a few of the study neighborhoods included the arrest and trial of two men who had executed five people in a drug-related incident, the murder of a woman and slashing of her mother and rape of her child, the robbery and critical wounding of an off-duty policeman, the bow-and-arrow slaying of a pregnant woman, the rape-murder of a 15-year-old girl by a drug dealer, the robbery and killing of a retired minister which sparked a wave of gun law interest, a family who caught a man raping an 11-year-old family member, the torture and rape of a woman and execution of her boyfriend, and several shootings outside of nightclubs.

We do not know if this level of serious crime and crime news is atypical of Baltimore or other cities. But salient levels of crime or at least disorder cues are a regrettable necessity of research on crime and, especially, fear of crime. Researchers in areas with less serious crime, crime news, or social and environmental disorder may not achieve the same results. It is important to note that these insights into the nature and possible impact of particular crimes and their news coverage come not from the quantitative portion of the news data, but from *qualitative* neighborhood-by-neighborhood news summaries, whose value should not be overlooked or underestimated.

Another important implication of these ecological assessment methods for theory, research, and action is their flexibility regarding content. As the present data demonstrate, all three methods lend themselves well to measuring community disorder. But there are many other ecological concepts that can be measured using these methods. More than half of the Block Environmental Inventory focuses on more positive or neutral characteristics of the environment not covered here, such as territoriality, beautification, and defensible space. Newspaper content analysis can, of course focus on any topic that is newsworthy and even ones that are not part of the "hard" news (e.g., violence in comics and movie advertising). For example, a methodology similar to the one presented here was used by the first author to evaluate both media and government treatment of different San Francisco neighborhoods (one wealthy, one poor) following the 1989 earthquake. With the advent of NEXIS and other news search services, the procedures for searching print media electronically have been made vastly more efficient.

Regarding surveys as an ecological method, the present and similar resident surveys have been aggregated to the block and neighborhood level to successfully measure all kinds of community social climate variables, such as citizen participation, neighboring, informal social control, sense of community, communitarianism, place attachments (Perkins et al., 1990), even aggregated anxiety and depression (Taylor & Perkins, 1994). But surveys are still probably better for measuring individual psychological constructs than for assessing community ecologies. For the latter, community psychologists should explore alternative quantitative *and* qualitative methods that are more commensurate with both the community level of analysis and the multifaceted (social, physical, political, and economic) human environment, such as direct and participant observation, and content analysis of media and other recorded communication.

APPENDIX A

The instrument also includes many items not used in the present analyses. For example, "territorial markers" (e.g., garden, yard decoration, other "personalizations," crime prevention signs) convey control over an area and a separation between one's self, family, or community and "outsiders," and are related to residents' perceptions of safety (Taylor et al., 1984), to their perception of less community disorder and crime problems (Perkins et al., 1992), and to more or less police reports of crime, depending upon the type of marker (Perkins et al., 1993). "Defensible space" describes features of the built environment, such as building size, street layout, width and lighting, sight lines for passive surveillance, and barriers to entry, that have been associated with modest, but real, reductions in crime (Perkins et al., 1993) and fear

(Newman & Franck, 1982; Taylor et al., 1984). Other studies have found defensible space features to have a limited influence on the residential social climate and thus fear levels (Merry, 1981) or to have some positive and some negative effects on perceived crime and disorder (Perkins et al., 1992). Nonresidential land use (corner stores, schools, etc.) has been found to encourage reported crime (Perkins et al., 1993) and observed incivilities (Taylor, Koons, Kurtz, Greene, & Perkins, 1995). Instructions and the latest version of the BEI may be obtained from the first author.

APPENDIX B

Assume we have a model where the outcome (Y) is fear of crime, and the individual-level predictor is perceived physical deterioration. Assume we have a group level predictor, in the form of a dummy variable W, indicating a high or low score on observed signs of incivility. HLM provides an individual-level model (Level I), and a group-level (Level II) model. The Level I model would be

$$Y_{ij} = \beta_{0j} + \beta_{1j}(X_{ij} - X_{.j}) + r_{ij} \tag{1}$$

where Y_{ij} = score of individual i in block j on fear of crime, β_{0j} = unique Y-intercept for each jth block, β_{1j} = unique slope for each jth block, $(X_{ij} - X_{.j})$ = each individual's perceived physical deterioration, after subtracting the average perceived physical deterioration in his/her block, and r_{ij} = the residual, unexplained portion of Y.

The model assumes (Bryk & Raudenbush, 1992, p. 12) that: r_{ij} is normally distributed, with homogeneous variance across blocks, and that the slopes (β_{1j}) and intercepts (β_{0j}) each have a bivariate normal distribution across blocks. A plausible hypothesis would be that those who perceive more deterioration will be more fearful.

The Level II model seeks to predict the block slopes and intercepts noted above. The two equations in the Level II model are as follows:

$$\beta_{0j} = \gamma_{00} + \gamma_{01}W_j + \mu_{0j} \tag{2}$$

$$\beta_{1j} = \gamma_{10} + \gamma_{11}W_j + \mu_{1j} \tag{3}$$

where γ_{00} = mean fear score in blocks where observed incivilities rates are below the median (i.e., the intercept in these blocks); γ_{01} = mean fear difference between blocks with observed incivilities levels below the median and those above the median; γ_{10} = average slope of fear on perceived physical deterioration in blocks where observed incivilities are below the median; γ_{11} = average *difference* in the slope of fear on perceived physical deterioration in blocks where observed incivilities are below the median versus those where it is above the median; μ_{0j} = unique effect of block j on average level of fear in a block *after* controlling for the differences on the outcome between low and high observed incivilities blocks (It captures between-block effects on the Y-intercept due to block differences other than observed incivilities.); and μ_{1j} = unique effect of Block j on the *slope* of fear on perceived physical deterioration *after controlling* for the effects that observed incivilities have on the slope. (It captures between block differences on the slope due to block differences other than incivilities.)

Substituting from Equation 2 and Equation 3 back into Equation 1, we derive the full *combined model*, that can be estimated with HLM using iterative maximum likelihood procedures.

$$Y_{ij} = \gamma_{00} + \gamma_{01}W_j + \gamma_{10}(X_{ij} - X_{.j}) + \gamma_{11}(X_{ij} - X_{.j})$$
$$+ \mu_{0j} + \mu_{1j}(X_{ij} - X_{.j}) + r_{ij} \tag{4}$$

In the current study, however, we have fixed the slope of Level I predictors, not allowing them to vary across blocks. We did this because we did not have enough cases per block. Raudenbush (1988) advises having at least 20 cases per group to efficiently model variations in slopes, which represent, in effect, interactions between the individual predictor and the group predictor. Further, in this study we do not have theoretical rationales for allowing specific slopes to vary. Therefore, we are assessing a reduced model, setting the Level II model of $\beta_{1j} = \gamma_{10}$, so the combined model is:

$$Y_{ij} = \gamma_{00} + \gamma_{01} W_j + \gamma_{10}(X_{ij} - X_{.j}) + \mu_{0j} + r_{ij} \tag{5}$$

and $\gamma 10$ is the slope of perceived physical deterioration on all blocks.

ACKNOWLEDGEMENTS

This research was supported by National Institute of Mental Health grants 1-R01-MH40842-01 and -02 from the Center for Violent and Antisocial Behavior, R.B.T., principal investigator, D.D.P., project director. R.B.T. also received support from grants IJ-CX-93-0022 and 94-IJ-CX-0018 from the National Institute of Justice during preparation of this manuscript. Opinions are solely those of the authors and do not reflect the opinions or official policies of the National Institute of Justice or the Department of Justice. This article benefitted in too many ways to list from the comments of Barbara B. Brown, Ron Davis, Marybeth Shinn, and anonymous reviewers on earlier drafts. Kenneth Maton and his students assisted in the collection of the on-site observational data. Jim Leflar and Sunil Madhugiri helped with the newspaper sampling and content analysis. D.D.P.'s students in Research Methods assisted in analyzing the interrater agreement of the newspaper content analysis procedure. Interviewing was carried out by Survey Research Associates of Baltimore.

REFERENCES

Babbie, E. (1995). *The practice of social research* (7th ed). Belmont, CA: Wadsworth.

Balkin, S. (1979). Victimization rates, safety, and fear of crime. *Social Problems, 26,* 343–350.

Bryk, A. S., & Raudenbush, S. W. (1987). Application of hierarchical linear models to assessing change. *Psychological Bulletin, 101,* 147–158.

Bryk, A. S., & Raudenbush, S. W. (1992). *Hierarchical linear models: Applications and data analysis methods.* Newbury Park, CA: Sage.

Bryk, A. S., & Thum, Y. M. (1989). The effects of high school on dropping out: An exploratory investigation. *American Educational Research Journal, 26,* 353–384.

Clarke, R., Ekblom, P., Hough, M., & Mayhew, P. (1985). Elderly victims of crime and exposure to risk. *Howard Journal of Criminal Justice, 24,* 1–9.

Covington, J., & Taylor, R. B. (1991). Fear of crime in urban residential neighborhoods; Implications of between- and within-neighborhood sources for current models. *Sociological Quarterly, 32,* 231–249.

Crenson, M. (1983). *Neighborhood politics*. Cambridge, MA: Harvard University Press.

Ditton, J., & Duffy, J. (1983). Bias in the newspaper reporting of crime news. *British Journal of Criminology, 23*, 159–165.

Dubow, F., McCabe, E., & Kaplan, G. (1979). *Reactions to crime: A critical review of the literature*. Washington, DC: U.S. Government Printing Office.

Ferraro, K. F. (1994). *Fear of crime: Interpreting victimization risk*. Albany: State University of New York Press.

Ferraro, K., & LaGrange, R. (1987). The measurement of fear of crime. *Sociological Inquiry, 57*, 70–101.

Garofalo, J., & Laub, J. (1978). The fear of crime: Broadening our perspective. *Victimology, 3*, 242–253.

Gomme, I. M. (1988). The role of experience in the production of fear of crime: A test of a causal model. *Canadian Journal of Criminology, 30*, 67–76.

Goodman, A. C., & Taylor, R. B. (1983). *The Baltimore Neighborhood Factbook*. Baltimore, MD: The Johns Hopkins University, Center for Metropolitan Planning and Research.

Greenberg, S. W., Rohe, W. M., & Williams, J. (1982). *Safe and secure neighborhoods: Physical characteristics and informal territorial control in high and low crime neighborhoods*. Washington, DC: U.S. Department of Justice.

Greene, J. R., & Taylor, R. B. (1988). Community-based policing and foot patrol: Issues of theory and evaluation. In J. R. Greene & S. D. Mastrofski (Eds.), *Community policing: Rhetoric or reality?* (pp. 195–224). New York: Praeger.

Hauser, P. M. (1974). Contextual analysis revisited. *Sociological Methods and Research, 2*, 365–375.

Hope, T., & Hough, M. (1988). Area, crime, and incivility: A profile from the British Crime Survey. In T. Hope & M. Shaw (Eds.), *Communities and crime reduction* (pp. 30–47). London: Her Majesty's Stationery Office.

Hunter, A. (1978, November). *Symbols of incivility*. Paper presented at the Annual Meeting of the American Society of Criminology, Dallas, TX.

Jaehnig, W. B., Weaver, D. H., & Fico, F. (1981). Reporting crime and fearing crime in three communities. *Journal of Communication, 31*, 88–96.

Kenny, D. A., & Lavoie, L. (1985). Separating individual and group effects. *Journal of Personality and Social Psychology, 48*, 339–348.

Kurtz, E., & Taylor, R. B. (1995). *Fear of crime: Testing interactions between individual and context*. Unpublished manuscript, Department of Criminal Justice, Temple University.

LaGrange, R. L., & Ferraro, K. F. (1989). Assessing age and gender differences in perceived risk and fear of crime. *Criminology, 27*, 697–719.

LaGrange, R. L., Ferraro, K. F., & Supancic, M. (1992). Perceived risk and fear of crime: Role of social and physical incivilities. *Journal of Research in Crime and Delinquency, 29*, 311–334.

Lawton, M. P., & Yaffe, S. (1980). Victimization and fear of crime in elderly public housing tenants. *Journal of Gerontology, 35*, 768–779.

Lewis, D. A., & Maxfield, M. (1980). Fear in the neighborhoods: An investigation of the impact of crime. *Journal of Research in Crime and Delinquency, 17*, 160–189.

Lewis, D. A., & Riger, S. (1986). Crime as stress: On the internalization of a social problem. In E. Seidman & J. Rappaport (Eds.), *Redefining social problems*. New York: Plenum Press.

Lewis, D. A., & Salem, G. (1985). *Fear of crime: Incivility and the production of a social problem*. New Brunswick, NJ: Transaction.

Liska, A. E., & Baccaglini, W. (1990). Feeling safe by comparison: Crime in the newspapers. *Social Problems, 37*, 360–374.

Liska, A. E., Sanchirico, A., & Reed, M. D. (1988). Fear of crime and constrained behavior: Estimating a reciprocal effects model. *Social Forces, 66*, 827–837.

Maxfield, M. G. (1987). *Incivilities and fear of crime in England and Wales and the United States: A comparative analysis.* Paper presented at the Annual Meeting of the American Society of Criminology, Montreal.

Melnicoe, S. (Ed.). (1987). Special Issue: Fear of Crime. *Crime and Delinquency, 33.*

Merry, S. E. (1981). *Urban danger: Life in a neighborhood of strangers.* Philadelphia: Temple University Press.

Mulvey, A., Turro, G., Cutter, T., & Pash, J. (1995). *Crime, communities and qualities of lives: Women and men in Lowell, 1982–1994.* Paper presented at the Biennial Conference on Community Research and Action, Chicago.

Newman, O., & Franck, K. (1982). The effects of building size on personal crime and fear of crime. *Population and Environment, 5*, 203–220.

Norris, F. H., & Kaniasty, K. (1991). The psychological experience of crime: A test of the mediating role of beliefs in explaining the distress of victims. *Journal of Social and Clinical Psychology, 10*, 239–261.

Norris, F. H., & Kaniasty, K. (1992). A longitudinal study of the effects of various crime prevention strategies on criminal victimization, fear of crime, and psychological distress. *American Journal of Community Psychology, 20*, 625–648.

O'Brien, R. M. (1985). *Crime and victimization data.* Beverly Hills: Sage.

O'Keefe, G. J., & Reid-Nash, K. (1987). Crime news and real-world blues: The effects of the media on social reality. *Communication Research, 14*, 147–163.

Ortega, S. T., & Myles, J. L. (1987). Race and gender effects on fear of crime: An interactive model with age. *Criminology, 25*, 133–152.

Pawson, E., & Banks, G. (1991). Rape and fear of violence in Christchurch. *Community Mental Health in New Zealand, 6*, 16–33.

Perkins, D. D., Florin, P., Rich, R. C., Wandersman, A., & Chavis, D. M. (1990). Participation and the social and physical environment of residential blocks: Crime and community context. *American Journal of Community Psychology, 18*, 83–115.

Perkins, D. D., Meeks, J. W., & Taylor, R. B. (1992). The physical environment of street blocks and resident perceptions of crime and disorder: Implications for theory and measurement. *Journal of Environmental Psychology, 12*, 21–34.

Perkins, D. D., Wandersman, A., Rich, R. C., & Taylor, R. B. (1993). The physical environment of street crime: Defensible space, territoriality and incivilities. *Journal of Environmental Psychology, 13*, 29–49.

Raudenbush, S. W. (1988). Educational applications of hierarchical linear models: A review. *Journal of Educational Statistics, 13*, 85–116.

Raudenbush, S. W., & Chan, W. (1992). Growth curve analysis in accelerate longitudinal designs. *Journal of Research in Crime and Delinquency, 29*, 387–411.

Raudenbush, S. W., & Chan, W. (1993). Application of a Hierarchical Linear Model to the study of adolescent deviance in an overlapping cohort design. *Journal of Consulting and Clinical Psychology, 61*, 941–951.

Riger, S., Gordon, M., & LeBailly, R. (1981). Community ties and urbanites' fear of crime: An ecological investigation. *American Journal of Community Psychology, 9*, 653–665.

Rosenbaum, D. P., Lewis, D. A., & Grant, J. A. (1986). Neighborhood-based crime prevention: Assessing the efficacy of community organizing in Chicago. In D. Rosenbaum (Ed.), *Community Crime Prevention: Does it work?* (pp. 109–133). Beverly Hills: Sage.

Sampson, R. J. (1987). Urban black violence: The effect of male joblessness and family disruption. *American Journal of Sociology, 93*, 348–382.

Skogan, W. (1990). *Disorder and decline.* New York: Free Press.

Skogan, W., Cook, F., Antunes, G., & Cook, T. D. (1978). Criminal victimization of the elderly: The physical and economic consequences. *Gerontologist, 18*, 339–349.

Skogan, W., & Maxfield, M. (1981). *Coping with crime: Individual and neighborhood reactions.* Beverly Hills: Sage.

Smith, S. J. (1984). Crime in the news. *British Journal of Criminology, 24*, 289–295.

Sparks, G. G., & Ogles, R. M. (1990). The difference between fear of victimization and the probability of being victimized: Implications for cultivation. *Journal of Broadcasting and Electronic Media, 34*, 351–358.

Steward, D., Perkins, D. D., & Brown, B. B. (1995, June 15). *Community social ties and fear of crime.* Presented at the Biennial Conference on Community Research & Action, Chicago.

Taylor, R. B. (1987). Toward an environmental psychology of disorder: Delinquency, crime, and fear of crime. In D. Stokols & I. Altman (Eds.), *Handbook of environmental psychology* (Vol. 2, pp. 951–986). New York: Wiley.

Taylor, R. B. (1995, July). *Responses to disorder in Minneapolis-St. Paul: Relative impacts of neighborhood structure, crime, and physical deterioration.* Unpublished final report (94-IJ-CX-0018) to the National Institute of Justice. Department of Criminal Justice, Temple University.

Taylor, R. B. (1996). Neighborhood responses to disorder and local attachments: The systemic model of attachment, social disorganization, and neighborhood use value. *Sociological Forum, 11*, 41–74.

Taylor, R. B., & Covington, J. (1993). Community structural change and fear of crime. *Social Problems, 40*, 374–397.

Taylor, R. B., Gottfredson, S. D., & Brower, S. (1984). Block crime and fear: Defensible space, local social ties, and territorial functioning. *Journal of Crime and Delinquency, 21*, 303–331.

Taylor, R. B., Gottfredson, S. D. & Brower, S. D. (1985). Attachment to place: Discriminant validity, and impacts of disorder and diversity. *American Journal of Community Psychology, 13*, 525–542.

Taylor, R. B., & Hale, M. (1986). Testing alternative models of fear of crime. *Journal of Criminal Law and Criminology, 77*, 151–189.

Taylor, R. B., Koons, B. A., Kurtz, E. M., Greene, J. R., & Perkins, D. D. (1995). Street blocks with more nonresidential land use have more physical deterioration: Evidence from Baltimore and Philadelphia. *Urban Affairs Review, 31*, 120–136.

Taylor, R. B., & Perkins, D. D. (1994). *The impact of block-level fear and citizen participation on changes in anxiety and depression: A stress and coping framework.* Unpublished manuscript.

Taylor, R. B., & Shumaker, S. (1990). Local crime as a natural hazard: Implications for understanding the relationship between disorder and fear. *American Journal of Community Psychology, 18*, 619–641.

Taylor, R. B., Shumaker, S., & Gottfredson, S. (1985). Neighborhood-level links between physical features and local sentiments. *Journal of Architectural Planning and Research, 2*, 261–275.

Tyler, T. R. (1984). Assessing the risk of crime victimization: The integration of personal victimization experience and socially transmitted information. *Journal of Social Issues, 40*, 27–38.

Williams, P., & Dickinson, J. (1993). Fear of crime: Read all about it? The relationship between newspaper crime reporting and fear of crime. *British Journal of Criminology, 33*, 33–56.

Wilson, J. Q. (1975). *Thinking about crime.* New York: Basic Books.

Wilson, J. Q., & Kelling, C. (1982, March). The police and neighborhood safety: Broken windows. *Atlantic, 127*, 29–38.

6

Detecting "Cracks" in Mental Health Service Systems: Application of Network Analytic Techniques

Mark Tausig

This paper argued that problems of coordination and integration of community mental health systems are best approached from a network perspective in which all linkages between agencies are considered simultaneously. Structural coordination and integration can be assessed through the analysis of these linkages. The utility of this approach was demonstrated by deriving a typology of system "cracks" from network analytic constructs. A network analysis of a community mental health service network was then generated to illustrate how these cracks can be empirically identified. It is suggested that mental health planners will find both the network analytic approach and the typology of cracks useful for addressing problems of coordination and integration.

In one form or another, the fragmentation of health and human services in the community has been identified as a major impediment to effective service delivery (Agranoff & Pattakos, Cumming, 1967; Leopold & Schein, 1975; Tessler & Goldman, 1982; Turner & TenHoor, 1978). Historically, attempts to coordinate services among agencies have relied upon voluntary

Originally published in the *American Journal of Community Psychology, 15*(3) (1987): 337–351.

Ecological Research to Promote Social Change: Methodological *Advances from Community Psychology*, edited by Tracey A. Revenson et al. Kluwer Academic/Plenum Publishers, New York, 2002.

mechanisms that have sought to maintain agency autonomy while facilitating coordinated activity in areas where there is agreement (Litwak & Rothman, 1970). These voluntary coordination mechanisms have generally not proven effective (Warren, 1973). The failure to create better coordinated services has been attributed to excessive autonomy of service agencies (attempts to preserve prerogatives about problem definition, intervention, priority, and client disposition) and to patterns of funding (Agranoff & Pattakos, 1979; Greenley & Kirk, 1973; Levine, 1974).

Attention has now shifted to explicit, directed attempts to coordinate services, for instance Community Support Programs for the adult chronic mentally ill client (Turner & TenHoor, 1978). The goal of efforts to coordinate the activities of community organizations such as the NIMH Community Support Program is in part to create an organized network of services (Turner & TenHoor, 1978). This goal is based on assumptions that the needs of clients, in this case the chronic mentally ill, extend to a wide variety of community human services, that a stable structure of services is necessary for long-term planning, and that lines of responsibility need to be clarified (Tessler & Goldman, 1982). These assumptions and the results of programming based on these assumptions require assessment. Indeed, as Sauber (1977) noted, there is a strong interest among planners and practitioners in developing methods for measuring the level of system integration for these purposes. I believe that network analysis may offer considerable help.

Interorganizational theory and analysis, with its focus on the origins, patterns, and consequences of interaction between complex organizations has found a natural object of study in the assessment of human service delivery systems (Baker & O'Brien, 1971; Litwak & Hylton, 1962; Tausig & Townsend, 1982; Van de Ven, Walker & Liston, 1979; Warren, Rose, & Bergunder, 1974). One of the latest developments in the interorganizational research field is the increasing use of network analytic procedures to measure and assess the performance of interagency coalitions (Alba, 1982; Knoke & Kuklinski, 1982; Wellman, 1983). This work, however, has concentrated on the development of theory and method rather than on how these procedures can be used to inform policy and programmatic issues in the delivery of community-based services.

In this chapter, I attempt to illustrate one way in which developments in interorganizational analysis can be applied usefully to just such policy and programming issues. In particular, I wish to show how the meaning of "structure" in network analytic theory can be used to define and locate possible "cracks" in the pattern of relationships existing among a set of community service providers.

The network perspective examines all interactions between organizations in a specified population of organizations (e.g., community mental health providers). The entire pattern of interorganizational relations is taken into account in order to describe the structure of the network. Thus, an interorganizational network can be defined as "the pattern of interrelationships among organizations that are meshed together as a social system to attain collective and self-interest goals or to resolve specific problems for a target population" (Van de Ven, 1976). The regularities in the pattern of relations between organizations provides the structure of the network. In turn, the extent to which these interactions serve to coordinate the activities of organizations in the network can be determined (Whetten, 1981).

The importance of using this level of analysis for assessing coordination lies in the fact that the action of a particular organization can be examined in terms of its effect on all other organizations in the network. This approach is the only one that provides information concerning coordination and integration at the community level. Coordination means the degree to which the network of organizations as a whole manages community resource flows, including clients, information, and money. The map or image of the network which is generated by network analysis represents the structure of relations between community agencies. The description and assessment of these patterns is the object of network analyses and are in turn of special interest to planners and programmers.

NETWORK ANALYTIC PROCEDURES

The use of network analytic procedures results in products which are of substantial importance to those interested in determining community-level coordination and integration. In the typical network analysis the researcher determines the boundary separating a network from the remainder of its organizational environment (generally using geographic or functional criteria, Laumann, Galaskiewicz, & Marsden, 1978). The flow of client, funding, and information resources between all members of the network are then determined using some form of cluster analysis (see Morrissey, Hall, & Lindsey, 1982, for a comprehensive outline of measures and dimensions) to provide the basis for assessing the pattern of resource flows in the network.

Next, relevant bases for interaction are used to construct the complete pattern of relations in the network. The researcher may represent these patterns in terms of either similar relations to the same other actors (structural equivalence, in a sense, they are substitutable for one another) or in terms of local density of interaction (cohesion or cliques) (Burt, 1983; Sondquist, 1980). Whether structural equivalence or cliques form the basis for identifying actors who ought to be considered to occupy similar network positions, these network positions can be described further in terms of the pattern of relations between positions (Alba & Gutman, 1972; Burt, 1977a; White, Boorman, & Breiger, 1976). This is the final network description in an analytic sense.

The analysis of these patterns permits us to literally draw a picture (in this case the picture is called a digraph, directed graph) of the network of interorganizational relations represented in the system. Neither the analysis nor the digraph gives the degree of coordination directly. They do, however, identify the extent of interaction and the patterns of dependence and autonomy made possible by the specific pattern of resource exchanges. For instance, if the network analysis revealed that a particular set of direct service provider relied on a single source for client referrals, then we would infer that these agencies were dependent on the single referral source. If multiple unrelated referral sources were present instead, then the degree of dependence on a single source is reduced and service providers would be described as autonomous with respect to client referral sources.

DETECTING CRACKS IN THE NETWORK

The term *cracks* is a catchall representing missing services, inaccessible services, administrative oversight, inappropriate referrals, and missing information, among other things. In short, cracks are indicators of structural gaps in the service system but, because cracks can mean so many different things, this notion has little utility for planners and programmers. However, since network analysis provides us with the structure of a given network, it may also be able to provide more specific indicators of types of cracks and their possible locations in the network. I am careful to say possible, because a missing linkage in the network structure cannot be assessed outside of the network context. Moreover, since network analysis is descriptive, those who employ the method must have some notion of where cracks may appear. The analysis becomes an assessment tool. Network analysis, then, is only a stage in a more complex analysis. In this case, the structural description of the network can only point to the possible existence of a crack or cracks.

Types of Cracks

At least three types of cracks can be derived logically from network analytic concepts:

> *Type 1*: Unpatterned relations between organizations in the service system.

Type 2: Absence of direct or indirect linkages between sectors of the system.

Type 3: Conflicted or unsatisfactory linkages between elements of the system.

Unpatterned Relations (Type 1). If network planners expect that a common referral pathway from criminal justice agencies to direct mental health providers should exist, then the inability to detect a group of criminal justice agencies with structurally equivalent links to mental health providers may indicate the failure to establish such a patterned relationship. The absence of an expected cluster means that the organizations that constitute this service area do not have similar relations with other actors in the mental health service system. Relations between these service providers and others in the network are not collectively systematic; whatever contacts are made are ad hoc in nature and unreliable. While failure to observe such links does not automatically imply that a client cannot be referred from a criminal justice agency to a mental health service agency, it does suggest that, in system terms, these referrals are relatively unsystematic and costly. Thus a failure to observe a particular cluster may provide an indication of a Type 1 crack (see Figure 1). In network analytic terms, the presence of more than one organization that provides identical or similar services (overlapping or duplicating) is not as important as whether these separate services have a common pattern of relations with other positions in the network (see Landau, 1969, for a justification of redundancy in a system).

Absence of Linkages Between Clusters (Type 2). Type 2 cracks are detectable when one attempts to examine the relationships among various service clusters that are intended to have systematic direct and/or indirect links. If, for instance, inpatient clusters and outpatient clusters are not linked, this absence may indicate a general system inability to coordinate these services. If there are neither direct nor indirect linkages between the inpatient and outpatient clusters, then the system may be said to be unable to provide coordinated follow-up for discharged patients requiring continued outpatient service (see Figure 1).

Conflicted or Unsatisfactory Links (Type 3). Type 3 cracks are detectable by analyzing the "relational" or affective content of interactions (Burt, 1980). This is a separate analysis which evaluates the content of the detected cluster relations. Thus, while a linkage may exist between clusters, the relationship may not fulfill its designated function. For instance, Hall, Clark, Giordano, Johnson, and Van Rockel (1977) suggested that high levels of conflict can exist between agencies whose linkage is mandated as opposed to voluntary. Although Warren et al. (1974) also noted that coordination can be achieved through conflict, the appearance of conflict

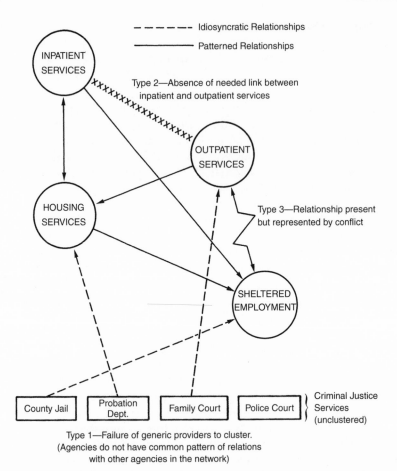

Figure 1. Hypothetical digraph of mental health services network illustrating location of network cracks.

should be investigated as a possible crack. Type 3 cracks arise, for instance, where a relationship between clustered outpatient services and sheltered employment services exists but is characterized by conflict or lack of cooperation. Regardless of the existence of the linkage, the poor quality of the link may mean that it is used to resolve conflict rather than for the purpose for which it was originally intended (see Figure 1).

In all of the cases, the existence of cracks in the system is suggested only indirectly by a network analysis. It may be the case that a missing linkage or linkage based primarily on competitive relations is functional for the network. Therefore, the network analytic solution generates only a clue to the true existence of cracks in the system. Its strength lies in its capacity to suggest where and what types of cracks may be present in a given network of interactions.

AN ILLUSTRATION

Data and Procedures

Forty-five agencies in an upstate New York county were selected for inclusion in this study. The agencies comprised a complete list of public and private organizations that have direct contact with adult chronic mentally ill individuals in the county. Although each of the 45 agencies deals with the adult mental patient, no presumption was made that the agency had a defined program for handling such individuals. For instance, criminal justice or family service agencies regularly come in contact with adult mental patients, yet may not have internal program capabilities to handle such clients. In the Spring of 1980 the agency directors of all 45 agencies were asked to complete an extensive questionnaire pertaining to their relations with other agencies. Data collected from directors of all 45 agencies were analyzed.

The basis for identifying network clusters was a single item, identical to the one used by Van de Ven et al. (1979): "From the list (45 agencies), select and write the names of up to five agencies that your organization was most directly involved with during the last six months."

In addition to information concerning the degree of involvement between agencies (those with whom the agency was most involved), information on five bases for interaction were also obtained. These bases included the exchanges of clients, funds, information, the presence of a legal mandate, and the need to settle disputes. This latter basis for interaction was used to identify Type 3 (conflict-based) cracks. Respondents could report multiple bases for interaction.

The 45 × 45 choice matrix generated by responses to the initial question was analyzed using the STRUCTURE Program developed by Burt (1977b) in order to discern structurally equivalent clusters. The data were treated as nonsymmetric choices (no assumption of reciprocity) and euclidean distances between actor agencies were computed. The program outputs a table of social role distances (a computation of exactly how similar the pattern of relations of actors are to one another) based on the algorithm suggested by Johnson (1967, p. 248). The table indicates criterion distances that must be satisfied in order to place agencies within a "cluster" with other agencies (Burt, 1977a; Equation 6).

The STRUCTURE program was then used to examine cluster inter-relations as well. The cluster memberships of all actors were specified and matrices based on reported exchanges of clients, information, and funds were analyzed to establish density of interaction between clusters.

Results

Twenty-two agencies were identified by the STRUCTURE program as members of clusters ranging in size from two to six agencies per cluster. In addition, three "broker" positions (single agencies that receive from one set of agencies and choose another set) were identified. The agencies constituting these clusters and brokerage positions are listed in Table I.

The results of the analysis of bases for interaction between clusters are depicted in Fig. 2 which represents the presence and direction of interactions among the seven clusters of agencies and three brokers. It may be seen that a distinct "mental health" grouping of clusters is linked to a distinct "social services" grouping of clusters through the brokerage position of the Department of Social Services. Thus, within the network of agencies handling the mentally ill, a two-tiered system has evolved which separates the delivery of mental health services from the delivery of related social services.

Table I. Clusters Derived from Analysis of Agency Choices

Cluster 1: Retardation Services	Cluster 5: Family services
State developmental center	Family counseling service 1
Private retardation association	Family counseling service 2
Private housing for retarded adults	Cluster 6: Street Agencies
Association for learning disabled	Health center
Cluster 2: Mental health services	Hot line
Residence 1	Outreach 1
Residence 2	Outreach 2
Outpatient clinic	Cluster 7: Charity services
Case management and halfway house	Day program
Social club	Day program and residence
Sheltered workshop	Broker positions
Cluster 3: Rehabilitation services	Private hospital psychiatric
State vocational rehabilitation project	outpatient unit
YMCA	Country Mental Health Board
Cluster 4: health services	Department of Social Services
City Department of Health	
Visiting Nurses Association	

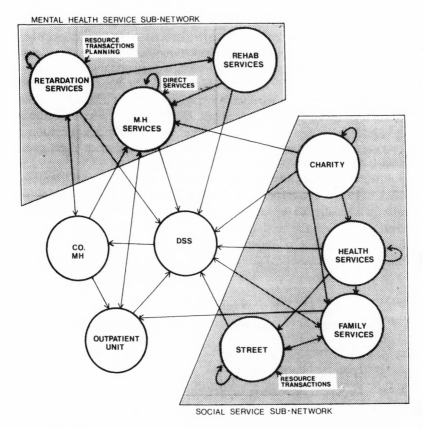

Figure 2. Diagrammatic representation of cluster and broker network interactions.

Type 1 Cracks

Of the 45 agencies in this network, 20 did not appear in any structurally equivalent cluster. Each of these 20 agencies therefore, has a unique set of relations to all other agencies in the network. The absence of patterned relationships between these organizations and other network agencies suggests that Type 1 cracks might be present in the network. It is possible that each of the unclustered organizations performs a unique function within the network and that, therefore, they are intentionally not structurally equivalent with any other network actors. Nevertheless, this result strongly suggests that such cracks do exist. The absence of common patterns of relations where they should or could be expected to exist can indicate a lack of system integration. In system terms, the network with unclustered actors is more complex and, therefore, requires a higher degree of centralization and formalization to achieve the same level of coordination as a less complex network (Van de Ven & Ferry, 1980).

Table II lists the 20 agencies that failed to cluster. Unlike the clustered agencies listed in Table I, the arangement of these services under categorical headings is strictly for the sake of argument. There is no statistical basis for the groupings. Yet the groupings are pertinent to the identification of Type 1 cracks. For example, all inpatient services, though dealing with similar client needs, are not systematically related to other positions (e.g., mental health services) in the network. This suggests that discharged clients from different inpatient services will not necessarily be referred to the mental health outpatient services cluster (there is no common relationship to the mental health cluster in Table I) if they are referred at all. Outpatient

**Table II. Unclusters Agencies Grouped by
Generic Service Function**

Inpatient services
    Private hospital inpatient unit
    State hospital inpatient unit
    State Mental Health Regional Administration

Criminal justice services
    County jail
    Family court
    Police court
    Probation department
    Legal advocacy group

Housing
    Private housing agency 1
    Private housing agency 2

Community services
    Adult day care
    City mission
    City Mental Health Clinic
    City Community Action Program

Federal
    CETA
    Office of the Aging

Local planning/support services
    Human Services Planning Council
    United Way
    YMCA
    Alcoholism program

services received will depend on the idiosyncratic relations established by each inpatient service with other agencies in the network.

Type 2 Cracks

Type 2 cracks are suggested by the absence of intercluster relationships. Each cluster represents (in this particular network) a category of service in the network. The absence of a direct tie between clusters, then, may indicate a barrier to the use of services in the other sector. Figure 2 can also be used to identify these types of cracks.

For example, clients receiving retardation services my find it difficult to acquire mental health services. Although the individual agencies represented in the mental health services cluster demonstrate systematic patterns of interaction with other agencies in the larger network, there is no direct link between retardation and mental health services. The absence of this direct connection may indicate a Type 2 crack. Whereas a client in an unclustered agency (symptomatic of Type 1 cracks) may face an arbitrary referral process, the client in a clustered agency may face structural barriers to receiving needed services simply because the requisite connection is not present. From the point of view of a comprehensive service system, this type of crack demonstrates a lack of integration of different services.

Type 3 Cracks

Type 3 cracks occur when a relationship between organizations in the network is characterized by conflict rather than the exchange of clients, information, or funds. These conflictive relationships may be at the cost of services to the client.

In order to locate this type of crack we must examine the basis for relationships rather than the structure of relationships. In this case, we inspect the direct relations between clusters or between clusters and unclustered agencies in the network in terms of the affective content of ties (need to settle disputes).

In Table III we see evidence that settling disputes can occupy a substantial portion of the interactions between clusters, brokers, and unclustered groups. (Since agencies could report other bases of interaction, these numbers must be treated as indicating relative rather than absolute levels of conflict.)

The unclustered groups of inpatient services and federal programs report dispute settlement as a reason for interaction in 80% of their contacts.

**Table III. Percentage of Relationships in Which Attempts to
Settle Disputes are Reported**

	No. of Agencies	Possible relationships	No. of disputed relationships	% of all possible relationships
Clusters				
Retardation services	4	20	8	40
Mental health services	6	30	9	30
Rehabilitation services	2	10	0	0
Health services	2	10	1	10
Family services	2	10	1	10
Street agencies	4	20	4	20
Charity agencies	2	10	0	0
Brokers				
County mental health	1	5	2	40
Dept. of social services	1	5	0	0
Private outpatient service	1	5	1	20
Groups (unclustered)				
Criminal justice services	5	25	10	40
Inpatient services	3	15	12	80
Housing services	2	10	0	0
Community services	4	20	3	15
Federal programs	2	10	8	80
Planning/special services	4	20	11	55

Other analyses indicate that these disputed relationships are concentrated
in contacts between the mental health cluster and the inpatient services
cluster and between the Federal programs and family and health services.
Particularly for the inpatient–mental health relationship, conflict plays a
major and negative role. It is interesting to note that four of the six unclustered groups report 40% or more of their relationships to be disputatious.
These levels of conflict may explain the failure to detect common patterns
of interaction among these agencies (Type 1 cracks) (or vice versa).

Among clustered agencies with organized patterns of relations, the
level of conflict is generally lower. Retardation services report a relatively
high level of conflict and, as we pointed out, they do not have direct access
to mental health services (Type 2 cracks). Conflicts between the mental
health service cluster and other clusters are also somewhat high. Some of
this conflict is reciprocal to the unclustered inpatient agencies but some is
based on relationships with other clustered actors.

In sum, Type 3 cracks may be derivative of Type 1 and Type 2 cracks
but there can also be other reasons for conflict. Where formal, legally

binding relationships have been established, conflict may be high despite patterned relationships (Hall et al., 1977). In these data, the number of mandated relationships was too small to assess this possibility.

CONCLUSION

At the outset of this chapter I suggested that network analyses of the interorganizational structure of community-based organizations are theoretically and methodologically suited to examining issues of coordination and integration among such organizations. The intent of this paper has been to indicate how the use of network methods can be applied to address the long-standing problem of system fragmentation among community service agencies. In this case I have shown how the rubric of "cracks in the system" can be analytically specified by applying network logic. The aim is not so much to build a well-defined notion of cracks as to illustrate the potential utility of applying network constructs to the general problem of interest.

With its strengths, network approaches also have their limitations. A cross-sectional network analysis cannot explain how patterns developed or emerged (a longitudinal design might) nor can the analysis take into account external determinants of community organization such as sources of program funding, community power relations, and statutory and regulatory constraints once network boundaries have been drawn. The problem of how to "bound" the network affects the obtained patterns and the sorts of inferences that can be drawn from an analysis. As yet, network analysis cannot be used to relate structural conditions to client outcomes. And, as in the example here, interpretation of results depends in part on a priori expectations concerning how network relations should appear.

Despite these limitations, the value of this approach is substantial. Underlying programs to structure community organizations are fundamental assumptions about the virtues of formalized and centralized systems which should be tested. In many cases network analytic techniques can evaluate these assumptions.

Attempts to improve coordination and integration of community services have relied generally on methods that have not recognized the interconnected nature of all providers, planners, and funders, etc. Needs assessments, case management strategies, and core services plans are based on creating dyadic or organization–set relationships rather than true network patterns. Therefore, these types of procedures are limited in the type of information they can provide. For instance, the network analysis reported here indicates the existence of separate mental health and social service subnetworks that are not well integrated. The barriers to more complete integration are recognizable in the network analysis but may not be with other forms of analysis.

Cracks in the system have not been analytically distinguished before. Yet for the mental health programmer these distinctions may be important in developing planning strategies. Van de Ven and Ferry (1980) suggested that systematic interorganizational relations are promoted by awareness on the part of agency directors of other agency programs and also by inducements (financial, in particular) for them to commit some of their organizational resources to reaching system-wide goals. The correction of Type 1 cracks may follow from efforts to promote such awareness and to supply inducements. Type 2 cracks may be related, among other ways, to questions about which organizations have legal responsibility for which clients. For example, in New York State, clients in the mental retardation and developmental disabilities (MRDD) service sector face statutory and regulatory barriers in seeking access to mental health services not provided within MR/DD authorized agencies. Problems of conflict, Type 3 cracks, may alert planners to the danger of mandating relationships. The problems of maintaining a network may be as great as those related to its creation (Van de Ven, 1976).

Interorganizational theory has discovered fertile ground in the study of community mental health networks. In the process it is beginning to clarify the heretofore elusive meaning of integration and coordination. At the same time the use of network analytic techniques is beginning to demonstrate its usefulness for locating sources of malintegration and disorganization. Although the approach of this paper was illustrative, it is also indicative of the value of employing a network approach to the study of this crucial problem.

ACKNOWLEDGEMENTS

This research was partially supported by a grant from the NIMH Community Support Program, Contract #278-78-007. The author would like to thank Dr. Ernest J. Townsend for making the data available and Dr. David Bass for helpful comments on an earlier draft.

REFERENCES

Agranoff, R., & Pattakos, A. (1979). Dimensions of services integration: Service delivery, program linkages, policy management, organizational structure, *Human Service Monograph Series 13, Project Share*. Washington, DC: U.S. Government Printing Office.

Alba, R. D. (1982). Taking stock of network analysis: A decade's results. In S. B. Bacharach (Ed.), *Research in the sociology of organizations* (Vol. 1, pp. 39–74). Greenwich, CT: JAI Press.

Alba, R. D., & Gutmann, M. P. (1972, May). SOCK: A sociometric analysis system. *Behavioral Science, 17*, 326.

Baker, F., & O'Brien, G. (1971). Intersystems relations and coordination of human service organizations. *American Journal of Public Health, 61*, 130–137.

Burt, R. S. (1983). Cohesion versus structural equivalence as a basis for network subgroups, In R. S. Burt, & M. J. Minor (Eds.), *Applied network analysis*. Beverly Hills: Sage.

Burt, R. S. (1980). Models of network structure. *Annual Review of Sociology, 6*, 79–141.

Burt, R. S. (1977b). *STRUCTURE: A computer program providing basic data for the analysis of empirical positions in a system of actors*. Berkeley: University of California, Berkeley Survey Research Center.

Burt, R. S. (1977a). Positions in multiple network systems, part one: A general conception of stratification and prestige in a system of actors case as a social typology. *Social Forces, 56*, 106–131.

Cumming, J. (1974). Elements of a comprehensive psychiatric service. *Psychiatric Quarterly, 48*, 473–482.

Greenley, J., & Kirk, S. (1973). Organizational characteristics of agencies and the distribution of services to applicants. *Journal of Health and Social Behavior, 14*, 70–79.

Hall, R. H., Clark, J. P., Giordano, P., Johnson, P., & Van Rockel, M. (1977). Patterns of interorganizational relationships. *Administrative Science Quarterly, 22*, 457–474.

Johnson, S. C. (1967). Hierarchical clustering schemes. *Psychometrika, 32*, 241–154.

Knoke, D., & Kuklinski, J. H. (1982). *Network analysis*. Beverly Hills: Sage.

Landau, M. (1969). Redundancy, rationality, and the problem of duplication and overlap. *Public Administration Review, 29*, 346–358.

Laumann, E. O., Galaskiewicz, J., & Marsden, P. V. (1978). Community structure as interorganizational linkages. *Annual Review of Scoiology, 4*, 455–484.

Leopold, E. A., & Schein, L. (1975). Missing links in the human service non-system. *Medical Care, 13*, 595–606.

Levine, S. (1974). Organizational and professional barriers to interagency planning. In H. Demone & D. Harshbarger (Eds.), *A handbook of human service organizations*. New York: Behavioral Publications.

Litwak, E., & Hylton, L. (1962, March). Interorganizational analysis: A hypothesis on coordinating agencies. *Administrative Science Quarterly, 5*, 583–610.

Litwak, E., & Rothman, J. (1970). Towards the theory and practice of coordination between formal organizations, In W. Rosengren & M. Lefton (Eds.), *Organization and clients*. Columbus, OH: Charles Merrill.

Morrissey, J. P., Hall, R. H., & Lindsey, M. L. (1982). *Interorganizational relations: A sourcebook of measures for mental health programs*. Washington DC: U.S. Department of Health and Human Services.

Sauber, S. R. (1977). The human services delivery system. *International Journal of Mental Health, 5*, 121–140.

Sondquist, J. A. (1980). Concepts and tactics in analyzing social network data. *Connections, 3*, 33–56.

Tausig, M., & Townsend, E. (1982). *Patterns of relations within a group of human service organizations*. Paper presented at the Conference on Organization Theory and Public Policy, State University of New York at Albany.

Tessler, R., & Goldman, H. (1982). *The chronically mentally ill: Assessing community support programs*. Cambridge, MA: Ballinger.

Turner, J., & TenHoor, W. (1978). The NIMH community support programs: Pilot approaches to a needed social reform. *Schizophrenia Bulletin, 4,* 319–408.

Van den Ven, A. H. (1976). A framework for organizational assessment. *Academy of Management Review, 1,* 64–78.

Van de Ven, A. H., & Ferry, D. L. (1980). *Measuring and assessing organizations.* New York: Wiley.

Van de Ven, A. H., Walker, G., & Liston, J. (1979). Coordination patterns within an inter-organizational network. *Human Relations, 32,* 19–36.

Warren, R. (1973). Comprehensive planning and coordination: Some functional aspects. *Social Problems, 20,* 355–364.

Warren, R. L., Rose, S. M., & Bergunder, A. F. (1974). *The structure of urban reform.* Lexingron, MA: Lexington Books.

Wellman, B. (1983). Network analysis: Some basic principles. In R. Collins (Ed.), *Sociological theory 1983.* San Francisco: Jossey-Bass.

Whetten, D. A. (1981). Interoganizational relations: A review of the field. *Journal of Higher Education, 52,* 1–28.

White, H. C. Boorman, S. A., & Breiger, R. L. (1976). Social structure from multiple networks. I. Blockmodels of roles and positions. *American Journal of Sociology, 81,* 730–780.

7

Social Support Processes in Early Childhood Friendship: A Comparative Study of Ecological Congruences in Enacted Support

Thomas A. Rizzo and William A. Corsaro

Examined congruences between children's friendships and classroom social ecologies in three distinct settings, and poses that such congruences or social adaptations are aptly characterized as a process of enacted social support; i.e., an interpersonal transaction involving the reduction or evasion of stress. Data were derived from Corsaro's recent ethnographics of children's friendship and peer culture in a University Preschool (Corsaro, 1985) and Head Start center (Corsaro, 1994), and from Rizzo's (1989) ethnography of friendship development among first-grade children. Despite vast differences across settings, the nature and activities of children's friendships appeared consistently linked with specific organizational features in their life-worlds and in this way may constitute significant interpersonal and individual adaptations to that world. In this view, friendship is best seen not as a static entity, which children appropriate in a consistent fashion, but as a general and malleable concept, which they modify and use in a collaborative fashion to address shared psychosocial concerns. Findings are related to research on the link between perceived and enacted support, and on the interplay between relational and social support processes.

Originally published in the *American Journal of Community Psychology*, *23*(3) (1995): 389–417.

Ecological Research to Promote Social Change: Methodological Advances from Community Psychology, edited by Tracey A. Revenson et al. Kluwer Academic/Plenum Publishers, New York, 2002.

Two significant advancements have occurred in social support research in the past decade. First, prompted by Barrera (1986), Heller and Swindle (1983), Sarason, Shearin, Pierce, and Sarason (1987), and others, researchers are making clearer distinctions between three facets of social support: *social embeddedness* (i.e., the extensivity and density of the social network), *perceived support* (i.e., appraisals of the availability and adequacy of supportive ties), and *enacted* (or *received*) *support* (i.e., the interpersonal transactions in which aid is dispensed). The second advance, spurred by Brown (1979), Coyne and DeLongis (1986), B. Gottlieb (1985, 1988), Hobfoll and Stokes (1988), and Thoits (1982, 1986), among others, is that researchers have an increased interest in the processes of support; that is, the system or series of events leading to the provision of support. The upshot is that investigators are developing methodologies which allow them to study specific facets of support in a time-sensitive fashion in their everyday contexts (cf. Montgomery & Duck, 1991).

One notable exception to this progress has been research on enacted support where the primary methods of measurement are still based on self-report (Barrera, 1986; B. Gottlieb, 1985, 1988). Moreover, since these measures correlate poorly with measures of perceived support and perceived stress, interest in the area appears to be waning: Investigators are increasingly exposing the view that people's *recall* of interactive events constitutes the primary data for their appraisals of social support, and thus that perceived support is the ultimate arbiter in the social support complex (cf. Hobfoll & Stokes, 1988; Leatham & Duck, 1990; Sarason et al., 1991; Wethington & Kessler, 1986). On the other hand, several studies have shown that *behavioral* measures of enacted support produce (Lindner, Sarason, & Sarason, 1988; Sarason & Sarason, 1986) or are positively correlated with (Heller & Lakey, 1985; Lakey & Heller, 1988; Procidano & Heller, 1983) enhanced performance on various laboratory tasks. Lakey and Heller (1988) also reported that these behavioral measures may *not* correlate with perceived stress or perceived support. Such findings suggest not only that enacted support is a viable component in the social support constellation, but that self-report measures may be relatively insensitive to mechanisms of enacted support.

This study is concerned with the processes of enacted support as they occur in young children's everyday interactions with friends. In particular, we were intrigued by Hobfoll's (1985; Hobfoll, Kelso, & Peterson, 1989) thesis of ecological congruences; that is, that the processes of social support are best studied as the fit between a given resource or set of resources and the emotional and task requirements for individuals in specific settings. In this view, stress is derived from the emotional and task requirements facing individuals, and may be evaded or mediated by their psychosocial resources.

Our position is that congruences between individuals' personal relationships and specific features in their ecosystems may represent a dynamic upshot of a broader developmental process of adaptation; and, like all developmental adaptations (G. Gottlieb, 1992), the conservation of these congruences would hinge upon their *functional* benefits—which in the present case are aptly conceptualized as enacted social support. Given this orientation, our aims are (a) to identify how the nature and activities of children's friendships appear linked with specific organizational features in their classroom, and (b) to evaluate whether and how such congruences may constitute significant interpersonal and individual adaptations to that environment.

The study poses two formidable methodological challenges. First is the identification of the emotional and task requirements of a setting. The second challenge is to identify how members' personal relations may have adapted to these requirements, and to depict general patterns in this dynamic process. Our solution was to employ data from three separate ethnographies of young children's peer relations and interaction at school. Rizzo, Corsaro, and Bates (1992) have underscored the links between the principles of ethnographic investigation and social constructionism (cf. Berger & Luckmann, 1966/1967; Gergen, 1985), and shown how such methods enable researchers to address the subjective nature of human experience. Specifically, Rizzo et al. described how central features of the ethnographic method such as attention to field entry, prolonged engagement in the setting, triangulation of information sources, and negative case analysis allow researchers to generate the detailed, historical, and ecologically sensitive chronologies that are necessary for an improved understanding of human action and development (Bronfenbrenner, 1977; Gergen & Morawski, 1980). Thus, each of the three ethnographies in this report involved direct observations of young children in everyday peer activities, provided detailed analyses of the social-ecological conditions surrounding the children's interactions, and included rich descriptions of the verbal, nonverbal, and circumstantial (e.g., prior interactive history) factors that constitute and affect their communication. The fact that we compare ethnographic data from three disparate settings (see below) is crucial to our focus on general processes of enacted support: We are not only able to identify potential linkages between the nature and activities of children's friendships and specific features in their ecosystems within individual settings, but we can identify qualities and patterns that are common *across* settings and thereby devise statements that are increasingly generalizable.

There is one final comment. Given our focus on the *processes* of enacted support vis-à-vis the study of congruences between the nature and activities of children's friendships and specific features in their ecosystems in three disparate settings, direct comparisons of distinct friendship behaviors and characteristics were not possible. As we show below, "friendship" and "friendship behaviors" appeared uniquely constituted by setting. For example, best friend-type relationships were predominant in only one of the three settings studied (i.e., first grade), and thus "conventional" friendship behaviors, such as helping, sharing, loyalty, and so forth, were most pertinent to this group. In the other two settings friendship relations were less exclusive, but there were differences in the nature and use of friendship in peer culture and interaction. On the other hand, meaningful commonalities were identified in the *functions* of friendship across settings. We argue that these functional similarities transcend the idiosyncracies in friendship behaviors and characteristics, and that they appear critical for understanding enacted support in young children's friendships. To highlight these commonalities in the functional processes of friendship, we first depict the social ecology, peer relations and friendship patterns, and apparent ecological congruences in each setting, and then address general theoretical implications of these observations.

METHODS

Ethnographic Contexts and Participants

The data for this report are derived from three separate ethnographies (see Corsaro, 1985, 1994; and Rizzo, 1989, for details not provided below). The first study involved two groups of children ages 3 to 5 years attending preschool at a university child study center in a large metropolitan city in the West. These children were predominately white and from families of upper to middle socioeconomic status (SES). We call this center "University Preschool." The second study involved two classes of 4- and 5-year-olds attending a Head Start program located in a large Midwestern city. These children were predominately African American and from families of lower SES. The third study involved a class of public school first graders (i.e., children ages 6 to 7 years) in a small university city in the Midwest. Most of the children were white and from families of working to middle SES (the school did *not* in general serve the university community).

Data Collection and Analysis

Corsaro conducted the investigations at University Preschool (Corsaro, 1985) and at Head Start (Corsaro, 1994), Rizzo conducted the study of first-grade children (Rizzo, 1989). Field entry and data collection were accomplished in similar fashion in all three studies. Both investigators were participant observers throughout the studies and utilized a "reactive" mode of field entry (cf. Corsaro, 1985). That is, we began the studies as "interested observers" allowing the children to react to us, define us, and gradually draw us into their activities. As the study progressed we increasingly adopted the role of a "peripheral participant." That is, we entered the ecological area, moved when necessary, responded when addressed, and occasionally offered verbal contributions when they seemed appropriate. We did not, however, attempt to initiate or terminate an episode, repair disrupted activity, settle disputes, or coordinate or direct activity. In short, we tried to become a part of the activity without affecting the nature or flow of peer episodes.

Corsaro's (1985) definition of an interactive episode was employed as the sampling unit in all three studies. Interactive episodes are those sequences of behavior that begin with the acknowledged presence of two or more interactants in an ecological area and the overt attempt(s) to arrive at a shared meaning of ongoing or emerging activity. Episodes end with physical movement of interactants from the area which results in the termination of the originally initiated activity. Similarly, participant observation followed the same general routine. During or shortly after an interactive episode, investigators wrote a general description of its contents in the form of a running record. In addition to the running record, Rizzo audiotaped virtually all interactions and Corsaro videotaped selected interactions. At the end of the school day, investigators reviewed the running record and audio or videotape for each interactive episode and devised a field note which consisted of the running record, all background material and details not included in the running record, and various notes of theoretical, methodological, and personal significance. Each field note was then cataloged so that investigators would have ready access to complete and accurate chronologies. Last, the priorities for subsequent data collection were determined (see below).

In all three studies sampling decisions were both representative and theoretical. Since it is impossible to record all interaction in a given setting, ethnographers often attempt to insure representativeness by collecting data across several dimensions, including people, places, time, and activities (cf. Denzin, 1977; Schatzman & Strauss, 1973). As is customary in such studies, each investigator drew up an initial inventory of the range and number of elements in each of the dimensions in the early phase of the study, and then modified this inventory as needed at various points in data collection. Second, each investigator routinely presented samples of their field notes to the schoolteachers, and asked for their perceptions regarding the representativeness of the data as typical or significant phenomena in school.

In addition to representativeness, sampling procedures in ethnographic research should have theoretical relevance. Data collection and data analysis are conducted reiteratively: As hypotheses arise through analysis, new procedures are devised and the appropriate data collected. In this way newly collected data extend emerging theoretical formulations by filling in gaps, posing additional issues, and so forth. One result of this process is that the same labels or constructs (i.e., "friendship," "social ecology," "enacted support," and "ecological congruence") refer to different-looking phenomena in different settings. With regard to friendship and social ecology, we have—to the best of our abilities—reflected the predominant concepts and concerns of the research participants. In these cases we worked to generate increasingly accurate interpretations (hypotheses) via the logic and procedures of abductory induction and indefinite triangulation (see below; but also see Rizzo et al., 1992). With regard to enacted support and ecological congruence, we worked deductively from a priori theoretical postulates in ecological psychology and social support. In these cases, we sought to apply extant theoretical constructs in three disparate settings. Both of these measurements processes (i.e., inductive and deductive categorization, respectively) and phenomena (i.e., phenotypic heterogeneity and situationally defined entities, respectively) are integral to all empirical sciences (cf. Duncan, 1984; Polkinghorne, 1983), and they are comparable to the objectives of familiar procedures, such as construct validation and exploratory and confirmatory factor analyses.

Although participant observation and audio- or videotaping were the primary methods of data collection, parent and schoolteacher interviews were also used in the three studies. The principal aims in these interviews were to obtain background and other information on the children (parental concerns, the children's reported concerns at school, the children's playmates and play characteristics at home and in the neighborhood, etc.) which would serve multiple interpretive functions, including broadening the context from which our interpretations were generated, clarifying apparent inconsistencies and idiosyncrasies, triangulating emerging hypotheses, and estimating our obtrusiveness in the setting.

Validity Issues in Data Collection, Analysis, and Interpretation in Interpretive Research

The process, techniques, and evaluative criteria of interpretive research have been described more fully elsewhere (Rizzo et al., 1992; see also Gaskins, Miller, & Corsaro, 1992; Mischler, 1990). The basic objectives, however, are to produce accurate interpretations of the participants' actions, and to generate formal, generalizable hypotheses from these interpretations.

Both of these objectives are accomplished via the general logic and procedures of *abductory induction* (C. Pierce's 1940 study was cited in Buchler, 1955) and *indefinite triangulation* (Cicourel, 1974; Denzin, 1977). In abductory induction, researchers use their total knowledge of the culture and of the interactive history of specific participants to generate several viable interpretations of their behavior. These interpretations are then evaluated and/or elaborated by posing auxiliary hypotheses and collecting additional data. In indefinite triangulation, the final "evidence" of the abductory induction is itself subjected to this same sort of analysis: the new data extending the emerging theoretical formulation or prompting a reformulation. Through this continuous process of eliminating or elaborating all viable interpretations, scientists arrive at a final, most accurate interpretation and simultaneously embed this interpretation in a dense network of corroborative evidence. Interpretations become increasingly accurate and convincing because of the number and scope of alternative interpretations and substantive issues considered, and because of the insight, creativity, and thoroughness exhibited by the investigators as they pursued these various objectives.

Although important differences exist between quantitative and interpretive research, the methodologies are similar in the ultimate evaluations of the validity and generalizability of findings. Regardless of methodology, validity must be evaluated vis-à-vis existing knowledge: with the understanding that "existing knowledge" is dynamic, as discussed by Toulmin (1972) and Polanyi (1962), among others. According to these philosophers, a study's validity is to be judged on the basis of the scientist's insight, rigor, and integrity during the investigation, on a consideration of the consistency of findings within and across studies, and ultimately in the light of future studies. With regard to the present report, we have published detailed accounts of the research process for two of the three studies herein (cf. Corsaro, 1985, chapter 1; and Rizzo, 1989, chapter 2); the Head Start data are new (but see Corsaro, 1994). We have also used these same datasets for articles on related topics, including disputes among peers and friends (Corsaro & Rizzo, 1990; Rizzo, 1992), friendship development (Rizzo, 1989), peer culture (Corsaro, 1985), childhood socialization (Corsaro, 1992; Corsaro & Rizzo, 1988), and the development of social concepts (Rizzo & Corsaro, 1988). The depth and breadth of these topics speak to the efficacy of our "indefinite triangulation" and captures the nature of generalizability in interpretive research. The fact that our findings in these diverse areas are readily integrated with the extant literatures also speaks to the validity of our observations. Finally, we emphasize that the current manuscript involves three studies conducted in quite diverse settings. This diversity in settings bolsters the potential validity and generalizability of our findings: The phenomenon of ecological congruences between the nature and activities of the children's friendships and predominant social-ecological features in their classrooms is likely to be quite robust. Whether the functional significance of these congruences is accurately or fully characterized by the concept of "enacted support" appears worthy of further consideration.

ANALYSIS AND DISCUSSION

University Preschool

The Social Ecology at University Preschool

The principal educational objective of the teachers at the University Preschool was to foster the children's cognitive and social development through informal learning experiences. Simply put, the teachers provided the children with a wide variety of educative materials, encouraged them to explore these materials, and then supported and enriched their experiences through teacher–child interaction. Thus, for a good deal of the school day the children were free to choose their playmates and activities. A second notable feature of the social ecology at University Preschool was a general concern for the needs, rights, and feelings of others. This concern was manifested in the teachers' discourse styles with the children as well as in their strategies for intervening in the children's free play activities. For example, the teachers regularly entered the children's peer activities to settle disputes, to enforce school rules, and to build on the significance of the ongoing play. Overall, these interventions displayed a pattern of adult–child culture contact in which children are encouraged to reflect upon the social significance of their everyday activities. Through a series of often leading questions the teachers encourage the children to articulate the general values of sharing and individual rights with situational features of the particular interactive event (Corsaro & Schwarz, 1991).

In relation to these socioecological characteristics, the children demonstrated two major, interrelated concerns: *social participation* (i.e., that the children rarely engaged in solitary play and when children found themselves alone they consistently attempted to gain entry into one of the ongoing peer episodes), and the *protection of interactive space* (i.e., the tendency for children involved in an ongoing play episode to resist the access attempts of other children). To better understand these concerns, Corsaro looked at the nature of children's peer play in the nursery school. He found that the vast majority of peer play episodes were of relatively short duration (approximately 84% of the episodes he recorded were less than 10 minutes long) and that termination was typically abrupt. In short, peer interaction was fragile in that termination could occur without warning at any time, and the predominate mode of leave-taking (simple movement from the play area) most often precluded any possible negotiation to continue the activity. Therefore, the children often found themselves with playmates one minute and alone the next. Upon finding themselves alone children could choose from a range of options that included solitary play, entry into a teacher-directed activity, or attempt to gain access to an ongoing peer episode. In such circumstances the children most often attempted to gain access to peer play, but when they did they frequently encountered resistance.

In response to such resistance, the children developed a wide variety of access strategies. The most successful strategies were nonverbal entry (i.e., entering a play area without verbal marking and observing what was happening), and producing a variant of ongoing behavior. Although initial access attempts were frequently ignored or resisted, if children persisted and employed a sequence of strategies, group entry was more likely (over 75% successful).

Peer Relations and Friendship at University Preschool

Corsaro analyzed both the nature of the children's social contacts and their use of the concept of friendship (i.e., their spontaneous references to friendship). Specifically he performed a microsociolinguistic analysis of 129 videotaped episodes of the children's peer play. Regarding the structure of their social contacts, it was found that the vast majority of the children (19 of 23 in one group, 22 of 25 in the other) did not form stable and exclusive relationships, but instead played with several (4 to 7) peers on a regular basis. Given the social ecology and peer culture at University Preschool (i.e., the fragility of peer interaction, the multiple possibilities for disruption of peer play, and the difficulty of gaining access to play groups), we suggest that the children may have developed stable relations with several playmates as a way to maximize the probability of gaining access and maintaining established and shared activities.

Regarding the use of the concept "friend," it was found that the children spontaneously referred to friendship (a) to gain access to ongoing play; (b) to protect shared activities from intruders; and (c) to build solidarity and mutual trust in the play group during ongoing activities (see Corsaro, 1985, chapter 4 for examples). In addition, in about 8% of their spontaneous references to friendship, the children attempted to use friendship as a means of social control, most especially during disputes regarding the nature of play. These disputes consisted of complaints about the way an act is carried out, imperatives to stop inappropriate behavior, or disagreements about the extension of the play frame (see Corsaro & Rizzo, 1990). In such instances the children invoked friendship in an effort to get their way. Consider the following example from field notes.

> Jenny and Betty are seated at a worktable with several other children drawing pictures.
> Jenny tells Betty that she is copying her picture. Betty says: "I am not!" which leads Jenny to claim: "Yes you are, you always copy me." Betty then replies, "I do not and if you keep saying that, then I don't like you any more and you're not my friend." "OK," says Jenny, "I won't say it any more."

What was most interesting about this and similar cases was the effectiveness of the "denial of friendship" strategy. The children took such threats very seriously; often giving in immediately or becoming upset and going to a teacher for comfort. The use of the strategy was, however, somewhat of a double-edged sword. Children on the receiving end in one instance could quickly turn things around and issue similar threats of their own in the next. Consider the following example from a videotaped episode.

> Peter tries to get Graham to move over next to him while they are playing with other children around a sandbox.
> Peter: Graham—if you play over here where I am, I'll be your friend.
> Graham: I wanna play over here.
> Peter: Then I'm not gonna be your friend.
> Graham: I'm not—I'm not gonna let—I'm gonna tell my Mom to not let you—
> Peter: All right, I'll come over there.

In sum, friendship at University Preschool is quite different from that commonly associated with older children and adults (cf. Selman, 1981; Youniss & Smoller, 1985). These friendships were not particularly stable, nor were they based on enduring personal characteristics. Rather, for the children at University Preschool, friendship served specific integrative functions such as gaining access to, building solidarity and mutual trust in, and protecting the interactive space of play groups. In addition, the children sometimes used the denial of friendship as a strategy to regulate or alter ongoing play.

Discussion

We see at least two important congruences between prominent patterns in the children's peer relations and interactions and specific organizational features (including the teachers' educational philosophy and discourse styles) of the school and peer culture. First, developing stable relations with several playmates (as opposed to one or two "best friends") appears to mediate well between the children's desire for social participation, their transitory interests in play activities, and the tendency for children in ongoing play to protect their interactive space from intruders because it afforded them a wider range of potential play groups. Second, the children used the concept of friendship in an effort to deal with *practical* problems encountered in being a member of and participating in a peer culture. Most of the time they used friendship to inject desired properties (e.g., stability, reciprocity, acceptance, trust) into their interactions with peers or to protect their interactive space. At other times, friendship—or the denial of friendship—proved to be an effective means of social control.

Whether such congruences constitute a form of enacted support is of course a more subjective judgment. We think the two major, interrelated concerns of social participation and protection of interactive space represent key emotional and task demands for the children in University Preschool, and that these demands helped spur the development of numerous access and resistance strategies (cf. Corsaro, 1985). The fact that friendship was frequently invoked in these efforts not only suggests that the children viewed friendship as a psychosocial resource but it also speaks to the adaptive efficacy or positive reinforcement value of such efforts.

Head Start

The Social Ecology at Head Start

The Head Start center is best described as a small community that emphasizes collective values and provides something approaching an "extended family" for the children. In a normal day at the center the children come into contact with a wide range of adults: teachers and teaching assistants in the nine classrooms, bus drivers, administrative staff, social workers and speech therapists, custodians, and cooks. Although the children spend the overwhelming majority of their time at the center with the teacher and assistant in their particular classrooms, they know all the adults' last names and frequently exchange greetings and playful talk with them everyday. These adults also knew all of the children and would call out to them by name when they entered classrooms or passed them in the hallways. Overall the social relations between adults and children at the center were very similar to the type of highly communal and verbal public life described by Heath (1983, 1989) in her work in a working-class African American community in North Carolina.

The school day at Head Start was short compared to the University Preschool. The children were at the center around 3.5 hours (in morning or afternoon sessions) Mondays through Thursdays. The teachers and children spent a majority of this time in required activities in line with the Head Start curriculum. These activities included having a snack and a full lunch, engaging in formal exercises to enhance language, reading, and cognitive skills, and reading stories or having discussions in line with weekly themes during circle time. The children also made two to three group trips to lavatories (which were located outside the classroom) each day. Finally, each class (either alone or with others) made frequent field trips into the community over the course of the school term (e.g., visits to the children's museum, airport, post office, zoo, and a local department store to see seasonal exhibits). As a result of these more structured activities the children had a relatively limited amount of time for free play (about 1 hour each school day) in one of the activity centers in the classroom, gym, or outside playground.

The Head Start teachers interactive and language styles with the children sought to encourage the development of self-esteem through individual contributions to and support of the group. The teachers discourse styles included a number of direct and indirect methods of social control, good-natured teasing and challenging, and displays of affection. The teachers were hesitant about intervening in children's activities during free play and seldom reacted positively to children's complaints about the behavior of their peers during free play. Instead, the teachers would often send children back to settle disputes on their own. When particular groups of children became overly disruptive or noisy during free play, the teachers often responded with reprimands expressed in the form of rhetorical questions or declarative sentences ("Who's making all that noise over there?," "You boys better not be fighting," "Is that Steven I hear crying?"). Since these indirect strategies were usually successful, the teachers rarely had to physically enter the children's play space to intervene (Corsaro, 1994).

Peer Relations and Friendship at Head Start

We do not have space to describe adequately the rich peer culture of the Head Start children. Instead, we note that the vast majority of these children (17 of 19 in one group, 16 of 16 in the other), like those in University Preschool, formed stable relations with several peers (vs. exclusive "best friend" relations). In addition, we focus on a particular and unique aspect of the Head Start children's language styles—that is, oppositional or competitive talk—which was closely related to friendship processes in the peer culture. Like the somewhat older inner-city African American children studied by Goodwin (1990; also see Goodwin & Goodwin (1987);

Mitchell-Kernan & Kernan, 1977), the Head Start children constructed social identities, cultivated and refined friendships, and both maintained and transformed the social order of the peer culture through opposition and confrontation.

Peer interaction and play routines were peppered with oppositional talk like: "Why you following me like that for?," "What you think you're doing boy?" and "Get that block out the way!" On most occasions such talk was not taken as insulting, and was accepted as part of the verbal enrichment of everyday play routines. Consider the following exchange that took place while two girls were playing in the sandbox.

> Pam: Hey, girl don't use that little ol' thing [scoop], use this big one.
> Brenda: [Takes the bigger scoop] OK.
> Brenda: What's a matter with you girl, that's too much sugar in that cake!
> Pam: No it ain't.
> Brenda: I said it is, girl.

In addition to producing this stylized oppositional talk in brief exchanges, the Head Start children also engaged in more extended debates. Although the source of the extensive debates was often related to competitive relations among the participants, the debates themselves revealed much about the children's knowledge of the world and also served as arenas for displaying self and building group solidarity. Consider the following example.

> Several children are seated at a table eating lunch: Roger, Jerome, Darren, Andre, Laura, Ryan, Alysha, and Diana. The researcher, Bill, is also seated at the table. A teacher sits nearby at a serving table and addresses the children from time to time. Roger and Jerome are talking about a television program called "Hard Copy" when the following sequence occurs.
>
> 1 Roger (to Jerome): I saw somebody on Hard Copy who had a bullet through the back of his head.
> 2 Jerome: I'm getting—I'm getting Hard Copy in the back of my head.
> 3 Roger: You can't get that word in the back of your head.
> 4 Jerome: OK, (inaudible) in the back of my head.
> 5 Roger: Can't get that word either.
> 6 Jerome: Yea I can.
> 7 Roger: Nah-uh (inaudible).
> 8 Jerome: (inaudible).
> 9 Roger: (inaudible).
>   [Apparently Jerome has claimed he saw another program (not Hard Copy) in line 8 that we have been unable to transcribe due to background noise.]
> 10 Jerome: It comes on every night.

11   Roger: We watch that channel and it don't come on our T.V. We got
      eight channels. And we got that channel, but when we watch that
      channel that don't even come on ... What channel it come on?
12   Jerome: H.B.O.
13   Roger: We watch H.B.O.
14   Jerome: It comes on cable.
15   Roger: We have cable.
16   Laura: We got cable too, for real.
17   Ryan: We do too.
18   Darren: We do too.
19   Jerome (to Darren): //Don't (inaudible) Darren.
20   Roger: //I got the biggest cable. I got the biggest cable.
21   Jerome: I got the little—[holding his hands close together].
22   Teacher: I thought all cable was the same.
23   Bill: [Laughs] So did I.
24   Jerome: (They ain't either.) My cable's this big [holds one hand under
      the table and the other above his head].
25   Laura: Nah-Uh.
26   Roger: My cable's 'bout this big. [holds hands about a foot apart]
27   Alysha: //(Jesus is) bigger than everybody.//
28   Darren: //My—My cable's like this //big [holds one hand about two
      feet above the table. [Ryan also holds one hand up way above the
      table, but he does not say anything]
29   Laura: Marvin's head is bigger (than anybody's) [Marvin is a child at
      the other table].
30   Jerome (to Alysha): I'm bigger than (Jesus).
31   Alysha: Nah uh. //Jesus// is bigger than everybody.
32   Teacher: //Y'all got to stop.//
33   Jerome (to Alysha): My cousin's bigger than Jesus. //My cousin's big-
      ger than Jesus. My cousin's is that big [again holds hands very far
      apart.] Yeah.//

38   Alysha (to Jerome): But he don't do—this. [reaches as far up as she
      can]. He's this big.
39   Jerome: My cousin's this //big [reaches up].
40   Teacher: //Alysha, //get through so you can drink your milk today.
41   Andre: He's this big. [holds hand far above table]
42   Jerome (to Andre): Who? Who?
43   Andre: Jesus.
44   Jerome: I'm this big—I'm this big [indicates very small]. (inaudible)
      I'm this little [holds his hands to the sides of his head and then brings
      them forward showing how little he is].

This sequence is representative of the types of competitive peer talk
that occur routinely at the Head Start center. At various times the debate
involved several children and, as the participants pursued different individual

agendas, a range of topics (e.g., specific television shows, cable systems, religious beliefs). Most important, however, are that (a) participation in such competitive talk provided the children the opportunity to display their knowledge about the world, build a general peer group identity, and fashion friendship alliances; and (b) friendship was *not* used as a divisive strategy, *rather* friendship alliances were generally maintained within the peer group and often served as catalysts for group activities (see Goodwin, 1990, for similar observations among groups of preadolescent African American boys and girls). In this case, Roger and Jerome have a history of trying to outdo one another in their displays of knowledge of media events including television and movies. In many ways their shared knowledge of the media, desire to display that knowledge, and enjoyment of competitive talk was the main basis of their friendship. Similarly, we know from interviews with the teachers and Alysha's mother that Alysha often attends church services with her mother and grandmother. Thus, as the debate evolved into competitive talk about size, Alysha drew upon this knowledge to assert that "Jesus is bigger than everybody" (line 27). In doing so Alysha not only entered into the valued activity of competitive talk in peer culture, but her contribution extended the debate by engaging new material (i.e., religious beliefs; lines 30–44) and participants (i.e., Andre; lines 41 and 43). Moreover, in this case the group's identity may have been underscored not only by their collective production of a valued cultural activity but by their shared cultural and religious values, as Andre and then Jerome (line 44) resonate to Alysha's statements about Jesus.

Discussion

Overall, the children's friendship relations appear to reflect a number of interrelated aspects of their lives and the Head Start program's curriculum and staff. First, there is the challenging circumstances of the children's families, neighborhoods and communities. The teachers were aware of the dangers and challenges associated with raising children in poverty, and they encouraged them to be both independent (especially in peer relations where they were expected to stick up for themselves) and respectful of others (most especially adult caretakers). Second, the limited amount of time the children spent in the program (due to an inadequate level of funding) and the specific educational requirements associated with the compensatory objective of Head Start restricted the children's opportunities for unstructured peer play. Finally, there was a clear demarcation of adults and children in the Head Start center. The children had both rights and obligations, but the teachers were clearly in charge. Overall, the teachers' discourse style encouraged the children to be responsible, active, and assertive members of their particular classes and the Head Start community more generally.

In relation to these factors it appears that the children relied on an oppositional style in friendship relations that has been observed in several studies of peer interaction among inner-city African American children (cf. Goodwin, 1990; Labov, 1972; Mitchell-Kernan & Kernan, 1977). However, the children Corsaro observed clearly refined and expanded the style in the Head Start program. While they were concerned about establishing friendships and often referred to each other as friends, they seldom used the verbal denial of friendship as a strategy to control the behavior of their peers. Rather friends were expected *both to compete and to support each other* in the peer culture of the Head Start center.

The children's valuing of competitive but supportive relations is in line with much work on African American language and communicative styles (Abrahams, 1970, 1975; Goodwin, 1990; Ogbu, 1988). For example, the folklorist Roger Abrahams (1975) has argued that among African Americans, opposition and conflict "tend to be viewed as constant contrarieties, antagonism that cannot be eliminated and in fact may be used to effect a larger sense of cultural affirmation of community through a dramatization of opposing forces (p. 63)." As we saw in the earlier examples, oppositions among the Head Start children were often reacted to in kind, and the overall tenor of exchanges was playful banter. As Corsaro (1994, p. 22) has argued in earlier work, this verbal dueling sends two messages: (a) that a particular child could hold his or her own and not be easily intimidated, and (b) that participation in oppositional talk signified allegiance to the values and concerns of the peer culture.

Children seldom escalated oppositional talk to the level of physical aggression or ran to the teachers to complain. In fact, skilled and clever oppositions or retorts were often indicated as such with appreciative laughter and comments, like "Good one" or "You sure got him good" by the audience, and at times even the target child. Ultimately what emerged among the Head Start children were assertive and competitive friendship relations that led to mutual respect and group solidarity.

How might such congruences effect enacted support? We assert that the Head Start mission of fostering individual competencies and self-esteem while cultivating mutual respect and a group identity constitute prominent emotional and task demands for the children at Head Start. The children also appeared challenged by the confrontational and competitive nature of the social discourse, even as they participated in and collectively produced such talk themselves. In this context, developing stable relations with several playmates and maintaining these alliances *within* the peer group appeared to pose a synergy between group affiliation, identity, and support on one hand; and individual and relational interests, competencies, and concerns on the other.

First Grade

The Social Ecology of First Grade

As is typical of first-grade classrooms, the teacher's primary educational objective was to develop each child's abilities in a broad range of school subjects; the school day was highly structured and segmented by subject; there was an overarching emphasis on schoolwork; and peer play was limited to two or three 15- to 20-minute recess periods per day. In addition, the transitions from classroom activities to recess were abrupt and required the children to organize their play–participants and activities—quickly, because they would soon have to stop playing and return to classroom work.

In relation to these social-ecological characteristics, the children demonstrated two principal concerns: social participation (i.e., to interact with others) and schoolwork. To wit, they invested considerable time and energy establishing and maintaining peer contact, and separation from peers via time-out procedures, revoking recess privileges, and so forth, were loathed punishments. The children's genuine interest in school activities was evident in their myriad reconstructions of school-like scenarios during free time, and in their frequent demonstrations and proclamations of their abilities to peers, teachers, and the researcher.

In addition to these primary concerns, the children became increasingly interested in establishing enduring friendships with specific classmates as the year progressed. Rizzo noted a general trend toward selecting classmates as playmates during recess, and that the majority of children (17 of 19) established a reasonably stable (longer than 1 week) friendship with a classmate in the first 5 months of the school year (see below). Most important for the present purposes is how the social ecology may have influenced the children's friendships. First, the social ecology appears to abet the first graders' *concern for friendship* in three ways: (a) For most children, playmates from previous classes and from the neighborhood were not in their current class. Thus, the early part of the school year involved the disruption of these previous relationships and a concern for establishing new relationships. (b) Given the severe time constraints on recess, previously established play patterns were not feasible and the children needed to redirect this desire toward more plausible alternatives (i.e., peer relations and schoolwork. (c) Schoolwork was a new and inescapable concern for the children: Finding someone to help with this work and sharing one's accomplishments with peers undoubtedly eased some of the tensions associated with these newly encountered demands.

The social ecology also appeared to influence *which children became friends*. Not only did 17 of the 19 children establish a reasonably stable friendship with a classmate (see below), but 50% (10 of 20) of these relationships involved children in the same reading-ability group, and 46% (i.e., 6 of the 13 relationships with sufficient data on their initial interactions) involved children whose school desks were adjacent in the initial stages of their friendship.[1] The principal factors behind this effect appeared to be (a) the children whom one could interact with in a relatively consistent manner were determined by the class roster, and within classes by desk proximity and ability group; (b) a major function and benefit of having friends in school was that they could facilitate schoolwork: Children who were in the same classroom and ability group were in the best position to provide this help because they were doing the same work themselves; and (c) one way the children built solidarity in their friendships was by highlighting similar attributes: Peers in the same class and ability group were perceived by the children to be more similar than peers in different classes and ability groups.

Finally, the social ecology influenced the *activities of friendship*; that is, what the children did with their friends. Schoolwork was an important concern for the children, and friends addressed this concern by making helping, sharing, and work-related ego reinforcement three of the more frequent displays of friendship in school. Certainly, the frequency of these activities reflects the fact that the children spent most of their school day doing schoolwork. More important, however, is that these findings illustrate that friends and friendship in first-grade were responsive to these social-ecological demands. These children were not simply looking to play with their friends, rather, they understood that friendship was vital to other concerns and pursuits as well.

Peer Relations and Friendship in First Grade

Perhaps the most important aspect of the first-grade children's experiences with friendship was that they worked, with some success, at establishing enduring friendships. Indeed, 34 friendships were observed

---

[1] There were insufficient data on the initial interactions of two friendships because they involved children who were judged by their kindergarten teacher to be friends or frequent playmates in the previous year. A third friendship was not included because it involved neighbors. Finally, four friendships began very early in the study when data collection was focused on more global considerations.

over the 5-month study, all of which involved the *mutual recognition of friendship* (i.e., the written or verbal acknowledgment of friendship by both children), *time together* (i.e., establishing a pattern of interacting with each other whenever the opportunity existed), and *continuity* (i.e., the number of consecutive days in which the children maintained the first two criteria). Of the 34 friendships, 14 lasted less than 1 week, 12 lasted longer than 1 week but less than 1 month, and 8 lasted several months. Since there were 19 children in the class, the 34 observed friendships represent 20% of all possible pairings (34 of 171). All but two children were involved in at least one friendship that endured longer than 1 week.

A second important aspect of first-grade children's experiences with friendship is the complexity of these relations and interactions. Interactions among first-grade friends contained frequent displays of sharing, helping, ego reinforcement, loyalty, similarity, and intimacy. In fact, when the children noticed shortcomings in their friend's behavior, they frequently initiated disputes with their friend in an apparent attempt to induce the necessary changes in his or her behavior. Most important, however, are Rizzo's (1989, 1992) observations that no friendship ended as a result of a dispute, and that disputes about the responsibilities of friendship appeared to be aimed at *improving* the relationship. Consider the following example from field notes.

> Doreen and Mary are working together at a table in the back of the classroom. Sharon walks over to her friend, Doreen.
> 1 Sharon (to Doreen): I have all my work done and I have my calendar done too.
> 2 Doreen: So, my calendar is all done. I was the first one done with my calendar.
> 3 Sharon: So.
> 4 Doreen: Sharon, you always have to say "so." That's all you ever should say.
> 5 Sharon: No I don't. I don't always say so.
> 6 Doreen: Help me I want, I have to find 2 more. Will you help me?
> 7 Sharon: What are they?
> 8 Doreen: I don't know. See, I have 3 more to do.
> 9 Sharon: I'll have—I'll help ya'. I have all my work done.
> 10 Doreen: OK.
> [Doreen and Sharon finish Doreen's work together. Mary leaves]

When interpreting this excerpt it is important to know that the children often looked to each other, and especially to friends, for acknowledgment of their accomplishments (labeled work-related ego reinforcement). Thus, Sharon's comment in line 1 should be interpreted as looking for support and not bragging. When Doreen fails to acknowledge Sharon's work in line

2, however, Sharon is probably offended and retaliates in line 3 by devaluing Doreen's work. Doreen's response in line 4 is effective because it places Sharon's behavior in a larger context. In essence, Doreen is claiming that Sharon's current lack of concern, and thus the cause of the present dispute, is not an isolated instance but is becoming a pattern with Sharon. Such a statement may also reflect Doreen's growing uncertainty about the relationship and thereby constitute a "secret test" (cf. Baxter & Wilmot, 1984) of Sharon's commitment to the relationship (see below). Sharon disagrees with Doreen's assessment in line 5 and is eager to disprove it. By line 6 Doreen feels secure enough to ask Sharon for help and the two girls begin an amiable interaction.

In sum, friendships in first grade were relatively stable and their interactions contained frequent displays of reciprocal helping, sharing, ego reinforcement, loyalty, intimacy, and so forth. The finding that three of these displays involved schoolwork (i.e., helping, sharing, and work-related ego reinforcement) suggests that the children were not simply looking to play with their friends, but understood that friendship was vital to other concerns as well. In addition, the findings that friends in first grade frequently disputed the responsibilities of friendship and that such disputes appeared aimed at improving (vs. terminating) the relationship, suggest that the children understood that friendships require effort and negotiation to maintain and develop. At the same time, however, these disputes highlight the negative or stress-inducing effects of social support vis-à-vis friendship and directly parallel observations by Rook (1984), Braiker and Kelley (1979), and others, concerning such effects in the supportive relationships of adults (see below).

Discussion

As in the two earlier studies, the nature and activities of the children's friendships appears well adapted to the prevailing socioecological conditions. Establishing enduring friendships with specific classmates is an effective strategy for mediating the demands of schoolwork in that friends routinely help, share, and reinforce each other's school performances. Indeed, even friendship composition appears to be influenced by social-ecological factors that favor friendships among classmates with similar abilities. Enduring friendships also appear instrumental in maximizing play during recess in that they help counter the frequent and abrupt transitions from schoolwork to recess, and the severe time limits on recess. Obviously, to the extent that school performance and social participation represent genuine emotional and task demands for the first-grade children, then these myriad instances and processes by which friends helped mediate these demands constitute bona fide examples of enacted support.

GENERAL DISCUSSION

Our aim was to discern some of the processes of enacted support in young children's friendships vis-à-vis the concept of ecological congruences (Hobfoll, 1985; Hobfoll et al., 1989). Central to this objective was the identification of a setting's emotional and task requirements, and of how members' interpersonal relations may have adapted to such requirements. To this end, we examined ethnographic data of young children's peer relations and interactions in three disparate settings: a preschool of predominately white children from families of upper- to middle SES (University Preschool); a preschool of predominantly African American children from families of lower SES (Head Start); and a public school first grade of predominantly white children from families of working to middle SES (First Grade).

In each of these social ecologies we found links between the nature and activities of children's friendships and prevailing features in their life-worlds (Table I). At University Preschool, for example, developing stable relations with several playmates appeared to mediate well between the children's desire for social participation, their transitory interests in play activities, and the tendency for children in ongoing play to protect their interactive space from intruders because it afforded them a wide range of potential playgroups. Similarly, the children used friendship to protect their ongoing play activities by invoking it to both build solidarity among play partners and resist intruders. At Head Start, friendships provided the children with a forum by which to demonstrate and develop their individual competencies and interests while simultaneously affirming their participation and identity in the larger group and culture. This was accomplished by both the children's offering of their individual knowledge and abilities to the group, and by their participation in a shared and symbolic cultural activity (i.e., oppositional talk). Finally, in first grade establishing enduring friendships with specific classmates appeared to mediate well between the children's (a) desire for social participation and the restrictive conditions of their free play, and (b) their need to produce increasingly individualized work assignments (via ability groups) and specific children's opportunity and capabilities to help with and appreciate this work.

Regardless of these apparent differences, in all of the settings friendship appeared to serve certain integrative functions for the children and in this way may constitute significant interpersonal and individual adaptations to their world. In this view friendship is not a static entity that children

Table I. Ecological Congruences in Three Disparate Settings

Classroom	Emotional/task demands	Children's concerns	Nature of friendships	Functions of friendships
University Preschool	Foster individual competencies and respect for others; ample opportunities for free play but peer activities are fragile and short-lived; teachers readily intervene in peer conflicts	Social participation; protection of interactive space	Multiple partners; friendships detached from peer group	Maximize access to peer play; protect ongoing peer activities
Head Start	Foster individual competencies and group identity; limited opportunities for free play; teachers encourage childen to resolve peer conflicts by themselves	Social acceptance; respect for skilled participation in a peer culture symbolized by oppositional or competitive talk	Multiple partners; friendships maintained within peer group	Friends support and compete with each other; skills in oppositional talk valued in individual friendships and symbolic of shared peer culture
First Grade	Academic achievement and production of schoolwork; limited opportunities for free play with abrupt transitions in and out of play; teacher readily intervenes in peer conflicts	Social participation; school work; enduring friendships	Stable relations with one or two peers; friendships detached from peer group	Facilitate schoolwork; maximize free play

appropriate in a consistent fashion. Rather it is best seen as a general and malleable concept which they modify and use in a collaborative fashion to address shared psychosocial concerns, challenges, and needs. More directly, we assert the theoretical significance of what might otherwise be construed as individual differences in friendship styles: The differences in the nature and activities of friendship which we observed at University Preschool, Head Start, and in first grade were not mere nuances in style but effective adaptations to the prevailing social-ecological demands of each setting.

In line with Hobfoll (1985; Hobfoll et al., 1989), Cutrona (1990), and others, we think the processes by which such ecological congruences are defined and practiced in everyday interaction constitute a primary source of enacted support, and that this is one reason why friendship is an important concern for all children despite the considerable differences in its constitution. Moreover, the present findings may provide insight into the general incongruence between perceived support and enacted support (cf. Wethington & Kessler, 1986). First, the processes by which people's personal relationships adapt to the prevailing social ecology appear to be quite subtle, and thus may not be readily acknowledged during reflection (see Moos & Mitchell, 1982; Pearlin & Schooler, 1979, for similar observations). Second, this incongruence may be further exacerbated in young children due to their immature skills and general disinclination for reflective thought. As a consequence, both adults' and especially young children's reflective appraisals of the availability and adequacy of supportive relationships (perceived support) may not be well grounded in their everyday experiences. In this view, perceived support and enacted support may not only represent distinct entities in the social support constellation but may operate via largely separate mechanisms; that is, perceived support may *not* be the ultimate arbiter of social support, since the processes and effects of enacted support would not necessarily be filtered through perceived support. Further research on both the developmental and social support prospects of this thesis seems warranted.

On a separate issue, our finding that in each setting friendship had negative (or stress-inducing) and positive (or stress-reducing/avoiding) effects is consistent with the current emphasis on viewing social support in a context of personal relationships which are themselves dynamic and multifaceted (Duck, 1990; Schulz & Tompkins, 1990).[2] Several studies have

---

[2] This emphasis on the interplay between social support and personal relationships should be distinguished from the vast literature on the effects of social support on psychological factors such as self-esteem, feelings of dependency, and so forth (see Fisher, Goff, Nadler, & Chinsky, 1988, for a review). While such effects will presumably reverberate in the relationship, they have not been addressed in this literature to date.

described the negative effects of these relationships, as well as the dynamic interplay between relationship development and social support. For instance, from adolescence onward, people do not necessarily perceive their close and supportive relationships as being low in interpersonal conflict (Berndt & Perry, 1986; Braiker & Kelley, 1979; Rook, 1984). Although children may not share this perception (Berndt & Perry, 1986)—no doubt due to their immature capacities for reflection, such conflicts are nonetheless common in their interactions with friends (see above and Shantz, 1987, for a review of relevant studies). Thus, for people of all ages, social support and stress appear inextricably linked.

Other studies have addressed the complex interplay between processes of social support and processes of relationship development. For example, Hobfoll, Nadler, and Lieberman (1986), Reis (1984, 1990), and others have reported a positive correlation between interpersonal intimacy and satisfaction with social support; Clark (1983) and Thoits (1985) have suggested that people may seek support in an effort to foster a closer relationship with the support provider; and Wiseman (1986) has shown that attempts to develop a friendship are sometimes misperceived as requests for support which are inappropriate and exploitative, and thereby lead to the disruption of the relationship. From this perspective Rizzo's (1989, 1992) findings that first-grade friends' disputes over the responsibilities of friendship appeared critical to the development of their relationship not only parallels the reports of interpersonal conflict in the supportive relationships of adults (e.g., Braiker & Kelley, 1979; Rook, 1984), but may explicate some of the causal relations among stress, social support, and personal relationships. These findings suggest that stress is a natural and perhaps necessary consequence of friendship development during childhood. Thus, while their friendships may be originally created and adapted to address extant challenges in the social ecology vis-à-vis enacted support, the maintenance and further development of these relationships engenders new challenges and stress, which in turn alters the social ecology and perhaps the future course of their relationships.

Whether such a scheme holds beyond childhood is an empirical issue; however, several investigators have raised comparable hypotheses with regard to adults (cf. Berger, 1988; Duck, 1988; LaGaipa, 1990). Each of these authors has noted that stress is likely to be engendered by feelings of uncertainty in developing relationships and by common uncertainty-reduction mechanisms. For example, Baxter and Wilmot (1984) identified several indirect "secret test" strategies which people employ to reduce relational uncertainties, including so-called *endurance tests* (i.e., exaggerating one's need to determine the partner's upper limits of commitment), *separation tests* (i.e., introducing physical separation to determine whether the partner's affection will endure), and *triangle tests* (i.e., creating a real or fictitious rival to determine whether the partner will become jealous). While the intent of such tactics may be to allay concerns about the nature of the relationship, they are likely to be stressful for the partner (cf. Mills & Clark, 1986).

We have two final comments which have been prompted by the queries of several colleagues. First, they have wondered whether the observed differences in friendship behaviors and patterns can be ascribed to differences in the social ecologies of the three settings, as opposed to extrasetting factors such as neighborhood, cultural, and socioeconomic differences in participants. Certainly, the classroom ecologies and friendship styles are both reflections of and embedded within the larger contexts of neighborhood and culture: The apparent congruences between the two local concerns may be epiphenomena. As with any observational study, we cannot claim conclusively that stress reduction or evasion actually occurred. Given our prolonged and continuous observation of the children in their natural environments however, we can state that these effects were likely.

A related issue is whether the construct of ecological congruence is usefully extended beyond the local ecology.[3] If classroom processes are viewed as distillates of larger neighborhood and cultural processes (cf. Bronfenbrenner, 1977), then the ramifications of forging such local congruences or "social adaptations" may extend far beyond our parochial concerns for enacted support. In this case, the present studies of congruences between children's friendships and their classroom ecologies may not only delineate a process of enacted social support, but they may illuminate a more general process by which pervasive community factors (i.e., sociocultural practices, demographic variables, social policies) affect children's daily interactions and subsequent development. Obviously, such considerations diverge significantly from Hobfoll's (1985; Hobfoll et al., 1989) original notion of ecological congruence and our particular datasets. Nonetheless, they underscore the generative potential of interpretive research: To address these issues one needs to link microethnographies of the sort presented herein with contemporaneous, interdisciplinary studies of the enveloping communities and governing policies.

The second concern of colleagues involves the process and product of ethnographic/interpretive research. They have argued that this and other interpretive studies do not comport well with the hypothesis-testing basis of contemporary psychological research. To wit, we have not worked to disprove extant theory vis-à-vis refutation of derivative hypotheses, as per

[3] This possibility was suggested by Dr. Trickett.

Popper (1972). Instead, our findings and report are intended as partial *explications* of the theoretical concepts and possibilities of friendship, enacted support, social-ecology, and ecological congruences. Our response is twofold. First, we note that neither quantitative nor interpretive methodology produces certain knowledge: Their contribution and efficacy is derived from the fact that they produce alternative perspectives on a problem (Feyerabend, 1970; Polking-home, 1983). Kuhn (1962/1970) and other historians of science have observed that the advent of a new or alternative perspective has often (but not always) marked the beginning of a rapid accumulation of knowledge and insight. Second, we stress the need for theory generation as well as theory testing in science (Glaser & Strauss, 1967; Reichenbach, 1951). In this regard, we hope that the current expositions of enacted support (a) revitalize interest in a concept that is falling from grace not because of empirical refutation but because of methodological difficulties and systemic neglect; and (b) serve as a caveat to conventional wisdom which is increasingly espousing perceived support as the ultimate arbiter in the social support complex.

CONCLUSION

We stress the efficacy of ethnographic research in developmental and social psychology, as well as the processes of enacted support in young children's friendships. By examining children's lives *in context* we were able not only to identify some the challenges and stressors which affect children on a daily basis but we were allowed to observe their successful adaptations to these conditions and to discern patterns in these adaptations. Such methodological and substantive concerns should be seen as extensions of existing trends in social and community psychology toward more naturalistic and interpretive inquiry (cf. Tolan, Keys, Chertok, & Jason, 1990). In particular, we show how the nature and activities of children's friendships appear linked with predominant socioecological features in their classrooms, and argue that the processes by which such ecological congruences are defined and practiced in everyday interaction constitute a primary influence on the interpersonal transactions in which aid is dispensed.

ACKNOWLEDGMENTS

Dr. Christopher Keys, Dr. Edison Trickett, and two anonymous reviewers are thanked for their comments on an earlier version of this manuscript. Portions of this manuscript were presented at the biennial meetings of the Society for Research in Child Development, Seattle, April 18–20, 1991.

REFERENCES

Abrahams, R. (1970). *Deep down in the jungle: Negro narrative folklore from the streets of Philadelphia*. Chicago: Aldine.

Abrahams, R. (1975). Negotiating respect: Patterns of presentation among Black women. In C. R. Farrer (Ed.), *Women and folklore*. Austin: University of Texas Press.

Barrera, M., Jr. (1986). Distinctions between social support concepts, measures, and models. *American Journal of Community Psychology, 14*, 413–445.

Baxter, L., & Wilmot, W. (1984). Secret tests: Social strategies for acquiring information about the state of the relationship. *Human Communication Research, 11*, 171–201.

Berger, C. (1988). Uncertainty and information exchange in developing relationships. In S. Duck (Ed.), *Handbook of personal relationships*. New York: Wiley.

Berger, P., & Luckmann, T. (1966/1967). *The social construction of reality*. Garden City, NY: Doubleday.

Berndt, T., & Perry, T. B. (1986). Children's perceptions of friendships as supportive relationships. *Developmental Psychology, 22*, 640–648.

Braiker, H., & Kelly, H. (1979). Conflict in the development of close relationships. In R. Burgess & T. Huston (Eds.), *Social exchange in developing relationships*. New York: Academic Press.

Bronfenbrenner, U. (1977). Toward an experimental ecology of human development. *American Psychologist, 32*, 513–532.

Brown, G. (1979). A three-factor causal model of depression. In J. Barrett (Ed.), *Stress and mental disorder*. New York: Raven.

Buchler, J. (Ed.). (1955). *Philosophical writings of Pierce*. New York: Dover.

Cicourel, A. (1974). *Cognitive sociology: Language and meaning in social interaction*. New York: Free Press.

Clark, M. (1983). Some implications of close social bonds for help-seeking. In J. Fisher, A. Nadler, & B. DePaulo (Eds.), *New directions in helping: Vol. 1. Recipients' reaction to aid*. New York: Praeger.

Corsaro, W. (1985). *Friendship and peer culture in the early years*. Norwood, NJ: Ablex.

Corsaro, W. A. (1992). Interpretive reproduction in children's peer cultures. *Social Psychology Quarterly, 55*, 160–177.

Corsaro, W. (1994). Discussion, debate and friendship: peer discourse in nursery schools in the United States and Italy. *Sociology of Education, 67*, 1–26.

Corsaro, W., & Rizzo, T. (1988). *Discussione* and friendship: Socialization processes in the peer culture of Italian nursery school children. *American Sociological Review, 53*, 879–894.

Corsaro, W., & Rizzo, T. (1990). Disputes in the peer culture of American and Italian nursery school children. In A. Grimshaw (Ed.), *Conflict talk*. New York: Cambridge University Press.

Corsaro, W., & Schwarz, K. (1991). Peer play and socialization in two cultures: implications for research and practice. In M. Almy, B. Scales, & S. Ervin-Tripp (Eds.), *Play and the social context of development in early care and education*. New York: Teachers College Press.

Coyne, J., & DeLongis, A. (1986). Going beyond social support: The role of social relationships in adaptation. *Journal of Consulting and Clinical Psychology, 54*, 454–460.

Cutrona, C. (1990). Stress and social support—in search of optimal matching. *Journal of Social and Clinical Psychology, 9*, 3–14.

Denzin, N. (1977). *The research act*. Chicago: Aldine.

Duck, S. (1988). *Relating to others*. Chicago: Dorsey.

Duck, S. (1990). (Ed.). *Personal relationships and social support*. London: Sage.

Duncan, O. D. (1984). *Notes on social measurement: Historical and critical.* New York: Sage.

Feyerabend, P. (1970). How to be a good empiricist—A plea for tolerance in matters episte-mological. In B. Brody (Ed.), *Readings in the philosophy of science.* Englewood Cliffs, NJ: Prentice-Hall.

Fisher, J., Goff, B., Nadler, A., & Chinsky, J. (1988). Social psychological influences on help seeking and support from peers. In B. Gottlieb (Ed.), *Marshalling social support: Formats, processes, and effects.* Newbury Park, CA: Sage.

Gaskins, S., Miller, P. J., & Corsaro, W. A. (1992). Theoretical and methodological perspec-tives in the interpretive study of children. In W. A. Corsaro & P. J. Miller (Eds.), *New directions for child development: Interpretive approaches to children's socialization* (No. 58). San Francisco: Jossey-Bass.

Gergen, K. (1985). The social constructionist movement in modern psychology. *American Psychologist, 40,* 266–275.

Gergen, K., & Morawski, J. (1980). An alternative metatheory for social psychology. In L. Wheeler (Ed.), *Review of personality and social psychology.* San Francisco: Sage.

Glaser, B., & Strauss, A. (1967). *The discovery of grounded theory: Strategies for qualitative research.* New York: Aldine.

Goodwin, M. H. (1990). *He-said-she-said: talk as social organization among Black children.* Bloomington: Indiana University Press.

Goodwin, M. H., & Goodwin, C. (1987). Children's arguing. In S. Phillips, S. Steele, & C. Tanz (Eds.), *Language, gender, and sex in a comparative perspective.* New York: Cambridge University Press.

Gottlieb, B. (1985). Social support and the study of personal relationships. *Journal of Social and Personal Relationships, 2,* 351–375.

Gottlieb, B. (1988). Support interventions: a typology and agenda for research. In S. Duck (Ed.), *Handbook of personal relationships.* New York: Wiley.

Gottlieb, G. (1992). *Individual development and evolution: The genesis of novel behavior.* New York: Oxford University Press.

Heath, S. B. (1983). *Ways with words: Language, life and work in communities and classrooms.* New York: Cambridge University Press.

Heath, S. B. (1989). Oral and literate traditions among black Americans living in poverty. *American Psychologist, 44,* 367–373.

Heller, K., & Lakey, B. (1985). Perceived support and social interaction among friends and confidants. In I. Sarason & B. Sarason (Eds.), *Social support: Theory, research and appli-cations.* Dordrecht, The Netherlands: Martinus Nijhoff.

Heller, K., & Swindle, R., Jr. (1983). Social networks, perceived support, and coping with stress. In R. Felner, L. Jason, N. Moritsugu, & S. Farber (Eds.), *Preventive psychology: theory, research, and practice.* New York: Pergamon.

Hobfoll, S. (1985). Limitations of social support in the stress process. In I. Sarason & B. Sarason (Eds.), *Social support: Theory, research, and applications.* Dordrecht, The Netherlands: Martinus Nijhoff.

Hobfoll, S., Kelso, D., & Peterson, W. (1989). When are support systems, support systems: A study of Skid Row. In S. Einstein (Ed.), *Drugs and alcohol use: Issues and factors.* New York: Plenum Press.

Hobfoll, S., Nadler, A., & Lieberman, J. (1986). Satisfaction with social support during crisis: Intimacy and self-esteem as critical determinants. *Journal of Personality and Social Psychology, 51,* 296–304.

Hobfoll, S., & Stokes, J. (1988). The process and mechanics of social support. In S. Duck (Ed.), *Handbook of personal relationships.* New York: Wiley.

Kuhn, T. (1970). *The structure of scientific revolutions* (2nd ed.). Chicago: University of Chicago Press. (Original work published 1962.)

Labov, W. (1972). *Language in the inner-city: Studies in the Black English vernacular.* Philadelphia: University of Pennsylvania Press.

LaGaipa, J. (1990). The negative effects of informal social support systems. In S. Duck (Ed.), *Personal relationships and social support.* London: Sage.

Lakey, B., & Heller, K. (1988). Social support from a friend, perceived support, and social problem solving. *American Journal of Community Psychology, 16*, 811–824.

Leatham, G., & Duck, S. (1990). Conversations with friends and the dynamics of social support. In S. Duck (Ed.), *Personal relationships and social support.* Newbury Park, CA: Sage.

Lindner, K., Sarason, I., & Sarason, B. (1988). Assessed life stress and experimentally provided social support. In P. Defares (Ed.), *Stress and anxiety* (Vol. 11). Washington, DC: Hemisphere.

Mills, J., & Clark, M. (1986). Communications that should lead to perceived exploitation in communal and exchange relationships. *Journal of Social and Clinical Psychology, 4*, 225–234.

Mischler, E. G. (1990). Validation in inquiry-guided research: The role of exemplars in narrative studies. *Harvard Educational Review, 60*, 415–442.

Mitchell-Kernan, C., & Kernan, K. (1977). Pragmatics of directive choice among children. In S. Ervin-Tripp & C. Mitchell-Kernan (Eds.), *Child discourse.* New York: Academic Press.

Montgomery, B., & Duck, S. (1991). (Eds.), *Studying interpersonal interaction.* New York: Guilford.

Moos, R., & Mitchell, R. (1982). Social network resources and adaptation: A conceptual framework. In T. Wills (Ed.), *Basic processes in helping relationships.* New York: Academic Press.

Obgu, J. U. (1988). Cultural diversity and human development. In D. T. Slaughter (Ed.), *Black children and poverty: A developmental perspective.* San Francisco: Jossey-Bass.

Pearlin, L., & Schooler, C. (1979). Some extensions of "the structure of coping," a reply to comments by Marshall and Gore. *Journal of Health and Social Behavior, 20*, 202–205.

Polanyi, M. (1962). *Personal knowledge.* Chicago: University of Chicago Press.

Polkinghorne, D. (1983). *Methodology for the human sciences: Systems of inquiry.* Albany State University of New York Press.

Popper, K. (1972). *Objective knowledge.* Oxford: Clarendon Press.

Procidano, M., & Heller, K. (1983). Measures of perceived social support from friends and from family: Three validation studies. *American Journal of Community Psychology, 11*, 1–24.

Reichenbach, H. (1951). *The rise of scientific philosophy.* Berkeley: University of California Press.

Reis, H. (1984). Social interaction and well-being. In S. Duck (Ed.), *Personal relationships: Vol. 5, Repairing personal relationships.* New York: Academic Press.

Reis, H. (1990). The role of intimacy in interpersonal relations. *Journal of Social and Clinical Psychology, 9*, 15–30.

Rizzo, T. (1989). *Friendship development among children in school.* Norwood, NJ: Ablex.

Rizzo, T. (1992). The role of conflict in children's friendship development. In W. Corsaro, & P. Miller (Eds.), *New directions for child development: Interpretive approaches to children's socialization.* San Francisco: Jossey-Bass.

Rizzo, T., & Corsaro, W. (1988). Toward a better understanding of Vygotsky's process of internalization: Its role in the development of the concept of friendship. *Developmental Review, 8*, 219–237.

Rizzo, T., Corsaro, W., & Bates, J. (1992). Ethnographic methods and interpretive analysis: Expanding the methodological options of psychologists. *Developmental Review, 12*, 101–123.

Rook, K. (1984). The negative side of social interaction: Impact on psychological well-being. *Journal of Personality and Social Psychology, 46*, 1097–1108.

Sarason, B., Pierce, G., Shearin, E., Sarason, I., Waltz, J., & Poppe, L. (1991). Perceived social support and working models of self and actual others. *Journal of Personality and Social Psychology, 60*, 273–287.

Sarason, B., Shearin, E., Pierce, G., & Sarason, I. (1987). Interrelations of social support measures: Theoretical and practical implications. *Journal of Personality and Social Psychology, 52*, 813–832.

Sarason, I., & Sarason, B. (1986). Experimentally provided social support. *Journal of Personality and Social Psychology, 50*, 1222–1225.

Schatzman, L., & Strauss, A. (1973). *Field research: Strategies for a natural sociology.* Englewood Cliffs, NJ: Prentice-Hall.

Schulz, R., & Tomkins, C. (1990). Life events and changes in social relationships: Examples, mechanisms and measurement. *Journal of Social and Clinical Psychology, 9*, 69–77.

Selman, R. (1981). The child as a friendship philosopher: A case study in the growth of interpersonal understanding. In S. Asher & J. Gottman (Eds.), *The development of children's friendship.* New York: Cambridge University Press.

Shantz, C. (1987). Conflicts among children. *Child Development, 58*, 283–305.

Thoits, P. (1982). Conceptual, methodological, and theoretical problems in studying social support as a buffer against life stress. *Journal of Health and Social Behavior, 23*, 145–159.

Thoits, P. (1985). Social support and psychological well-being: Theoretical possibilities. In I. Sarason & B. Sarason (Eds.), *Social support: Theory, research, and applications.* Dordrecht, The Netherlands: Martinus Nijhoff.

Thoits, P. (1986). Social support as coping assistance. *Journal of Consulting and Clinical Psychology, 54*, 416–423.

Tolan, P., Keys, C., Chertok, F., & Jason, L. A. (1990). *Researching community psychology: Issues of theory and methods.* Washington, DC: American Psychological Association.

Toulmin, S. (1972). *Human understanding.* Princeton, NJ: Princeton University Press.

Wethington, E., & Kessler, R. (1986). Perceived support, received support, and adjustment to stressful life events. *Journal of Health and Social Behavior, 27*, 78–89.

Wiseman, J. (1986). Friendship: Bonds and binds in a voluntary relationship. *Journal of Social and Personal Relationships, 3*, 191–211.

Youniss, J., & Smoller, J. (1985). *Adolescent relations with mothers, fathers, and friends.* Chicago: University of Chicago Press.

8

Setting Phenotypes in a Mutual Help Organization: Expanding Behavior Setting Theory

Douglas A. Luke, Julian Rappaport, and Edward Seidman

Expands Barker's theory of behavior settings by proposing an additional method of classifying settings based on their functional/behavioral aspects—the setting phenotype. Although behavior setting theory has been widely hailed as a revolutionary contribution to behavioral science, it has had limited impact on general psychology. This may be due in part to a reliance on a purely structural method of classifying behavior settings—the setting genotype. Behavioral data were collected from 510 meetings of 13 self-help groups from a mutual help organization for persons with problems in living. A cluster analysis was performed to uncover meaningful behavioral patterns among the groups. Four phenotypes were identified: personal, impersonal, small talk, and advising. Mutual help group phenotype was found to be related to a set of setting characteristics as well as to overall rated change of group members. The results are discussed in light of the significance of the phenotype construct for making behavior setting theory more relevant for social scientists.

The legacy of the person–environment debate is an appreciation by social scientists of the importance of both person and place in understanding human behavior (Bandura, 1978; Bem & Funder, 1978; Pervin, 1987).

Originally published in the *American Journal of Community Psychology, 19*(1) (1991): 147–167.

Ecological Research to Promote Social Change: Methodological Advances from Community Psychology, edited by Tracey A. Revenson et al. Kluwer Academic/Plenum Publishers, New York, 2002.

Despite this awareness, systematic study of the relationship between people and settings has been both rare and had only isolated impact on mainstream psychology (see Barker, 1978; Bronfenbrenner, 1979; and Moos, 1984, for notable exceptions). The major reason stems from a psychological world view which tends to see behavior and settings as independent entities; although they may interact with each other, usually in a unidirectional fashion, they are rarely seen as parts of a larger whole (Altman & Rogoff, 1987). An additional reason is the complexity associated with environmental assessment.

Barker's theory of behavior settings (1968, 1978) was hailed as a potentially revolutionary eco-behavioral theory upon first introduction (Wicker, 1987). For the most part, however, behavior setting theory has not had the expected impact on the work of community psychologists and others (Kaminski, 1983; Perkins, Burns, Perry, & Nielsen, 1988). In this article we discuss one possible reason for this lack of impact, and present the results of a study designed to expand the theory of behavior settings. Specifically, we examine behavioral regularities among various groups of a particular mutual help organization in order to uncover consistent and meaningful behavior patterns.

CLASSIFICATION OF SETTINGS BASED ON BEHAVIOR EPISODES

Barker's theory of behavior settings is an important attempt to understand the psychology of human behavior in other than intrapsychic or person-centered terms. A behavior setting is a small-scale social system which is both physically and temporally bounded. It is made up of both people (actors) and inanimate objects with which the people interact (behavior objects). Within the setting, the setting program is carried out. The program is a sequence of person–environment interactions (behavior episodes) which form the essential functions of the setting.

Barker provides explicit criteria by which behavior settings are identified and classified, primarily with the use of the Behavior Setting Survey (Barker, 1968; Barker & Schoggen, 1973; Barker & Wright, 1955; Schoggen, 1989). The Behavior Setting Survey is used to identify all the behavior settings within a large, heterogeneous social system, such as a town or a large medical center. To ascertain the number of different types of behavior settings within a system, settings are grouped into *genotypes*. A genotype is made up of settings whose components (actors and physical objects) are similar enough so that they can be exchanged without greatly disturbing the sequence of behavior episodes of any of the settings (Barker, 1968). More specifically, for two settings to belong to the same genotype, persons most responsible for carrying out the setting program (i.e., the leaders) must be able to enter the other setting and perform the same setting program without delay (Schoggen, 1989).

Genotypes represent a simple but coarse-grained taxonomy of settings (Kaminski, 1983; Moos, 1983). For example, "Plays, Concerts, and Programs" is a behavior setting genotype that occurs within a high school (Barker & Gump, 1964). This genotype includes such settings as music festivals, pep rallies, school assemblies, fashion shows, and school plays. Although these settings all take place in the auditorium or gymnasium and the participants are all high school students, there is presumably a fair amount of behavioral variability between the different settings.

The concept of genotype is most useful when one wants to distinguish among different types of settings within a larger social system, such as a town, high school, or large corporation (see, for example, Price & Blashfield, 1975). Many social scientists, however, are interested in smaller, more homogeneous systems. They pose questions concerned with the behavioral patterns within a particular genotype. For example, how do students act differently in a pep rally as compared to a school assembly? Or, what are the differences within the genotype of "Psychological Treatment Session" in a community mental health center?

To answer questions like these, one must look within genotypes. For example, the behavior settings "Group Therapy," "Individual Adult Therapy," and "Crisis Intervention" all would belong to the genotype "Psychological Treatment Session" in a typical mental health center. Structurally these settings share common objects and actors. It would not be uncommon for these settings to share the same leaders (therapists). However, important behavioral differences exist among these settings. Crisis intervention sessions would have different clients, last fewer sessions, and have a different therapeutic focus than group therapy sessions.

These three settings display consistent and meaningful intragenotype behavioral variability. It is consistent in that the behavioral differences are stable across time and different examples of the same behavior setting. The variability is meaningful in that the behavioral differences have confirmable consequences for the persons who inhabit the settings. A crisis intervention client has a very different therapeutic experience than a group therapy client.

Thus, while the settings of the genotype "Psychological Treatment Session" are structurally similar, they may differ in the behavior episodes internal to these settings. We refer to this level of classification as setting *phenotypes.* A phenotype is defined by settings that share the same geno-type, but differ meaningfully and consistently in the behavior episodes within particular settings. Meaningful differences are those that are inter-pretable and related to setting characteristics in theoretically interesting ways. Consistent differences are those that are relatively stable over time and found in more than one location. If only one of the locations within a genotype exhibits a particular behavior pattern, or the behavior pattern only occurs once, then it would not qualify as a setting phenotype.

The definition of phenotype is dependent on the behavior episodes that occur in settings and not on the actors or physical components. Furthermore, the phenotype classification is not based on setting partici-pants' perceptions, as are ratings of social climate (Moos, 1973), but on meaningful and consistent behavioral patterns that are, or can be, observed by others. These behavioral patterns may influence participants' percep-tions of social climate (e.g., Toro, Rappaport, & Seidman, 1987; Toro et al., 1988), but phenotypes refer to the actual patterns of observed behavior.

The use of setting phenotypes as well as genotypes would make a taxonomy of settings less coarse, increase its ecological validity, and perhaps augment the usefulness of behavior setting theory to general psychology, which is often concerned with understanding behavioral differ-ences in similar settings.

BEHAVIOR SETTING FACETS

Settings have a life-cycle, they come into being, develop, and some-times die; generally these temporal aspects of behavior settings have been ignored (Kaminski, 1983; Koch, 1986; Wicker, 1987). Similarly, settings are usually viewed as isolated islands, the external context and connections with other settings are seldom examined. Wicker (1987) pointed out these limitations and presented a more dynamic framework of behavior setting theory. The important features of a behavior setting are categorized into one of three *setting facets:* resources, internal dynamics, and context. In addition, behavior settings are viewed in relation to their temporal stage.

Setting resources include the people, behavior objects, physical space, and information to which the setting has access. Quantity and quality of these resources are both important. For example, a setting often needs a certain minimal number of people to function, but even if there are enough people, they must also have the requisite abilities (e.g., intelligence, strength, psychological health).

Internal dynamics include personal cognitions and motives, functional activities, social processes, growth, and stability. Much of the early research in this area dealt with the theory of underpopulation (Schoggen, 1989; Wicker, 1983).[1] If a setting has fewer people to fill its roles than is optimal, the setting is considered underpopulated. The setting then exerts considerable influence on the members; they work harder, fill more roles, and participate in more varied activities in an attempt to carry out the program of the setting. Studies of underpopulated settings have shown that members of these settings feel more responsible, feel better about their work, feel more important, experience more pressure, and feel more insecure about their jobs (Wicker, 1983).

The larger context within which settings exist is also an important influence on the behaviors within settings. Contextual characteristics include political, legal, and economic conditions; setting history; and links between settings and either other settings or larger organizational or social units.

Barker's early treatment of behavior setting theory considered settings as stable, unchanging entities (Wicker, 1987). Current researchers realize that settings continually come into existence, grow, stabilize, decline, and finally die. Sarason (1972) provided some rich descriptions of the precariousness of newly formed settings. Wicker and King (1988) and Stokols and Shumaker (1981) reported some preliminary work on the developmental stages of behavior settings. Although not aimed at behavior settings per se, Katz and Kahn (1978) developed a detailed developmental theory of organizations. A general finding from the above work is that the interactions between people and their immediate environments change over time. A setting places different demands on its members at different points in its life cycle.

CONTEXT OF STUDY

This study was conducted as part of a longitudinal evaluation of GROW, Inc., a mutual help organization for persons with a history of serious problems in living (see Rappaport et al., 1985, for details of the larger study). GROW is a highly structured organization that communicates its ideology of growth through "caring and sharing" via its leadership, social events, well-developed literature, and formally structured group meetings. The typical group has eight members ($M = 7.84$, ranging from 3 to 19) who meet weekly. They discuss their personal lives, provide support and guidance, and develop friendship networks. The groups all follow a formal "group method" (GROW, 1982) that structures much of the meeting time.

---

[1] Previous authors have used the term "undermanning" when referring to this work. We encourage others to follow the lead of Perkins, Burns, Perry, and Nielsen (1988) and Schoggen (1989), and adopt the nonsexist word "underpopulation."

There is very little known about what behaviors actually take place in the behavior settings of mutual help organizations. Typically, professionals have been excluded or permitted only restricted observational procedures (Levy, 1984; Roberts et al., in press). Our involvement with this organization provides us with a unique opportunity to explore in a more detailed fashion a taxonomy of behavior settings because we were permitted to record actual ongoing behavior during the meetings.

Each GROW *meeting* takes place at a particular location, which is a specific place and a single time. A GROW *group* is composed of a series of meetings which take place at a specific location over many occasions. Each GROW group represents a different example of the same behavior setting genotype—a mutual help group. A GROW group satisfies the definition of genotype in that the actors and physical structures can be exchanged between settings without serious difficulty. Each group shares the same ideology, meeting elements, similar physical resources; leaders and members are all trained to follow the same "GROW Program." Indeed, GROW members and leaders are often able to shift from one group to another with no problem. This satisfies the operational definition of genotype as described above. Nevertheless, wide behavioral variations may exist between different GROW groups.

Given that the groups are all of the same genotype one might expect certain behavioral consistencies across the various settings. To the extent that the lion's share of the behavioral variance across settings is explained by the genotype "mutual help group" the theory of behavior settings may be adequate. However, if there is also systematic behavioral differences between these settings, despite being of a common genotype, the concept of setting phenotype may be a useful addition to the theory.

Our task is threefold: (a) to describe the cross-group differences and consistencies in behavior episodes within the GROW organization (i.e., to elaborate on a taxonomy of behavior settings by exploring phenotypes within the genotype "mutual help groups"); (b) to ascertain the relationship between the behavior episode phenotypes and setting facets; and (c) to discover whether the identified phenotypes have meaningful consequences.

METHODS

Procedure

Over a $2\frac{1}{2}$-year period, 10 trained participant–observers attended and collected data from 510 meetings of 13 different GROW groups in central Illinois. Each group met at a different location.[2] The average number of observations per group is 39 with a range of 17 to 71.

Participants

During the data collection period, a minimum of 799 different people attended at least one meeting of the 13 central Illinois GROW groups. They ranged in age from 15 to 85 ($M = 39$), tended to be female (60%), white (97%), single (73%), and a majority had at least some education beyond high school (60%). A slight majority have had at least one psychiatric hospitalization in the past (55%), while approximately three quarters of GROW members have received some form of formal inpatient or outpatient treatment for psychological problems. Approximately one third of the individuals who first come to a GROW meeting attend only one or two meetings, another third attend for 3 to 4 months, and the final third are members of GROW for longer than 4 months. Persons come to GROW for a variety of reasons: some with a history of psychotic episodes, some for their depression or anxiety, some to deal with family problems, many are lonely, and some are simply curious.

Measures

Behavior Settings and Genotypes

The K-21 Scale is used to determine the degree of interdependence between pairs of settings (Barker, 1968; Schoggen, 1989). If interdependence exceeds a prespecified criteria (usually 21), the two settings are considered separate behavior settings. A K index of less than 21 indicates that the pair of settings actually belong to the same behavior setting. The K-21 Scale is made up of seven subscales assessing different aspects of interdependence: behavioral consequences, inhabitant, leadership, spatial, temporal, behavior objects, and behavior mechanisms. Two of the three authors independently chose random pairs of GROW groups and completed the K-21 Scale for each group pair. For each pair both a conservative and a liberal set of criteria were used to determine subscale cutoffs. K-21 scores were then averaged across group pairs and raters.

---

[2] Data were collected from two other groups. In one we obtained observations from only five meetings. The other was made up exclusively of long-term institutionalized psychiatric patients. Because of the small number of repeated observations on the former group, and unique constellation of members in the latter group, both were dropped from the current analysis.

To determine if a set of behavior settings belong to the same setting geno-type, the Genotype Comparator is used (Schoggen, 1989). The Genotype Comparator is simply a table that facilitates the computation of time required for a setting leader to carry out the program of one setting in a different set-ting. If this time is low compared to the amount of time required to learn the program in the first place, then the two settings belong to the same genotype.

Behavior Episodes

In collaboration with the GROW organization, the Mutual Help Observation System (MHOS) was developed to record both verbal behav-ior and individual and meeting rating data from GROW meetings. The MHOS consists of the Behavioral Interaction Codes (BIC) and the Observer Rating Form (ORF). The BIC is an on-line observational coding system that is used to code talk during the meeting into one of 12 exhaus-tive and mutually exclusive categories. These BIC data are in the form of frequencies of occurrence for each of the 12 behavioral categories summa-rized at the meeting level. These data show marked positive skewness. Therefore, the normal deviate transformation (Guilford & Fruchter, 1978) was used to normalize the data.

Each observer was extensively trained and thereafter checked period-ically for reliability against a criterion videotape. This assured a minimum initial level of reliability as well as protecting against "drift" over time. To minimize the amount of intrusion, each GROW group had only one observer at any given time. However, most observers attended more than one group, and many groups had a series of different raters over time, thus preventing a perfect confounding of group and rater.

Cohen's kappa (1960) was used as the measure of rater reliability. The average kappa across all raters across the study was .73. In addition, kappa was calculated for each of the 12 behavioral codes. These, along with the descriptions of the 12 behaviors, are listed in Table I. For more information on the development of the MHOS and its psychometric characteristics, see Roberts et al. (1991). These verbal behaviors constitute our accounting of the behavior episodes within the 510 meetings of the 13 groups.

Setting Facets

Setting facets are those nonbehavioral variables that describe the structural and functional aspects of the groups at each location. Setting facet variables were obtained from the ORF and archival records of the GROW organization. The ORF complements the BIC's behavioral code with more global information about the group's activities, the members, and the meeting in general. Although traditional measures of reliability

Table I. Behavioral Interaction Code Categories and Reliabilities

Code description	Mean kappa
Small Talk: comments not relevant to the group's current task	.78
Impersonal Question: ask for general and impersonal factual information	.75
Personal Question: question which encourages another to reveal personal information	.65
Request for Help: request information or guidance from another	.67
Information Sharing: general and impersonal information	.69
Self-disclosure: provide personal information	.72
Group Process: alter or reflect on the group's direction	.87
Support: comment which is encouraging, approving, or offering tangible assistance	.85
Interpretation: analyze, evaluate, reconceptualize, challenge, or summarize another member's comments	.73
Guidance: specific suggestions, direction, or guidance about possible courses of action	.70
Agreement: agreement with another's opinion or feedback	.71
Negative: comment which disagrees, is resistant or defensive, or indicates disapproval	.62

were not assessed on the ORF, multiple raters were used for each group at multiple timepoints. This allows for an increased confidence in the obtained data.

Wicker's (1987) framework was employed to organize our selection of setting variables:

Resources. The psychological functioning of the group is seen as a critical resource for mutual help groups. At each meeting, the psychological functioning of each member was rated by the observers on a scale ranging from (1) *disturbed* to (4) *high functioning.* Scores are averaged across individuals within the meeting.

Internal Dynamics. Underpopulation is conceptualized as the critical internal dynamic. It is assessed indirectly in three ways. First, the *size* of the meeting was recorded simply as the number of people at the meeting. Every GROW meeting has a set number of roles to be filled by group members (e.g., meeting leader, records keeper, refreshment preparation). Therefore, fewer people should be an index of greater underpopulation. Second, average *communication density*, defined as the total number of direct communications coded on the BIC between members divided by the total number of possible relationships in that system (Knoke & Kuklinski, 1982), was calculated for each group. Density ranges from 0 to 1, 0 meaning nobody talked to anyone else, and 1 meaning everyone communicated directly with everyone else during the meeting (excluding instances where one person made a general comment to the whole group). Density is a measure of the connectedness of the system and is assumed to be an index of underpopulation. As the number of people in a GROW group increase relative to the number of roles it should be more difficult for any particular person to communicate directly with any other person, thus density should decrease. A third barometer of underpopulation is the average *level of participation*, as observed by the raters. Participation was scored on a scale of (0) *did not participate at all* to (4) *active participant*. As underpopulation increases, so should the level of participation for each member, since fewer people are available to fulfill the GROW roles.

Size of meeting, communication density, and average level of participation represent three related yet conceptually and methodologically distinct aspects of internal dynamics. Size is a structural measure, communication density is a psychosocial variable, and level of participation is an independently rated measure of dynamics.

Context. One of the main goals of GROW is to form "caring and sharing" communities. To attain this, GROW strongly encourages and supports contact among GROW members outside the normal weekly meetings. These are known as "12th-Step Contacts."[3] An important contextual variable for these mutual help goups is the extent to which the members are participating in 12th-step contacts outside the meeting, as reported during the weekly meetings.

Temporal Stages. During the time of this study the GROW organization was expanding throughout Illinois (Zimmerman et al., 1985). New groups were started over time. The temporal stage of a particular GROW group was simply measured as the *age of the setting*—number of months from initiation of the group to the end of data collection. All 13 GROW groups

---

[3] GROW is one example of a large number of mutual help organizations which are collectively known as "12 Step" organizations (e.g., Alcoholics Anonymous). The 12th step of personal growth is always concerned with carrying the organization's message to others.

were still in existence at this time, and thus differences in group age were due entirely to varying starting dates.

Grower Improvemnt Ratings

At the end of the study, all observers with firsthand knowledge of an individual GROW member rated on 15 scales the amount of change that individual had experienced. The scales assessed change in such areas as employment, independent living, friendships, depression, anxiety, spirituality, and incorporation of GROW philosophy. Each scale ranged from (1) *got much worse* to (7) *improved a lot*, with (4) in the middle, *no change*. Because of extremely high intercorrelations (alpha = .95), these ratings were totaled to obtain an overall change score for each of the individuals.

RESULTS

Identification of Within-Genotype Differences

The K-21 Scale was used to show that GROW groups are separate behavior settings and not simply aspects of one larger setting. When the K-21 Scale was completed for any given pair of GROW groups, an average interdependence score of 33 was obtained, ranging from 31 to 35 depending on the particular groups. This is well above the generally accepted cutoff of 21, meaning that the GROW groups are indeed separate behavior settings.

The Genotype Comparator was then used to determine if the 13 GROW groups belong to the same genotype. Group leaders usually take several months of GROW membership before they have adequately learned the GROW program. Once learned, it takes almost no time to carry out that program in other GROW groups. This indicates that the 13 GROW groups all belong to the same genotype.

To assess whether the 13 GROW settings are distinguishable based on their behavior episodes,[4] a one-way MANOVA for the 13 different GROW locations with 510 meetings was performed on the BIC data. The dependent variables were the 12 transformed BIC frequencies per meeting

---

[4] It may be argued that an empirical exploration of behavioral patterns is unnecessary because the K-21 Scale already has within it two subscales concerned with behavioral independence (behavioral consequences and behavioral mechanisms). However, these subscales are concerned only with a limited type of behavioral interdependence (e.g., do both settings have the same amounts of talking, observing, gross motor activity, etc.). The K-21 Scale makes no provision for assessing more sophisticated behavioral patterns that are consistent over time and have meaningful consequences for the setting inhabitants (e.g., personal questioning and self-disclosure).

per location. The multivariate F yielded a significant main effect for location, $F(144, 5810) = 9.29$; $p < .001$, suggesting that at least some locations are behaviorally distinguishable from other locations. That is, the 13 locations within the GROW mutual help genotype do not form a single homogeneous set. Each location may have variance that is not accounted for by being a member of the genotype. Consequently, behavior frequencies were aggregated across meetings within each location.

Identification of Setting Phenotypes

To explore similarities and differences among the 13 group locations, cluster analytic procedures were employed. Cluster analysis forms homogeneous groups of entities on the basis of similarities and dissimilarities among the entities with respect to measured characteristics. The goal of these methods is to form groups that simultaneously maximize the interclass differences and intraclass similarity. Thus, for the current study, a cluster represents a grouping of mutual help locations that produce similar behaviors, while different clusters represent different behavior patterns.

Ward's (1963) method of hierarchical cluster analysis was employed. Initially it considers each entity as a separate cluster. The two most similar entities or clusters are then merged forming a larger cluster and reducing the total number of clusters by one. This step is repeated, each time merging the two most similar clusters, until all entities have been merged into a single cluster. It yields a tree of N possible cluster partitions. Ward's method maximizes cluster homogeneity by minimizing the within-cluster error sum of squares.

There is no generally acceptable empirical rule for choosing the correct number of clusters. Instead, a combination of empirical rules of thumb and interpretability are usually used (Anderberg, 1973; Romesburg, 1984). A four-cluster solution suggested itself for a number of reasons. The four clusters are similar in size, which can aid interpretability. A more important reason is that the partitions containing the five-, six-, and seven-cluster solutions are all created by forming a cluster based on a single location that has split off from one of the four larger clusters. The fact that single split-offs appear only after the four-cluster solution suggests that the four clusters are fairly homogeneous, and may represent actual behavioral similarities. The final and most important reason for choosing the four-cluster solution is that the clusters are meaningful.

Table II presents the results of the cluster analysis of the 13 locations using the 12 transformed average BIC frequencies. The first cluster consists of three locations that are distinguished by meetings that have relatively

Table II. Hierarchical Cluster Solution—Ward's Method[a]

Small Talk	Impersonal Question	Personal Question	Request for Help	Information Sharing	Self-disclosure	Group Process	Support	Inter-pretation	Guidance	Agreement	Negative
				Cluster 1: Impersonal (3 groups)							
.22	.75	.28	.20	.78	.13	-.10	.10	.00	.28	-.02	.45
				Cluster 2: Personal (3 groups)							
-.39	-.18	.56	.33	-.56	.43	-.52	-.14	-.32	-.06	-.41	.19
				Cluster 3: Small Talk (3 groups)							
.39	-.35	-.22	.35	-.41	-.38	.06	-.13	-.25	-.31	-.47	.19
				Cluster 4: Advising (4 groups)							
.00	.03	.10	.37	.13	.09	.20	.10	.38	.30	.43	.04

[a]Because of skewed distributions, the raw behavior frequencies were transformed using the normal deviate transformation (Guilford & Fruchter, 1978).

higher frequencies of information giving, impersonal questions, and to a lesser extent, negative talk. In other words, they spend relatively more time dealing with the factual and informational components of their meetings, and in a somewhat negative fashion. This cluster is labeled *impersonal*. The second cluster is also based on three locations. It is relatively high in personal questions and self-disclosive behavior. Members share more personally with each other. On the other hand, they spend less time focusing on group process, are low in sharing information, agreement, small talk, and interpretation. This cluster is labeled *personal*. The three locations composing Cluster 3 have lower frequencies of most of the BIC behaviors relative to the other clusters. It is higher in small talk, low in agreement, information sharing, personal and impersonal questions, and self-disclosure. It is labeled *small talk*. The last cluster is based on four locations. It is high in agreement, interpretation, guidance, and group process. Additionally, these locations are more balanced in the personal/impersonal dimension of behaviors. This behavioral pattern is seen as less concerned with communication and more concerned with advising and guiding. This cluster is labeled *advising*.

The stability of this four-cluster solution was examined by using a variety of the split-half test. For each of the 13 groups, half of the meeting data were randomly chosen and subjected to the clustering procedure as described above. The same four-cluster solution emerged from this split-half test, suggesting that the clusters constitute a stable behavioral pattern.

These four behavior episode clusters are based on meaningful and stable behavioral differences between locations within the genotype of mutual help organization. Thus they are examples of setting phenotypes.

RELATIONSHIP OF PHENOTYPES AND SETTING FACETS

To determine whether these clusters of behavior episodes are related to setting facets, five one-way ANOVAS were performed. Table III presents the results of these analyses.

From Table III one can see that there was a significant difference between clusters on each of the five variables: level of psychological functioning (resource), meeting size, communication density, and level of participation (internal dynamics, i.e., underpopul8ation), and number of 12th-step contacts (context). The personal cluster members are lowest in psychological functioning and meeting size, higher in communication density and level of participation. For psychological functioning, meeting size, and density, the personal cluster differs significantly from the other three

Table III. Relationships Between Setting Characteristics and Cluster Solution (Phenotype)

Cluster	Setting characteristic cluster means				
	Level of psychological functioning	Meeting size	Communication density	Level of participation	No. of 12th-step contacts
1. Impersonal	3.00	8.45	0.75	2.85	0.44
2. Personal	2.69	6.04	0.84	2.97	0.34
3. Small talk	3.03	8.35	0.74	2.83	0.57
4. Advising	2.89	7.88	0.77	2.83	0.53
F	10.32	12.69	3.92	2.82	12.96
p	.0001	.0001	.009	.04	.0001
Multiple comparisons	2 < 1,3,4 4 < 3	2 < 1,3,4	2 > 1,3,4	2 > 4	1,2 < 3,4

and for participation, only from the advising cluster (Tukey multiple comparisons, see Miller, 1985). The personal, along with the impersonal clusters have fewer 12th-step contacts than the other two clusters. Thus, the personal cluster can be seen as a setting with members who are low in psychological functioning and who do not reach out beyond the group, but where inside the setting itself most everyone is communicated with and active in their participation.

The advising cluster members are also low in psychological functioning, particularly when contrasted with the members of the small talk cluster. However, the advising and small talk cluster members are alike in being high in 12th-step contacts as compared with the other two clusters.

Unlike the five previous variables, setting age was not measured at the meeting level. Each setting has only one value for its age, based on the date at which the group formed. The 13 groups examined in this study formed over a $4\frac{1}{2}$-year period. Relating the date of their formation to the behavior clusters revealed that the three groups making up the impersonal cluster also were the three groups most recently formed. The odds of this happening by chance are 0.003.[5]

These results suggest that the behavioral differences may be due to differences in setting facet characteristics. To rule out the possibility that the

---

[5] This probability is calculated as follows. We are interested in knowing how likely it is that a particular set of three groups has the last three starting dates, out of a pool of 13 groups. The probability of any of those three groups having the last starting date is 3/13. The probability of either of the remaining two groups having the next start date is 2/12. Finally, the probability of the third group having the next start date is 1/11. The total probability therefore is: $(3/13)*(2/12)*(1/11) = .00349$.

differences are simply due to individual demographics, a set of analyses was conducted relating the cluster solution to the following demographic variables: member age, sex, race, religion, marital status, and socioeconomic status. A chi-square test was done for the discrete variables, while ANOVAs were performed for the continuous variables. None of these variables were significantly related to the cluster solution.

MEANINGFUL CONSEQUENCES OF SETTING PHENOTYPES

After identifying the four setting phenotypes and linking them to a small number of setting facets, we wished to ascertain their predictive utility. A total change score from the GROW Improvement Ratings was obtained for 111 GROW members who had joined GROW after the study had commenced. This score was used as the dependent variable in a one-way ANOVA with the four clusters as the independent factor. Since each member attended for different lengths of time, attendance was used as a covariate. After controlling for attendance, the behavioral clusters still accounted for significant amount of the variance, $F(3, 106) = 3.20, p = .026$. A multiple classification analysis also demonstrated that the mean differences were in the expected directions. Members of the personal cluster are rated as improving the most, followed by the advising, and small talk clusters; and finally the members of the impersonal cluster are rated as improving the least. Tukey's multiple comparison test showed that the personal cluster was significantly different from the impersonal cluster on rated change ($p < .05$).

DISCUSSION

The data from this study are used to illustrate the usefulness of adding the concept of phenotype to Wicker's (1987) recent elaboration of Barker's (1968) theory of behavior settings. Our data suggest that setting genotypes do not always adequately account for the interesting variance between settings. The 13 groups we attended could exchange actors and components without severe difficulty; they are all of the genotype *mutual help group*. However, as we have shown, there are important and unique behavior patterns that exist within this same behavior setting genotype. Some groups exhibit more personal behavior, some more impersonal, some spend more time in small talk, and some are more advising than other groups within the same genotype. Thus, the 13 GROW groups in central Illinois constitute four unique phenotypes.

The highly structured GROW Program serves to constrain the amount of behavioral variability found among different GROW groups. However, it is not too surprising that differences were found. Each group meets in a different locale, has a unique history, with different members attending for varying reasons. Some groups were more organized than others, some more chaotic, and so on. During the study the participant/observers quickly developed a feel for the groups they were observing. Indeed, several of the observers were able to identify which group a set of data came from simply based on summary statistics. The concept of phenotypic differences was consistent with these institutions. In fact, qualitative descriptions of these groups matched quite closely their respective phenotype assignments. For example, one group was described by its observers as having terrible leadership, the meetings were often chaotic, and members had difficulty staying on task. Interpersonal helping was often inappropriate, and not much time was spent on interpersonal sharing. This group ended up in the "Small Talk" phenotype. Another quite different group was described as having sharp leaders who helped keep meetings on track. Members were very involved with each other, both in and out of the meetings. There was a lot of appropriate interpersonal helping, perhaps due to the fact that the group had a large number of long-term experienced GROW members—it was also called a "prototypic" GROW group. This group was part of the "Advising" phenotype. Thus, the phenotype classification empirically confirmed the more subjective experiences of the GROW observers.

More important than confirming researchers' expectations, the assessment of phenotypic variability can be very useful for furthering our understanding of mutual help groups, and subsequently feeding that information back to the groups themselves. For example, the data reported here suggest that despite the consistency of the GROW program across different groups, some types of groups result in more member improvement than others. Specifically, members attending the groups in the personal phenotype were rated as improving more than those attending the impersonal groups. Given that the personal groups were also seen as more underpopulated than others, GROW may want to consider limiting the size of groups in the future.

The relationship between phenotype and group age is another potentially useful finding. The groups constituting the impersonal phenotype were also the youngest groups to form. This suggests that it may take some time for new GROW groups and group members to fully learn the GROW program of interpersonal sharing and helping. GROW may want to pay a little more attention to new groups in order to help them adopt the program. Furthermore, this finding suggests that future research on mutual help consider the temporal aspects or the life cycles of groups (Maton, Leventhal, Madara, & Julien, 1989; Wicker & King, 1988).

At a more general level, a major advantage of the phenotype construct is that it may serve as a bridge between ecological psychology on the one hand, and the more individually oriented branches of psychology on the other. This research has been guided from the outset by a belief that people's behavior, and the settings within which people act, are interdependent aspects of a holistic system. This transactional viewpoint (Altman & Rogoff, 1987) assumes a simultaneous definition of behavior and setting: Just as the setting is determined by the behavior within the setting, behavior cannot be understood without taking its context into account. This approach has important implications for both ecological psychology and community psychology.

Introduction of the phenotype concept has two main advantages for ecological psychology: It reemphasizes the importance of behavioral variability among settings, and it allows behavior setting theory to be applied to smaller, more homogeneous social systems. Barker (1968) was always aware of the inseparability of the structural and functional aspects of behavior settings, what he called "behavior-and-milieu." For example, two of the seven K-21 subscales that are used to determine if two synomorphs are separate behavior settings focus on behavioral aspects. The other five focus on the inhabitant, physical, and temporal aspects of the settings. However, the treatment of the behavioral aspects of settings does not receive the same specificity that the structural aspects do. For example, the whole concept of genotype is based on the notion of interchangeability of actors without upsetting the program of the setting. Interchangeability and actors are well defined, but the description of setting program remains sketchy. Sometimes it is treated as the overall goals of the setting, sometimes as the sum of the behaviors that occur in the setting. This greater attention to the structural aspects of behavior settings results, as Perkins et al. pointed out (1988), in an overemphasis of form over function.

By introducing the concept of phenotype, more attention may be paid to the behavioral patterns that consistently occur in various settings. Because phenotypes are stable structures, which occur over time and across different settings, and are not due to the idiosyncratic contributions of particular individuals, they are firmly part of the preperceptual molar environment. Thus, we saw that the four GROW phenotypes were identifiable across many groups, despite the fact that group membership changed dramatically over time. Consideration of setting phenotypes may help to bring back the structural–functional balance of behavior setting theory.

The second problem addressed by the phenotype concept has to do with how behavior setting theory has been put into practice in the past. The Behavior Setting Survey has often been used to collect data on all the settings within large heterogeneous social systems such as hospitals, schools, and small towns (e.g., Barker & Gump, 1964; Barker & Schoggen, 1973; LeCompte, 1972; Price & Blashfield, 1975). The concept of genotype is most useful when applied across the wide variety of settings found in such systems. However, behavior setting theory has not heretofore provided a comparable guide when one wishes to examine setting characteristics in smaller, more homogeneous, social systems such as therapy sessions, mutual help groups, and the like. The phenotype concept is proposed specifically to address this need. This results in a hierarchical classification system of behavior settings, where settings with similar programs and actors belong to the same genotype, and within that genotype settings that show consistent and meaningful behavioral patterns belong to separate phenotypes.

Although hierarchical classification schemes are common in other fields, there are few examples of them in psychology (Pervin, 1978). A hierarchical taxonomy of behavior settings results in a more flexible, useful theory. One can use the genotype category for those questions dealing with comparisons across many different types of settings. However, when one is interested in a more fine-grained analysis of the behavioral functioning within a smaller set of more similar settings, the phenotype categozy will be most useful.

It is hoped that future research will apply the phenotype concept to different types of settings. This study, for example, was restricted to settings within a particular genotype. It would be interesting to examine phenotypes across different genotypes. For example, do other types of mutual help groups (Alcoholics Anonymous, Recovery) exhibit the same number and types of phenotypes as GROW does?

The phenotype concept also will be useful for the concerns of community psychologists. Social activists have always recognized the need to immerse themselves in the context of the group, community, organization, or culture they are trying to influence (Sarason, 1972). The identification of phenotypic groups may prove a valuable addition to the more subjective methods already used.

Related to this has been a spate of interest on the part of social scientists on the relationship between perceived environment and behavior. Forgas' *social episodes* (1979) and Schank and Abelson's *scripts* (1977) are noteworthy attempts to understand sequences of behavior that occur consistently in situations of everyday life. Like behavior setting theory, these approaches emphasize that much of human behavior is rooted in social contexts. Unlike more ecological theories, these efforts focus on the collectively stored cognitive representations of common behavioral patterns. Seidman's *social regularities* (1988) provide an additional noncognitive way to understand sequences of behavior that occur over time. In other words, they are portraits of everyday life. Phenotypes as defined here are meaningful and consistent patterns of behavior occurring in specific settings. As such they represent an operationalization of Seidman's social regularities construct.

The phenotype concept may prove to be an important link between ecological psychology and the social psychology of everyday situations by providing a common unit of analysis. The phenotype, as a set of meaningful and consistent behavioral patterns occurring in a specific context, is of interest to ecological, social, and community research scientists.

We hope that a classification system of behavior settings composed of both genotypes and phenotypes will make behavior setting theory more relevant to social scientists. Just as a purely intrapsychic approach to understanding human behavior has been found to be incomplete, we can say that trying to understand settings without taking individual behavior into account is similarly inadequate. The phenotype classification links behavior and settings inextricably, showing again that people and place are two sides of the same coin.

ACKNOWLEDGMENTS

Support for this research came from an NIMH grant (MH37390) awarded to Julian Rappaport and Edward Seidman. We thank Brian Luke, the associate editors, and three anonymous reviewers for comments on an earlier draft; also Julie Genz, Thomas Reischl, Linda Roberts, and the members of the GROW organization for making this study possible.

REFERENCES

Altman, I., & Rogoff, B. (1987). World views in psychology: Trait, interactional, organismic, and transactional perspectives. In D. Stokols & I. Altman, *The handbook of environmental psychology*. New York: Wiley.

Anderberg, M. R. (1973). *Cluster analysis for applications*. New York: Academic Press.

Bandura, A. (1978). The self system in reciprocal determinism. *American Psychologist, 33*, 344–358.

Barker, R. B. (1968). *Ecological psychology*. Stanford, CA: Stanford University Press.

Barker, R. B. (1978). *Habitats, environments, and human behavior*. San Francisco: Jossey-Bass.

Barker, R. G., & Gump, P. V. (1964). *Big school, small school: High school size and student behavior*. Stanford, CA: Stanford University Press.

Barker, R. G., & Schoggen, P. (1973). *Qualities of community life*. San Francisco: Jossey-Bass.

Barker, R. G., & Wright, H. F. (1955). *Midwest and its children*. New York: Harper & Row.

Bem, D. J., & Funder, D. C. (1978). Predicting more of the people more of the time: Assessing the personality of situations. *Psychological Review, 85*, 485–501.

Bronfenbrenner, U. (1979). *The ecology of human development: Experiments by nature and design*. Cambridge, MA: Harvard University Press.

Cohen, J. (1960). A coefficient of agreement for nominal scales. *Education and Psychological Measurement, 20*, 37–46.

Forgas, J. P. (1979). *Social episodes: The study of interaction routines*. New York: Academic Press.

GROW, Inc. (1982). *The program of growth to maturity* (4th ed.). Sydney, Australia: Author.

Guilford, J. P., & Fruchter, B. (1978). *Fundamental statistics in psychology and education* (6th ed.). New York: McGraw-Hill.

Kaminski, G. (1983). The enigma of ecological psychology. *Journal of Environmental Psychology, 3*, 85–94.

Katz, D., & Kahn, R. L. (1978). *The social psychology of organizations*. New York: Wiley.

Knoke, D., & Kuklinski, J. H. (1982). *Network analysis*. Beverly Hills, CA: Sage.

Koch, J. J. (1986). Behavior Setting und Forschungsmethodik Barkers: Einleitende Orientierung and einige kritische Anmerkungen [Barker's behavior setting and research methodology: Introductory orientation and several critical observations]. In G. Kaminski (Ed.), *Ordnung und Variabilität im Alltagsgeschehen* [Order and variability in everyday life] (pp. 33–43). Göttingen: Verlag für Psychologie.

LeCompte, W. E. (1972). The taxonomy of a treatment environment. *Archives of Physical Medicine and Rehabilitation, 53*, 109–114.

Levy, L. (1984). Issues in research and evaluation. In A. Gartner & F. Riessman (Eds.), *The self-help revolution* (pp. 155–172). New York: Human Sciences Press.

Maton, K. I., Leventhal, G. S., Madara, E. J., & Julien, M. (1989). Factor affecting the birth and death of mutual-help groups: The role of national affiliation, professional involvement, and member focal problem. *American Journal of Community Psychology, 17*, 643–671.

Miller, R. (1985). Multiple comparisons. In S. Kotz & N. L. Johnson (Eds.), *Encyclopedia of statistical sciences* (Vol. 5, pp. 679–689). New York: Wiley.

Moos, R. H. (1973). Conceptualization of human environments. *American Psychologist, 28*, 652–665.

Moos, R. H. (1983). Discussion of 'The enigma of ecological psychology,' by G. Kaminski. *Journal of Environmental Psychology, 3*, 173–183.

Moos, R. H. (1984). Context and coping: Toward a unifying conceptual framework. *American Journal of Community Psychology, 12*, 1–36.

Perkins, D. V., Burns, T. F., Perry, J. C., & Nielsen, K. P. (1988). Behavior setting theory and community psychology: An analysis and critique. *Journal of Community Psychology, 16*, 355–372.

Pervin, L. A. (1978). Definitions, measurements, and classifications of stimuli, situations, and environments. *Human Ecology, 6*, 71–105.

Pervin, L. A. (1987). Person-environment congruence in the light of the person-situation controversy. *Journal of Vocational Behavior, 31*, 222–230.

Price, R. H., & Blashfield, R. K. (1975). Explorations in the taxonomy of behavior settings. *American Journal of Community Psychology, 3*, 335–351.

Rappaport, J., Seidman, E., Toro, P., McFadden, L. S., Reischl, T. M., Roberts, L. J., Salem, D. A., Stein, C. H., & Zimmerman, M. A. (1985). Collaborative research with a self-help organization. *Social Policy, 15*, 12–24.

Roberts, L. J., Luke, D. A., Rappaport, J., Seidman, E., Toro, P., & Reischl, T. M. (1991). Charting uncharted terrain: A behavioral observation system for mutual help groups. *American Journal of Community Psychology, 19*, 715–737.

Romesburg, H. C. (1984). *Cluster analysis for researchers*. Belmont, CA: Lifetime Learning.

Sarason, S. B. (1972). *The creation of settings and the future societies.* San Francisco: Jossey-Bass.

Schank, R. C., & Abelson, R. P. (1977). *Scripts, plans, goals, and understanding: An inquiry into human knowledge structures.* Hillside, NJ: Erlbaum.

Schoggen, P. (1989). *Behavior settings: A revision and extension of Roger G. Barker's Ecological Psychology.* Stanford, CA: Stanford University Press.

Seidman, E. (1988). Back to the future, community psychology: Unfolding a theory of social intervention. *American Journal of Community Psychology, 16,* 3–24.

Stokols, D., & Shumaker, S. A. (1981). People in places: A transactional view of settings. In J. Harvey, *Cognition, social behavior and the environment.* Hillsdale, NJ: Erlbaum.

Toro, P. A., Rappaport, J., & Seidman, E. (1987). Social climate comparison of mutual help and psychotherapy groups. *Journal of Consulting and Clinical Psychology, 55,* 430–431.

Toro, P. A., Reischl, T. M., Zimmerman, M. A., Rappaport, J., Seidman, E., Luke, D. A., & Roberts, L. J. (1988). Professionals in mutual help groups: Impact on social climate and members' behavior. *Journal of Consulting and Clinical Psychology, 56,* 631–632.

Ward, Jr., J. H. (1963). Hierarchical grouping to optimise an objective function. *Journal of the American Statistical Association, 58,* 236–244.

Wicker, A. W. (1983). *An introduction to ecological psychology.* Monterey, CA: Brooks/Cole.

Wicker, A. W. (1987). Behavior settings reconsidered: Temporal stages, resources, internal dynamics, context. (pp. 613–653). In D. Stokols & I. Altman, *Handbook of environmental psychology.* New York: Wiley.

Wicker, A. W., & King, J. C. (1988). Life cycles of behavior settings. In J. E. McGrath (Ed.), *The social psychology of time* (pp. 182–200). Newbury Park, CA: Sage.

Zimmerman, M. A., McFadden, L. S., Toro, P. A., Salem, D. A., Reischl, T. M., Rappaport, J., & Seidman, E. (1985, May). *Expansion of a mutual help organization: The 'Johnny Appleseed' approach.* Paper presented at the meeting of the Midwestern Psychological Association, Chicago.

III

Culturally Anchored Research

Tracey A. Revenson

Community psychologists, as well as other social scientists, have argued that research methodology must be attuned to the unique aspects of culture, particularly with regard to action research and program development. In reality, however, research on nonmajority cultures has been dominated by the use of traditional methodologies, i.e., methodologies used in mainstream psychology that assume universal laws of behavior. Until recently, most studies—even in community psychology—compared a mainstream to a nonmainstream group and attributed any differences to ethnicity or culture. A number of community psychologists (e.g., Roosa & Gonzales, 2000; Sasao & Sue, 1993; Trickett, 1996) have called for the implementation of diverse and multiple methods to adequately understand context and culture.

This section opens with an essay prepared especially for this volume. Nearly 10 years ago, Seidman, Hughes, and Williams (1993) edited a special issue of the *American Journal of Community Psychology* on Culturally Anchored Methodology. For that issue, they crafted a conceptual article that laid out the tenets of a culturally anchored methodology (Hughes, Seidman & Williams, 1993) and elucidated practical guidelines that were suited to the unique aspects of studying cultural phenomena within communities. The focus was not how to measure culture, *per se*, but how to consider the impact of culture within intervention and social action research.

For this book, Diane Hughes and Edward Seidman provide a revision of that essay. One could call it an "update," as it draws upon studies that they and others have conducted since its original publication. But the authors revisit their original tenets with a more experienced set of eyes, being even more specific about how research must change. Their central theme remains the same: Culture intersects each and every phase of the

Tracey A. Revenson • Doctoral Program in Psychology, The Graduate Center of the City University of New York, New York, New York 10016-4309.

research enterprise—problem formulation, conceptualization, measurement, research design, data analysis, and interpretation—and thus, a culturally anchored approach cannot be selectively applied. Their chapter provides a critical analysis of the unexamined assumptions that underlie research with nonmainstream cultural groups, such as how ethnocentric biases may distort how the research problem is framed. Moreover, they provide examples of when and how (mis)assumptions may lead to erroneous research design choices and consequently, flawed conclusions (on which social programs might be based). Hughes and Seidman conclude with a set of guidelines to help researchers make deliberate decisions that will anchor their work in the culture in which it is based.

The two reprinted articles in this section expand upon Hughes and Seidman's discussion, focusing on two specific points in the research process: framing the question and operationalizing constructs. Relying solely on the published literature to define which constructs and measures are important is insufficient because, to date, divergent cultural mindscapes have not influenced conceptualization (or measurement) in a consequential fashion. Hughes and DuMont (1993) argue for focus groups as a critical tool for elucidating culturally relevant concepts for which little prior research or theory is available. Focus groups help researchers to see the phenomenon of interest through the participants' eyes and words; they also help us to understand participants' beliefs, values, and "blueprints for living."

The article by Mitchell and Beals (1997) considers the issues of construct equivalence and measurement equivalence (see also Knight, Virdin, Ocampo, & Roosa, 1994; Prelow, Tein, Roosa, & Wood, 2000; Seidman et al, 1995), as well as the dilemma of between- vs. within-subject designs. The extent to which a particular research program is culturally anchored depends not only on the relevance and meaning of the research constructs to the target population, but also on the appropriateness of the measurement procedures employed. Once a construct has been determined to mean the same thing across groups, it still needs to be determined whether the measures elicit the same response across groups. Without establishing the equivalence of measures, it is impossible to know whether any apparent differences are due to measurement artifacts, true substantive differences, or both (Knight, Virdin, Ocampo, & Roosa, 1994).

Mitchell and Beals (1997) set out to understand the constructs of "positive and problem behaviors" in Native American youth who resided in four different communities. Using factor analysis, they found that the content and structure of what constituted positive and problem behaviors differed across the four communities; that is, the structure of the concepts of positive and problem behavior were not equivalent across groups.

Thus, what was originally designed as a within-group study quickly became a between-group study. This led to dilemmas not only of construct equivalence and measurement equivalence, but also of construct relevance and interpretation: What aspects of Native American culture and community life might have affected the way that these behaviors were being viewed? How deep into "culture" must one dig to find its roots? The youth in the four communities came from over 50 tribes, suggesting that even the community level of analysis was too distal. By investigating the extent to which two or more groups differ from one another in the patterns of relationships among variables, and not just on an outcome measure, between-group studies can facilitate an understanding of how cultural and ecological contexts moderate relationships between predictor and criterion variables.

In sum, the three articles in this section continue to lay the groundwork for making community research truly culturally anchored. We still have a lot to learn about which aspects of culture affect the phenomena in which we are most interested, but it is apparent that ignoring the historic, economic, and social aspects of different cultures may limit our knowledge and our ability to create effective and culturally anchored interventions.

REFERENCES

Hughes, D. L., & DuMont, K. (1993). Using focus groups to facilitate culturally-anchored research. *American Journal of Community Psychology*, *21*, 775–806.

Hughes, D. L., & Seidman, E. (2002). In pursuit of a culturally anchored methodology. In T. A. Revenson, A. R. D'Augelli, S. E. French, D. L. Hughes, D. Livert, E. Seidman, M. Shinn, & H. Yoshikawa (Eds.), *Ecological Research to Promote Social Change: Methodological Advances from Community Psychology* (pp. 243–255). New York: Kluwer Academic/Plenum Publishers.

Hughes, D. L., Seidman, E., & Williams, N. (1993). Cultural phenomena and the research enterprise: Toward a culturally anchored methodology. *American Journal of Community Psychology*, *21*, 687–703.

Knight, G. P., Virdin, L. M., Ocampo, K. A., & Roosa, M. (1994). An examination of cross-ethnic equivalence of measures of negative life events and mental health among Hispanic and Anglo-American children. *American Journal of Community Psychology*, *22*, 767–783.

Mitchell, C. M., & Beals, J. (1997). The structure of problem and positive behavior among American Indian adolescents: Gender and community differences. *American Journal of Community Psychology*, *25*, 257–288.

Prelow, H. M., Tein, J., Roosa, M. W., & Wood, J. (2000). Do coping styles differ across sociocultural groups? The role of measurement equivalence in making this judgment. *American Journal of Community Psychology*, *28*, 225–244.

Roosa, M. W., & Gonzales, N. A. (2000). Minority issues in prevention. [Special Issue]. *American Journal of Community Psychology*, *28* (2).

Sasao, T., & Sue, S. (1993). Toward a culturally-anchored ecological framework of research in ethnic-cultural communities. *American Journal of Community Psychology*, *21*, 705–727.

Seidman, E., Allen, L., Aber, J. L., Mitchell, C., Feinman, J., Yoshikawa, H., Comtois, K. A., Golz, J., Miller, R. L., Ortiz-Torres, B., & Roper, G. C. (1995). Development and validation of adolecent-perceived microsystem scales: Social support, daily hassles, and involvement. *American Journal of Community Psychology, 23*, 355–388.

Seidman, E., Hughes, D. L., & Williams, N. (Eds.) (1993). Culturally anchored methodology. [Special Issue] *American Journal of Community Psychology, 21*(6).

Trickett, E. J. (1996). A future for community psychology: The contexts of diversity and the diversity of contexts. *American Journal of Community Psychology, 24*, 209–234.

9

In Pursuit of a Culturally Anchored Methodology

Diane L. Hughes and Edward Seidman

The need to represent and understand diverse cultural groups and populations, particularly those who are underserved or inappropriately served, has been a rallying cry for Community Psychology since its formal beginnings at the Swampscott Conference (Bennett, Anderson, Cooper, Hassol, Klein, & Rosenblum, 1966), where the importance of studying behavior in context was emphasized (Livert & Hughes, 2002). A central component of context is cultural—that is, all contexts, and the behaviors and interactions that take place within them, are infused with values, belief systems, and world-views that emanate from cultural phenomena. In this essay, we summarize the elements of a methodology in Community Psychology that recognizes that research processes are culturally embedded—what we term a *culturally anchored methodology*. In doing so, we draw heavily from our previous explication of components of such a methodology published in a special of the *American Journal of Community Psychology* devoted to the topic (Hughes, Seidman, & Williams, 1993).

Culture has been conceptualized and defined from a variety of perspectives. It is a concept that is applicable across standard social categories including race, gender, ethnicity, nationality, religious preference, sexual orientation, and disability status. Most conceptualizations of culture include external referents, such as customs, artifacts, and social institutions; and internal referents such as ideologies, belief systems, attitudes, expectations,

Diane L. Hughes ● Department of Psychology, New York University, New York, New York 10003   **Edward Seidman** ● Department of Psychology, New York University, New York, New York 10003.

Ecological Research to Promote Social Change: Methodological Advances from Community Psychology, edited by Tracey A. Revenson et al. Kluwer Academic/Plenum Publishers, New York, 2002.

and epistemologies. Although no single definition of culture is universally accepted by social scientists, we believe that we can elaborate a culturally anchored methodology without resolving such definitional quandaries. Three elements of culture, which emerge in most efforts to define it, are central in articulating such a methodology:

1. *All individuals develop in cultural context.* Cultural contexts supply blueprints for living that determine what is learned, the process through which learning occurs, and the rules for displaying competencies that are valued by group members. Thus, culture mediates and shapes all aspects of human behavior.

2. *Culturally based values, norms, beliefs, and behaviors are transmitted intergenerationally and are syntonic with demands of the context in which child rearing occurs.* Some aspects of culture are purposefully transmitted whereas others are simply absorbed by children throughout the course of their development (Boykin & Toms, 1985). Thus, the goal of research should be to understand how culturally distinct socialization processes are adaptive to local contexts.

3. *Culture is evidenced in patterns of behavior and social regularities among members of a population, as well as between the population and its larger ecological context.* This suggests the need for conceptualizing and operationalizing explanatory constructs beyond the individual level of analysis (Seidman, 1988). This is a more general challenge for community psychologists; a challenge that has been recognized since the field's inception (Reiff, 1968).

These elements of culture are relevant throughout all phases of the research process. They influence what researchers (choose to) observe, how researchers decide which problems are worthy of study, and which methods are appropriate for studying those problems. They influence the operationalization of constructs; respondents' interpretations of, and responses to, the research process itself (setting, stimulus materials, task demands); and the meanings that researchers attach to the data that they collect (Kuhn, 1962; Maruyama, 1983; Seidman, 1978).

Social scientists need to develop methodologies that acknowledge both researchers' and study participants' embeddedness in diverse cultural contexts. The diversity of populations studied (blacks, Latinos, rural populations, gay/lesbian populations), and the values and assumptions of Community Psychology (community strengths, empowerment, promotion of well-being) demand that we do so (Bernal & Enchautegui-de-Jesus, 1994; Rappaport, 1976; Trickett, 1996; Trickett, Watts, & Birman, 1993). Such culturally anchored methods should incorporate conceptual and empirical strategies that stem from different values, belief systems, behaviors, and social regularities among nonmainstream groups and communities. Hopefully, such strategies should reduce researchers' ethnocentric biases and contribute to a greater understanding of people within diverse cultural communities, e.g., the rhythms of community life and patterns of behavior, and the nature of the larger ecological context in which these are embedded. Such strategies should also help ensure that interventions are appropriate to the values and traditions of a group.

ELEMENTS OF A CULTURALLY ANCHORED METHODOLOGY

Culture influences research at each stage of the research process (Hughes, Seidman, & Williams, 1993). Using the stages of the research process as our organizing schema, we describe the intersection between cultural phenomena and the researcher's tasks, and provide current exemplars of culturally anchored research for each. We then suggest how a more culturally anchored methodology can be developed from existing methods and approaches.

Problem Formulation

The researcher is not an objective, detached entity. Rather, she frames research questions through the various cultural lenses that inform her worldview (Maruyama, 1983; Seidman, 1978, 1983). Cultural lenses are shaped by the researcher's own interests, experiences, and perspectives, as well as by an existing research literature that also is embedded in a particular (usually Western) cultural framework. To the extent that researchers' own cultural lenses differ from those used by the cultural group under study, researchers are more likely to utilize theories and variables that reflect their own—or the mainstream's—experiences rather than those of the target population. Systematic biases can emerge from this cultural ethnocentrism, resulting in distortions or misinterpretations of the group's experiences and in the formulation of the "wrong" problem or an "error of conceptualization" (Seidman, 1978). Errors of conceptualization often are multiply determined by a variety of unexamined premises and pressures. Mainstream societal values, the priorities of funding agencies, and the narrow focus of disciplinary paradigms each constrain the nature and formulation of social science questions and hypotheses.

Thus, researchers must exercise both caution and sensitivity in problem selection and formulation, particularly when they are examining questions regarding cultural groups and communities of which they are not a member. Multiple stakeholders—scientists, community participants, funders—should participate in this process, as they are likely to hold different underlying beliefs and models about a prespecified phenomenon of interest or, indeed, about what the phenomena of interest should be. Stakeholders need to examine the premises underlying the selection and formulation of research problems in order to generate alternative conceptualizations, questions, and constructs. Because choices at each stage of research are constrained by earlier choices (Seidman, 1978), the dialectic that emerges from a collaborative process in which multiple stakeholders participate is a critical component of culturally anchored research and must begin at the earliest stages of the research.

Population Definition

Traditionally, little attention has been paid to explicating group boundaries (that is, who is and who is not a member of a particular cultural group) or to identifying important within-group variations in experiences and relationships. Social science researchers typically use simple demographic markers or proxy variables (e.g., Hispanic, black, nationality) to define nonmainstream cultural groups. However, these broad demographic markers are insufficient to define any cultural group (Marin & Marin, 1991; Vega, 1992). The norms, values, and experiences of different cultural subgroups, for example, Dominicans and Puerto Ricans, may be as large as those between racial or ethnic groups (Bernal & Enchautegui-de-Jesus, 1994). Moreover, individuals may be members of multiple cultural groups (e.g., biracial individuals) or of other social groups (e.g., defined by socioeconomic, regional, or other factors) that condition the meaning of cultural categories. It is unlikely that simple proxy variables adequately capture the common blueprints for living or social regularities inherent in a cultural community (Betancourt & Lopez, 1993).

Concept and Measurement Development

The choice of constructs and the instruments used to measure them are subject to the same unwitting biases as the formulation of the problem. Concerns regarding the equivalence of constructs and measures across cultural groups have been discussed widely in numerous disciplines (e.g., cultural and cross-cultural psychology, anthropology). Several methodological concerns are of particular relevance to community psychologists.

The first concern occurs at the level of conceptualization and involves the definition of the constructs to be studied (*linguistic equivalence*). Not all constructs mean the same thing to members of all groups. If one accepts the argument that worldviews and meanings are culturally constructed, then we must also consider that different cultural groups attach different meanings to different concepts. Even broad umbrella constructs for the field—such as competence or well-being or social responsibility—can have different meanings across cultural groups. For example, Burton, Allison, and Obedillah (1995) quote from a 15-year-old, inner city African American talking about his teacher: "I take care of my mother and have raised my sisters. Then I come here and this know-nothing teacher treat me like I'm some dumb kid with no responsibilities ... Don't they understand I'm a man and I been a man longer than they been a woman" (p. 129). This youth's comments underscore critical differences in the meaning of competence between mainstream and nonmainstream populations.

Nor are all psychological concepts equally relevant across groups. That is, even when a construct is equivalent in meaning across groups, it may be more relevant to one group than to another. In fields that commonly study underrepresented groups, the bias that is most likely to emerge involves those constructs critical to a group's identity, experiences, or development. These constructs are commonly omitted from researchers' conceptual frameworks because they have not been identified or examined extensively in the available literature. Constructs such as ethnic identity, sexual orientation, racial socialization, discrimination—each central to understanding social processes both within and between ethnic minority populations within the United States—only recently have appeared in mainstream psychology, due to renewed interest in ethnic minority and immigrant populations. Such concepts have been peripheral at best, although not completely absent, in the literature on European American youth because they are not viewed as phenomena central to this group.

Thus, one element of a culturally anchored methodology is to identify, define, and operationalize concepts that are relevant to social processes and experiences for the particular cultural group(s) under study. Relying solely on the published literature to define which constructs and measures are important is insufficient because, to date, divergent cultural mindscapes have not influenced conceptualization (or measurement) in a consequential fashion. A number of scholars have called for the implementation of diverse and multiple methods to adequately understand context and culture (e.g., Trickett, 1996). As an example, Hughes and DuMont (1993, Chapter 10, this volume) illustrate how to use focus group interviews to elucidate culturally relevant concepts for which little prior research and theory is available. Methods from discourse analysis were adopted to code focus group dialogues about race-related socialization among African American dual-earner families. With these codes, the researchers were able to identify

consensual models about the constructs held by the focus group participants. These models were used to elaborate multiple dimensions of the
construct—some new to the researchers—that were used, in turn, as the
basis for generating survey items.

A second set of concerns occurs at the level of measurement and has
been referred to as *measurement equivalence*. The extent to which a particular research program is culturally anchored depends not only on the relevance and meaning of the research constructs to the target population, but
also on the appropriateness of the measurement procedures employed.
Once a construct has been determined to mean the same thing across
groups, the issue of whether the measures elicit the same responses across
groups still needs to be determined. Without establishing the equivalence
of measures, it is impossible to know whether any apparent differences are
due to measurement artifacts, true substantive differences, or both. Knight,
Virdin, Ocampo, and Roosa's (1994) elaboration of the types of equivalence illuminates this issue. At the same time, their study reminds us that
establishing equivalence requires sample sizes that are much larger than
those typically employed, because establishing equivalence requires the
researcher to support the null hypothesis in a test of differences between
groups rather than a failure to reject lack of equivalence at $p < .05$. Sufficient
sample sizes yield relatively narrow confidence intervals, which permit
researchers to demonstrate that the difference between two groups is either
zero, or is statistically significant but substantively meaningless.

Several aspects of measurement equivalence have been of particular
interest to cross-cultural researchers. *Scale equivalence* refers to the extent to
which response choices have similar meanings across cultural groups.
A number of studies suggest that between-group differences using particular scale formats may be a function of methodological artifacts rather
than meaningful differences. For instance, Bachman and O'Malley (1984)
demonstrated that African Americans were more likely than whites to use
extreme response choices on Likert-type scales; Hui and Triandis (1989)
found similar tendencies between Hispanic and non-Hispanic populations.
Ethnic and cultural differences in response sets can emerge either from
differing cultural norms for responding to stimuli or from differing abilities
to map subjectively-held internal states onto the rating categories that
researchers use. In the former instance, extreme or modest response styles
may be culturally sanctioned, influencing the scale points that respondents
endorse. In the latter instance, there are culturally-based differences in
respondents' abilities to evenly distribute subjectively-held experiences
across the entire range of response categories that researchers have provided.

Closely related to the issues of scale equivalence is the issue of *task
equivalence*. Task equivalence is the extent to which respondents' familiarity

with, or interpretation of, the assessment situation and task demands are similar across cultural groups. The beliefs that participants hold about what is expected or required of them in a research situation, and respondents' familiarity with task requirements, are critical determinants of what respondents actually do in response to task demands. Despite a long history of comparative studies of Western and non-Western, and schooled and non-schooled populations that have argued this point (e.g., Cole & Bruner, 1971; Cole, Gay, Glick, & Sharp, 1971; Laboratory of Comparative Human Cognition, 1983; Levine, 1989), contemporary psychologists rarely consider subtle sources of cultural or contextual influence on their interpretations of the research findings. Even seemingly benign research strategies, such as utilization of family dinner table conversations as a context for observing parent–child interaction, become suspect and misleading when they are applied to other cultural groups such as African-American families, as they impose traditional middle-class norms about family rhythms on a cultural group to whom such norms may not apply. Several ethnographic studies of black families (Heath, 1983; Ward, 1971) suggest a different normative pattern, in which daily family patterns do not include scheduled meal times—family members, friends, and relatives catch meals as they come and go throughout the course of the day. Moreover, dyadic interaction between mothers and children occurs relatively frequently, at least in southern and rural black families. Children are more often observers of adult interaction or are engaged in multiparty interactions with family, extended family, and fictive kin. Thus, the social context that researchers commonly use to observe family relations may be normative in some cultures but not in others. Only after researchers have determined that participants interpret the research setting and stimuli in the "expected" fashion, can they determine the extent to which observed group differences are true differences in the constructs assessed, rather than cultural differences in the interpretation of, or familiarity with, the research setting.

Within- versus Between-Group Research Designs

The utility of within- vs. between-group (comparative) designs is a pivotal research design issue for a culturally anchored methodology. The question of research design is already fixed, to some extent, by the definition of the research question. In within-group studies, researchers investigate phenomena of interest in the context of a single cultural community. In between-group studies, researchers investigate similarities and differences in phenomena across two or more cultural communities. Within-group designs have been criticized for their inability to determine the extent to which observed phenomena are unique to, or common across, cultural groups, but have been lauded for their attention to normative processes within a cultural group. Between-group studies have been criticized for encouraging a deficit orientation (one group is compared to a normative, "adjusted" group), adherence to a single universal standard, and inattention to the meaning of differences or their functional utility within particular cultural contexts (Howard & Scott, 1981).

Between- and within-group designs each have strengths and limitations; the decision about which to use ultimately depends on the overarching aims of the research project and the specific questions that it is intended to address. Between-group studies are most useful when they are theoretically grounded and used to illuminate social and psychological processes that occur both between *and* within groups. Maton and his colleagues' (1996) examination of cultural and contextual influences on support processes among African-American and Caucasian youths in varying contexts is a thoughtful example of the sorts of methods to which we refer. Rather than simply comparing outcomes between the two groups of youth, Maton et al. (1996) tested different predictions about the influence of support for the two groups of youth based on each group's sociocultural and historical values, as well as on the source of social support. Too often, only main effects models are tested (i.e., comparing two or more groups on a particular outcome variable), with no attention to the meaning of the observed differences or to the mediating processes through which they occur. Moreover, researchers rarely establish the equivalence of concepts, measures, and tasks across groups *before* interpreting the results. By investigating the extent to which two or more groups differ from one another in the patterns of relationships among variables, and not just on an outcome measure, between-group studies can facilitate an understanding of how cultural and ecological contexts moderate relationships between predictor and criterion variables.

For example, Mitchell and Beals (1997, Chapter 11, this volume) sampled adolescents from four different Native American communities made up of children from over 50 different tribes. Using structural equation modeling, they demonstrated the superiority of a two-factor model of positive and problem behavior, as opposed to a single factor model. More importantly, using a between-group analysis they discovered that the fit for the positive behavior construct was robust across all four Native American communities, and that substantial and important differences were evident in the item loadings for the problem behavior construct across the four communities. In our view, the next step for these authors, had they been aiming towards a culturally anchored perspective, would have been to search for the antecedents of these differences in item loadings within the cultures of the four Native American communities they studied.

A within-group study is the design of choice when either: (a) the design question is solely oriented toward a within-culture understanding, (b) conceptual equivalence across cultures is not possible, or (c) conceptual equivalence exists, but measurement equivalence does not. In the first instance, when researchers are simply interested in understanding phenomena within their unique cultural contexts, between-group designs are irrelevant to the research problem. The research program described by Hughes and Dumont (1993, Chapter 10, this volume) provides an illustration of the second instance, in which conceptual equivalence is lacking. Their research focuses on relationships between prejudice, discrimination, and child socialization within African-American families. Parallel phenomena are probably far less salient to nonminority groups, and thus, a between-group study would be inappropriate. In the third instance, hypothetical at this point, when a construct means the same thing to two or more groups (e.g., competence as the ability to function optimally in one's local environment) but the mapping of indicators to the construct is variant (different skills in different cultural contexts), between-group (comparative) studies inevitably promote the sort of deficit perspective that has traditionally characterized the literature on ethnic minority and other under-represented groups (French & D'Augelli, 2002; Howard & Scott, 1981).

Using Multiple Methods

A culturally anchored perspective draws attention to the ongoing debate regarding the relative utility of qualitative versus quantitative research methodologies. Qualitative research provides what anthropologists refer to as an *emic* perspective—one in which research questions emerge within the context of researchers' interactions within the group. In contrast, quantitative methods are most closely associated with the *etic* perspective, which relies on researchers' predetermined concepts and hypotheses. Combining the two methods enables researchers to learn about nonmainstream cultural groups and, at the same time, to utilize methodologies that are necessary for hypothesis testing. In recent years, the literature has begun to reflect just such a fruitful conjunction of methods (for example, see Campbell, 1995; Hines, 1993; Maton, 1993).

We feel it important to reiterate that for all good research, the method should emanate from the research questions (rather than the reverse), but this principle holds special import for culturally anchored research. We do not yet have an extensive knowledge base about psychological processes within nonmainstream cultures. Until we do, an approach is needed that provides the appropriate cultural lens for problem definition and concept/measurement development. Quantitative studies, however, maintain integrity according to traditional scientific criteria, and are needed both for building knowledge and maintaining a dialogue with other disciplines.

Data Analytic Strategies

As Rapkin and Luke (1993) point out, capturing the diversity of cultural phenomena may require methods of data analysis that can identify unique, rich, and meaningful descriptions of complex behavioral patterns. The search for statistical interactions between phenomena of interest and cultural/contextual variables is critical for the development of a culturally grounded knowledge base, because it encourages a focus on similarity and difference in processes as well as outcomes. Steinberg and his colleagues' (1995) finding that authoritative parenting has different effects on academic achievement depending on the youth's ethnic background, reminds us of both the danger of overgeneralization, and the opportunities for exploration and learning that emerge when well-established findings fail to hold across cultural contexts. Kaufman, Gregory, and Stephan (1990) found that when in the statistical minority in their classroom, Anglo children were perceived by teachers as responding with greater aggression and Hispanic children as responding with greater moodiness; these differences were attributed to cultural differences in conflict resolution styles. In this regard, however, it is critical to remember that in field research, unlike controlled laboratory or laboratory analogue studies, interaction effects are extremely difficult to detect, particularly when the interaction is not manifested in the form of a distinct crossover effect (McClelland & Judd, 1993). Researchers must compensate by obtaining large samples, over sampling extreme observations, or accepting higher rates of Type I errors (which will increase statistical power, Cohen, 1992) whenever these solutions are feasible.

ADVANCING A CULTURALLY ANCHORED METHODOLOGY

For those committed to the development and use of culturally anchored methods, we recommend the following guidelines:

1. Engage multiple and diverse stakeholders—community residents, power brokers, funders, scientists—in the formulation of the question or phenomenon of interest, salient constructs, definition of the population(s), design, and methods.

2. Make every effort to ensure that if you use only a single proxy variable to define a cultural group, it is a meaningful and valid one. Better yet, define the population with a rich nomological network of salient manifest indicators.
3. Establish both conceptual and measurement equivalence before conducting a between-group investigation. Even when a comparative study is contraindicated and a within-group study is undertaken, assure the meaningfulness of the concepts and the appropriateness and sensitivity of their measurement operations.
4. Employ a within-group design when it is isomorphic with the question(s) of interest.
5. Search for the underlying processes and mechanisms that shed the most light on the phenomena of interest.
6. Do not restrict your modes of measurement or data analysis techniques. Choose, combine, and develop new methods and techniques not only tailored to the question of interest but also to the cultural nuances of the population of concern.

With the evolution of a culturally anchored methodology, we can approximate the fulfillment of our promise to build a firmer base of knowledge about diverse cultural groups for the sake of both knowledge and action.

REFERENCES

Bachman, J. G., & O'Malley, P. M. (1984). Yea saying, nay saying, and going to extremes: Black-white differences in response styles. *Public Opinion Quarterly, 48*, 491–509.

Bennett, C. C., Anderson, L. S., Cooper, S., Hassol, L., Klein, D. C., & Rosenblum, G. (Eds.), (1966). *Community psychology: A report of the Boston conference on the education of psychologists for community mental health.* Boston: Boston University Press.

Bernal, G., & Enchautegui-de-Jesus, N. (1994). Latinos and Latinas in community psychology: A review of the literature. *American Journal of Community Psychology, 22*, 531–557.

Betancourt, H., & Lopez, S. R. (1993). The study of culture, ethnicity, and race in American Psychology. *American Psychologist, 48*, 629–637.

Boykin, A. W., & Toms, F. (1985). Black child socialization: A conceptual framework. In H. M. McAdoo & J. McAdoo (Eds.), *Black children: Social, educational, and parental environments* (pp. 33–51). Beverly Hills: Sage.

Burton, L. M., Allison, K. W., & Obedelliah, D. (1995). Social context and adolescence: Perspectives on development among inner-city African-American teens. In L. J. Crocker, & A. C. Crouter (Eds.), *Pathways through adolescence: Individual development in relation to social contexts* (pp. 119–138). Hillsdale, NJ: Lawrence Erlbaum Associates.

Campbell, D. T. (1995). The postpositivist, nonfoundational, hermeneutic epistemology exemplified in the works of Donald W. Fiske. In P. E. Shrout, & S. T. Fiske (Eds.), *Personality research, methods, and theory: A festschrift honoring Donald W. Fiske* (pp. 13–27). Hillsdale, NJ: Lawrence Erlbaum Associates.

Cohen, J. (1992). A power primer. *Psychological Bulletin, 112*, 155–159.

Cole, M., & Bruner, J. (1971). Cultural differences and inferences about psychological processes. *American Psychologist, 26,* 867–876.

Cole, M., Gay, J., Glick, J. A., & Sharp, D. W. (1971). *The cultural context of learning and thinking.* New York: Basic Books.

French, S. E., & D'Augelli, A. R. (2002). Diversity in community psychology. In T. A. Revenson, A. R. D'Augelli, S. E. French, D. L. Hughes, D. Livert, E. Seidman, M. Shinn, & H. Yoshikawa (Eds.), *A quarter century of community psychology: Readings from the American Journal of Community Psychology* (pp. 65–77). New York: Kluwer Academic/Plenum Publishers.

Heath, S. B. (1983). *Ways with words: Language, life, and work communities and classrooms.* Cambridge, England: Cambridge University Press.

Hines, A. M. (1993). Linking qualitative and quantitative methods in cross-cultural survey research: Techniques from cognitive science. *American Journal of Community Psychology, 21,* 729–746.

Howard, A., & Scott, R. A. (1981). The study of minority groups in complex societies. In R. H. Munroe, R. L. Munroe, & B. B. Whiting (Eds.), *Handbook of cross-cultural human development* (pp.113–152). New York: Guilford.

Hughes, D. L., & DuMont, K. (1993). Using focus groups to facilitate culturally anchored research. *American Journal of Community Psychology, 21,* 775–806.

Hughes, D. L., Seidman, E., & Williams, N. (1993). Cultural phenomena and the research enterprise: Toward a culturally-anchored methodology. *American Journal of Community Psychology, 21,* 687–704.

Hui, C. H., & Triandis, H. C. (1989). Effects of culture and response format on extreme response style. *Journal of Cross-Cultural Psychology, 20,* 296–309.

Kaufman, K., Gregory, W. L., & Stephan, W. G. (1990). Maladjustment in statistical minorities within ethnically balanced classrooms. *American Journal of Community Psychology, 18,* 757–765.

Knight, G. P., Virdin, L. M., Ocampo, K. A., & Roosa, M. (1994). An examination of cross-ethnic equivalence of measures of negative life events and mental health among Hispanic and Anglo-American children. *American Journal of Community Psychology, 22,* 767–783.

Kuhn, T. S. (1962). *The structure of scientific revolutions.* Chicago: The University of Chicago Press.

Laboratory of Comparative Cognition (1983). Culture and cognitive development. In P. H. Mussen (Ed.), *Handbook of Child Psychology, 4th Ed., Vol. 1* (pp. 296–356). New York: John Wiley.

Levine, R. A. (1989). Cultural environments in child development. In W. Damon (Ed.) *Child development today and tomorrow* (pp. 52–68). San Francisco: Jossey Bass.

Livert, D., & Hughes, D. L. (2002). The ecological paradigm: Persons in settings. In T. A. Revenson, A. R. D'Augelli, S. E. French, D. L. Hughes, D. Livert, E. Seidman, M. Shinn, & H. Yoshikawa (Eds.), *A quarter century of community psychology: Readings from the American Journal of Community Psychology* (pp. 51–63). New York: Kluwer Academic/Plenum Publishers.

Marin, G., & Marin, B. V. (1991). *Research with Hispanic populations.* Beverly Hills, CA: Sage.

Maruyama, M. (1983). Cross-cultural perspectives on social and community change. In E. Seidman (Ed.), *Handbook of social intervention* (pp. 33–47). Beverly Hills, CA: Sage.

Maton, K. I. (1993). A bridge between cultures: Linked ethnographic-empirical methodology for culture-anchored research. *American Journal of Community Psychology, 21,* 747–774.

Maton, K. I., Teti, D. M., Corns, K. M., Vieira-Baker, C. C., Lavine, J. R. (1996). Cultural specificity of support sources, correlates and contexts: Three studies of African-American and Caucasian youth. *American Journal of Community Psychology, 24,* 551–587.

McClelland, G. H., & Judd, C. M. (1993). Statistical difficulties of detecting interactions and moderator effects. *Psychological Bulletin, 114,* 376–390.

Mitchell, C. M., & Beals, J. (1997). The structure of problem and positive behavior among American Indian adolescents: Gender and community differences. *American Journal of Community Psychology, 25,* 257–288.

Rapkin, B. D., & Luke, D. A. (1993). Cluster analysis in community research: Epistemology and practice. *American Journal of Community Psychology, 21,* 247–277.

Rappaport, J. (1976). *Community psychology: Values, research, and action.* New York: Holt, Rinehart, and Winston.

Reiff, R. (1968). The need for a body of knowledge in Community Psychology. *American Psychologist, 23,* 524–531.

Seidman, E. (1978). Justice, values and social science: Unexamined premises. In R. J. Simon (Ed.), *Research in law and sociology* (pp. 175–200). Greenwich, CT: JAI Press.

Seidman, E. (1983). Unexamined premises of social problem-solving. In E. Seidman (Ed.). *Handbook of social intervention.* Beverly Hills, CA: Sage.

Seidman, E. (1988). Back to the future, community psychology: Unfolding a theory of social intervention. *American Journal of Community Psychology, 16,* 3–24.

Steinberg, L., Darling, N. E., Fletcher, A. C., Brown, B. B., & Dornbursch, S. M. (1995). Authoritative parenting and adolescent adjustment: An ecological journey. In P. Moen, G. H. Elder, & K. Luscher (Eds.), *Examining lives in context: Perspectives on the ecology of human development* (pp. 423–466). Washington, DC: American Psychological Association.

Trickett, E. J. (1996). A future for community psychology: The contexts of diversity and the diversity of contexts. *American Journal of Community Psychology, 24,* 209–234.

Trickett, E. J., Watts, R., & Birman, D. (1993). Human diversity and community psychology: Still hazy after all these years. *Journal of Community Psychology, 21,* 264–279.

Vega, W. A. (1992). Theoretical and pragmatic implications of cultural diversity for community research. *American Journal of Community Psychology, 20,* 375–391.

Ward, M. C. (1971). *Them children: A study in language and learning.* Prospect Heights, IL: Waveland Press.

10

Using Focus Groups to Facilitate Culturally Anchored Research

Diane L. Hughes and Kimberly DuMont

Scholars have acknowledged the need to anchor scientific knowledge about social and psychological processes in the norms, values, and experiences of the particular population under study. This article describes how focus groups can be incorporated into the planning stages of a research program to facilitate these goals. After a brief overview of the central components of focus group research, an example from a program of research involving dual-earner African American families is used to as an illustration. The article describes how (a) the identification of cultural knowledge and (b) access to the language participants use to think and talk about a topic can help researchers formulate a conceptual framework, identify important constructs, and develop appropriate instruments for assessing constructs. Some strengths and limitations of focus group research are discussed.

Community psychologists and other social scientists have underscored the limitations of traditional scientific paradigms for research with diverse cultural groups. For instance, Bronfenbrenner's (1979) discussion of the "social address" model and Howard and Scott's (1981) discussion of "deficiency formulations" each criticize the comparative frameworks, which

Originally published in the *American Journal of Community Psychology, 21*(6) (1993): 775–806.

Ecological Research to Promote Social Change: Methodological Advances from Community Psychology, edited by Tracey A. Revenson et al. Kluwer Academic/Plenum Publishers, New York, 2002.

dominate the literature on ethnic minorities in the United States. They argue that comparative frameworks simply describe between-group differences on particular outcome variables of interest, providing little insight into the range of social and psychological processes that occur within a cultural group. Other scholars have questioned the validity of studies utilizing constructs and measures developed in one cultural group to understand phenomenon in another (Boykin, 1979). Cultural norms, values, and experiences influence the relevance of a set of constructs to respondents, the range of behaviors and ideas that are valid indicators of the constructs, and how respondents interpret items employed to assess them (Hui & Triandis, 1989; Marsella & Kameoka, 1989). Inattention to these sorts of issues can undermine the accuracy of scientific knowledge about both intragroup processes and between-group similarities and differences.

These criticisms underscore the need for improved strategies for research on social and psychological processes within diverse populations. For social research to be good science, sound scientific methods must be merged with knowledge of, and respect for, a group's spirit. However, such a union requires conceptual and methodological tools. These tools should facilitate researchers' knowledge about the experiences and perspectives of the group under study, as well as the development of research instruments that are useful and relevant.

Focus group research is one qualitative method that can be used as such a tool. Focus groups are in-depth group interviews employing relatively homogenous groups to provide information around topics specified by researchers. They have several strengths that make them particularly useful for facilitating research that reflects the social realities of a cultural group. Focus groups provide researchers with direct access to the language and concepts participants use to structure their experiences and to think and talk about a designated topic. Within-group homogeneity prompts focus group participants to elaborate stories and themes that help researchers understand how participants structure and organize their social world. In their reliance on social interaction, focus groups can also help researchers identify cultural knowledge that is shared among group members as well as to appreciate the range of different experiences individuals within a group may have. Each of these brings researchers closer to a phenomenological understanding of a cultural group. Such an understanding can help investigators ask better research questions and develop the measures needed to study them.

In this regard, focus groups have advantages over quantitative and other qualitative methods that community psychologists commonly use. Unlike quantitative methods, they emphasize participants' perspectives and allow the researcher to explore the nuances and complexities of participants' attitudes and experiences. As well, they have unique strengths over other qualitative methods (Morgan, 1988; Morgan & Spanish, 1984). Unlike in-depth individual interviews, they permit researchers to observe social interaction between participants around specific topics (Morgan, 1988; Morgan & Krueger, 1993; Morgan & Spanish, 1984). Unlike naturalistic observational methods, they provide a mechanism by which the researcher can structure the content of such interaction. As Morgan (1988) noted, focus groups are neither as strong as participant observation in their ability to observe phenomena in naturalistic settings, nor as strong as in-depth individual interviews in providing a rich understanding of participants' knowledge, but they are better at *combining* these two goals than either of the two techniques alone. Therein, focus groups provide a body of material that differs in form and content from that provided by other research methods.

This article describes how focus groups can facilitate culturally sensitive research. In the sections that follow, a brief overview of the essential components of focus group research is provided. Then, using an example from a research program involving African American parents in dual-earner families, an illustration of how focus groups can facilitate culturally anchored research is provided.

ESSENTIALS OF FOCUS GROUP RESEARCH

A focus group study is designed to accomplish a particular research objective. Thus, careful attention to the central components of the method—including sample selection, instrumentation, and data analysis—helps ensure that the study's research objectives are met. This section briefly describes the central components of a focus group study.

The Sample

Focus groups are commonly conducted among a small nonrepresentative sample of participants who share one or more characteristics that are of interest to the researcher. The characteristics participants share may be demographic (e.g., age, ethnicity, gender), situational (e.g., employment status, health status), behavioral (e.g., substance abusers), ideological (e.g., political party membership), or any combination of these. The sample selection is purposive and based more on suitability and availability, rather than on representativeness (O'Brien, 1993). Thus, focus group samples are often small and nonrepresentative, allowing for in-depth description of phenomena but not for generalization to a larger population.

Each group is typically composed of 6 to 12 participants (Morgan, 1988; Stewart & Shamdasani, 1990). Within this range, appropriate group size depends upon the aims of the study. Small groups facilitate in-depth exploration of issues, since participants each have more time to share their experiences and perspectives. Larger groups are appropriate when the aim of the research is to collect a breadth of experiences and perspectives, since each participant's experiences and perspectives are unique (Morgan, 1988).

In designing a focus group study, the composition of the group requires special attention. Many researchers suggest that groups be composed of strangers, since groups composed of acquaintances are more likely to focus on a narrow set of concerns (Basch, 1987; Stewart & Shamdasani, 1990). More important, intragroup homogeneity is believed to facilitate rapport among respondents (Knodel, 1993; Morgan, 1988; Stewart & Shamdasani, 1990). Participants with similar characteristics may more easily identify with each others experiences (Knodel, 1993; Morgan, 1988). Homogeneity also reduces the likelihood of mixing participants who have sharp differences in opinions or behaviors (Knodel, 1993). Finally, heterogeneity can result in social status differences within a group. Lower status participants may defer to the perspectives of higher status participants (Knodel, 1993; Morgan, 1988; Stewart & Shamdasani, 1990), yielding biased focus group data. Thus, although focus groups may be used to compare and contrast different groups, researchers suggest that comparisons be made across homogenous groups rather than within heterogenous groups.

The number of groups needed to accomplish the aims of the study depends on the problem that is to be addressed and available time and resources. At a minimum, two groups are needed for each subset of the population the researcher intends to study, to ensure that the focus group data do not simply reflect the idiosyncracies of a particular group (Basch, 1987; Morgan, 1988). Some investigators recommend that researchers conduct focus groups until groups are producing redundant information (Krueger, 1988). This typically requires three to four groups per subset of the population under study.

The Interview Schedule

The typical instrument for a focus group study is a discussion guide. The guide establishes a set of issues for the group to discuss and is used to channel the discussion towards accomplishing the research objectives. The guide may be more or less structured, depending on the purposes of the study. Exploratory studies call for relatively unstructured discussion guides that specify the broad topics participants are to discuss but not the order in which topics are introduced. Unstructured discussion guides facilitate insight into participants' thinking by allowing them to discuss any dimension of a topic they wish. In contrast, structured discussion guides usually specify the order in which topics are introduced and include probes for specific types of information. They are most appropriate in studies designed to obtain information on a particular aspect of a topic. For example, in studies designed to compare differently defined groups, structured guides ensure that specific points are discussed or that similar points are discussed across groups (Krueger, 1988; Morgan, 1988; Stewart & Shamdasani, 1990).

In either case, the discussion guide should facilitate a synergistic discussion and interaction around a particular set of issues. Simply reading lists of questions to participants produces a tedious focus group session and encourages participants to talk to the moderator more so than to each other (Morgan, 1988; Stewart & Shamdasani, 1990). Morgan (1988) suggested, that researchers create discussion guides by first preparing a full list of questions and then organizing the list into an ordered set of topics (see also Stewart and Shamdasani, 1990, for an in-depth discussion of framing focus group questions). Generating a list of topics rather than a set of questions allows the moderator to use participants' experiences to probe or introduce new topics, facilitating a more fluid and natural discussion.

The Moderator

The moderator is the primary link between the goals of the research and the quality of the focus group data. The moderator channels the discussion to meet the objectives of the research, a role that involves several divergent skills (Krueger, 1988; Morgan, 1988). For instance, the moderator must create an atmosphere conducive to self-disclosure by building rapport within the group, conveying interpersonal sensitivity and diplomacy, and speaking in language that is comfortable to participants. The moderator must also manage group dynamics by encouraging quieter participants to share their perspectives and experiences, ensuring that outspoken participants do not bias the discussion, and encouraging respondents to elaborate perspectives that differ from the predominant one. At the same time, the moderator must remain neutral and nondirective: Leading probes and follow-up questions, as well as verbal and nonverbal cues, may signal participants to focus on certain aspects of a topic and not others. They also encourage participants to share experiences and attitudes believed to support the moderator's perspective.

The moderator's most important role is to track the focus group discussion in order to ensure that it flows smoothly and produces the desired information (Basch, 1987; Morgan, 1988). Such tracking involves storing perspectives and later using them to reintroduce a topic, introduce a new topic, or pursue an issue in greater depth. It also involves gauging when participants have adequately elaborated a theme and when more information is needed. Finally, tracking involves evaluating the extent to which there is consensus or disagreement among participants regarding a particular topic.

The Setting and Equipment

The physical setting for the focus group interview and the quality of audio taping equipment are critical to the success of each session and deserve special mention because they are so readily overlooked. Locations that are convenient and easy to find ensure adequate participation, saving the researcher time and money (Krueger, 1988; Basch, 1987). Since audiotapes are the primary form of data that focus group sessions produce the researcher should also take special care to ensure sound quality. Poorly recorded tapes result in large chunks of inaudible material. Inaudible material is difficult to transcribe, and valuable information may be lost in the process. Quality equipment is a worthwhile investment, since insensitive equipment is prone to miss softly spoken comments and to pick up background noise (Krueger, 1988).

The Focus Group Data

Focus group data consists of moderator notes and audiotapes from each focus group session. However, because the data consist of group dialogue, it is distinct from that derived from surveys or individual interviews. Accordingly, it is also more tedious to manage than that derived from individual interviews.

An important characteristic of focus group data is that groups, rather than individuals within groups, are the unit of analysis (Krueger, 1988; Morgan, 1988; Stewart & Shamdasani, 1990). That is, although identifying redundant experiences and perspectives within and across groups can provide some useful information, data from individuals within a single focus group session are not independent. Thus, it is important to remember that data from individuals within a focus group session cannot be treated in the same manner as data from individual interviews with the same number of respondents. Group participants cue each other to frame events in particular ways, and to focus on some aspects of a topic and not others. Thus, it is critical to look for convergence in emergent themes across a sample of focus groups, rather than across participants within a group, to draw accurate conclusions.

An additional characteristic of focus group data is that, unlike survey data, focus group data consist of words and, unlike in-depth individual interviews, focus group data consist of group dialogue. Thus, although focus group data can provide rich insight into the phenomenon under study, coding it is a time-consuming and sometimes ambiguous task. For instance, a single exchange may be quite long, containing numerous themes. Categorizing themes is a highly subjective endeavor, since the distinctions between them is often blurred. Further, different participants use different words to describe the same phenomenon; it can be difficult to judge the extent to which two participants are actually relaying similar perspectives and world views. Finally, in a group context, participants usually intend more than they actually say. Thus, the interpretation of participants dialogue requires researchers to tie the explicit content of a statement to its connotative meaning.

Researchers use many strategies to analyze focus group data. These range from simply listening to tapes, to using cut and paste techniques, to constructing hand-written charts and tables, to computerized text analysis. Computerized text analysis programs have made focus group research feasible for investigators with limited time and resources (Knodel, 1993; Stewart & Shamdasani, 1990). Among those commonly used are The Ethnograph (Seidel, Kjolseth, & Seymour, 1988), TEXTPACK V (Mohler & Zull, 1984), and the Key-Word-in Context Bibliographic Indexing Program (Popko, 1980). Decisions about the unit of analysis within transcripts (e.g., words, phrases, sentences, paragraphs, themes), the coding schemes employed, and the extent of analysis each depend upon the research objectives. In later sections we describe our approach to analysis of focus group data. Readers are referred to Krippendorf (1980), Miles and Huberman (1984), and Weber (1985) for a full treatment of content analysis. Stewart and Shamdasani (1990) and Morgan (1993) discuss the analysis of focus group data specifically.

This brief overview of the essentials of focus group research was intended to introduce unfamiliar readers to the technique. Several comprehensive accounts are available to those who may be interested in planning and conducting a focus group study (Krueger, 1988; Morgan, 1988, 1993; Stewart & Shamdasani, 1990).

A RESEARCH EXAMPLE

In this section, an example from a program of research examining work and parenting issues in African American families is used to illustrate how focus groups can facilitate culturally sensitive research. To begin, a brief overview of the larger research project is provided.

Overview of the Research

The program of research from which the example is taken investigates characteristics of parents' jobs as they influence child socialization in African American dual-earner families. In particular, the research examines the ways in which parents' efforts to orient their children towards race relations (termed *racial socialization*) may be influenced by a range of race-related stressors that they are likely to experience in their occupational roles (termed *racial job stressors*). The primary study consists of structured interviews with a community-based sample of African American parents and their children.

The conceptual framework that guides the study is founded upon Kohn's research on relationships between occupational values and child-rearing practices (Kohn, 1969; Kohn & Schooler, 1973, 1978). Briefly, Kohn suggested that parents come to value skills and behaviors that enable them to function effectively in their occupational roles. In turn, they transmit these values to children in the process of socialization. It should be noted that Kohn's work focused primarily on how job autonomy and task complexity influence parents' disciplinary practices. However, in the present research program, it is hypothesized that the processes Kohn proposed may link parents' exposure to racial job stressors and their racial socialization practices. That is, African American parents continue to learn about modes of interracial contact, and about the structure and content of racial bias and discrimination, through their occupational experiences. In turn, African American parents may come to value particular ways of negotiating racial issues in the social world and transmit these values to their children in the process of socialization.

An important impetus behind this program of research is that the experiences, concerns, and perspectives of ethnic minority families have received little attention in the work–family literature, despite psychologists' increased interest in relationships between work and family (e.g., Crosby, 1987; Piotrkowski, 1979; Voydanoff, 1980). Thus, little is known about how the stressors associated with minority status in the workplace may influence family processes generally or about how such stressors shape parents' racial socialization practices in particular. In a similar manner, there is little empirical information about how African American parents' racial socialization practices are structured or about the factors that influence them. Thus, the quantitative study was designed to address these sorts of gaps in the social science literature.

When there is little prior research in an area, as is the case here, focus groups can be used to help the researcher to formulate a research model and to develop instruments that are appropriate to the population and phenomenon under study. Focus group dialogues allow researchers to capture the in-depth contextual detail that facilitates an understanding of a group's experiences and perspectives. Without such an understanding, the theoretical model guiding the research may be misspecified. For instance, researchers may overlook essential components of a groups experiences, resulting in interpretations that distort the social realities of the group. In addition, because focus groups give researchers direct access to participants' language and experiences, they can facilitate the development of survey instruments that reflect these and are therefore appropriate to the population and phenomenon under study (Wolff, Knodel, & Sittitrai, 1993).

The objectives of the focus groups conducted as part of the program of research parallel the particular strengths of focus group research described above. The primary goal of the focus groups was to understand, from participants' perspectives, how being African American shaped their experiences as workers and parents. A second objective was to develop instruments to assess two constructs that are central to the study: racial job stressors and racial socialization. After a brief description of how the focus groups were structured, the following section describes the ways in which focus groups facilitated these objectives.

Conducting the Focus Groups

Six focus groups were conducted among a total of 43 African American parents. Participants were recruited by telephone from communities in the New York Metropolitan area using a combination of snowball sampling and a data base provided by an ethnic marketing agency. Small groups, with six to eight participants per group, were organized in order to facilitate close rapport among participants and in-depth exploration of phenomenon.

In all groups, participants were full-time employed African American parents living in dual-earner families. However, since we were interested in exploring different kinds of occupational experiences, groups were homogeneous in terms of occupational category. As noted earlier, researchers warn against sharp intragroup differences in social status, as well as in the perspectives and experiences of group participants. Thus, in three of the groups, participants worked in blue-collar occupations as maintenance workers, hospital orderlies, food service workers, postal carriers, and so forth. These participants lived in homogenous middle-class African American communities. In the other three groups, participants held white-collar jobs as lawyers, marketing executives, engineers, bank managers, and so forth. Most of these participants lived in predominantly white upper middle-class communities. Although the intragroup homogeneity in occupational category was deliberate, the confounding of occupational category and neighborhood variables (e.g., ethnic homogeneity, social class) was unanticipated. The confound underscored the need to stratify the sample for the quantitative study by both occupational category and neighborhood ethnicity; this prompted us to develop strategies for doing so.

The moderator began each of the focus group sessions by describing the purposes of the session, providing ground rules for the discussion, and asking participants to introduce themselves. In particular, participants were told that the purpose of the group was to learn about their experiences as workers and as parents in order to identify issues that would be important to include in a larger study among African American parents.

After the opening statements, the moderator introduced the various topics for discussion, following a relatively structured discussion guide. The guide specified the order in which topics were introduced and specific topics that were to be covered in each group. The structured discussion guide facilitated a comparison of the themes and issues that emerged within the blue-collar and white-collar focus groups. As is common in focus group research, the discussion guide moved from the general to the specific in order to prevent premature narrowing of participants' dialogue. The guide specified an initial focus on work rewards and stresses and then narrowed in on topics related to race relations in the work environment. The structure of the discussion of parenting was similar; the guide specified an initial focus on the rewards and stresses of parenting and then narrowed in on special issues involved in parenting African American children. These sorts of general introductions put the topics of work and parenting on the table without cuing participants to our particular interest in race relations.

Each group discussion lasted about $1^{3}/_{4}$ hours. At the end of each discussion, the moderator distributed a set of items that had been generated to assess "racial job stressors" and "racial socialization." Participants were asked to complete the items and to comment on the clarity of item wording, as well as on the relevance of items to their experiences. Participants were also asked to discuss various strategies for recruiting subjects for the quantitative study. At the close of each session, the moderator thanked participants and they were given $35 as a token of appreciation for their time.

Understanding Race-Related Perspectives and Experiences

As mentioned previously, one goal in conducting the focus groups was to understand, from participants' perspectives, how being African American shaped their experiences as workers and parents. Although the discussion guide emanated from a particular conceptual framework, we were interested in the structure and content of racial bias, discrimination, and racial socialization, as these emerged in participants' own descriptions. Of particular interest was dialogue between participants in each of the focus group sessions, rather than between the moderator and each participant, about the meaning of race for participants' roles as workers and parents. Such dialogue allows researchers to view phenomenon through the lenses of group members, which can, in turn, facilitate their ability to frame relevant research questions and to identify particular concepts that are relevant to study.

The organization of the focus group data for this study was guided by an emerging literature on shared cultural knowledge. According to contemporary scholars, knowledge consists of concepts that individuals acquire by way of testing hypotheses about features of the social environment (Hecht, Collier, & Ribeau, 1993; Kreckel, 1981; Shweder & LeVine, 1984). Kreckel (1981) further distinguished between *common* knowledge and *shared* knowledge. In her view, common knowledge consists of similarities in concepts that individuals from similar cultural backgrounds acquire *separately*, due to similarities in socialization processes and to the increased likelihood that the process of hypothesis testing yields similar information. Shared knowledge emerges through social interaction as individuals test their constructions of the world through each other, identifying general principles that govern their common experiences. Shared knowledge cannot be held by individuals who have had no contact, even if their experiences are similar. As described in this section, we attempted to distinguish common knowledge that participants each brought to the group from shared knowledge that was negotiated and displayed during the course of group interaction. Redundant themes that emerged in participants' narratives within and across groups were classified as common knowledge. In contrast, consensual models that were developed within each group via participants' recognition of commonalities in their experiences and perspectives were classified as shared knowledge.

To facilitate the identification of common and shared knowledge, participants' narratives were categorized into one of three narrative forms—descriptive statements, stories, and abstract generalizations—using the framework Polanyi (1985) proposed for analyzing cultural stories. These three narrative forms each provide unique information that contribute to researchers' understanding of a phenomenon of interest. Though they are described separately, it is important to note that they were embedded in one another throughout the focus group transcripts.

Descriptive Statements

Descriptive statements are narratives in which participants characterize enduring actions or states of affairs that persist over time (Polanyi, 1985). The bulk of the focus group transcripts consisted of such descriptive statements. In response to queries made by the moderator and others in the group, participants described in detail the nature of their occupational roles; their relationships with supervisors, co-workers, and clients; their perspectives on race relations in their work environments; their child-rearing practices, experiences, and concerns; and their children's knowledge about and experiences with race-relations. These descriptive statements were most common during the first 40 minutes or so of each focus group session, as participants described to others their individuals experiences and points of view.

In coding descriptive statements, the goal was to identify patterns and redundancies in participants' reports about their environments, so as to elucidate participants' common knowledge. To facilitate this goal, the initial coding system grouped descriptive statements according to similarities in their surface content, using codes that were close to the words participants used. For instance, references to the need to go around people and events were grouped in a category labeled "going around." References to rules for advancement in the work place that change for African Americans were grouped in a category labeled "changed rules." The process of summarizing descriptive statements generated over 30 such codes. To illustrate the structure of the coding process and what it can yield, Table I contains examples of this first-level coding. Included in the table are categories that were mentioned more than once across two or more groups.

The first-level coding facilitated an understanding of participants' common knowledge regarding race relations by ordering text and providing a bird's-eye view of the content of descriptive statements. It permitted us to count the number of times a phrase or theme emerged within and across groups. For instance, Table I shows that having lower level positions and being paid less for equal work were mentioned by multiple participants in each of the blue-collar focus groups but were mentioned less often in the white-collar focus groups. The reverse is true for other phenomenon, such as different performance standards for blacks and blocked opportunities. Encountering stereotypes about blacks and efforts to teach children about

Table I. First-Level Coding and Pattern Coding of Participants' Descriptive Statements[a]

	Blue-collar groups					White-collar groups				
	1	2	3	Example		4	5	6	Example	
Racial phenomenon at work										
Blacks have less desirable assignments	1	2	2	They [managers] don't have whites doing those types of things [cleaning bed pans]. Those are the dirty jobs. Those are our jobs.		0	0	0		
Blacks have lower level positions	4	2	3	Most of us black people have like maintenance jobs but like the higher class white people, they have higher positions and they don't, like, put any minorities in those types of jobs they have.		0	0	0		
Blacks get paid less for equal work	4	3	4	When you start a job, sometimes you might think the position you came for, you getting paid this much money. And then you might hear this guy got hired in the same position you got hired in and his check might not be the same as yours but more, as a white person.		0	0	0		
Overt discrimination*	9	7	9			0	0	0		
Different standards for blacks	0	0	0			4	5	4	The mediocre white guys could rise to the top at my job. The people that they select for promotion—it's not because they're particularly great, talented, this or that. They weren't the best and the brightest. They were just OK. Then when it got to black people—see black	

Table I. Continued

	Blue-collar groups				White-collar groups			
	1	2	3	Example	4	5	6	Example
Perceives blocked opportunity	0	0	0		3	3	1	people had to be super-black. They had to be like superman, had to have all the people skills, be the best everything. In terms of promotional opportunities, I look at certain blacks that are qualified and look at the black woman who used to sit next to me. She was a vice president who I thought would get a promotion. I thought she was just that qualified. And they've moved her off the business. I tend to start thinking "What is my future here? Where can I go?"
Glass ceiling	1	1	0	There's a few blacks in powerful positions but there's glass ceilings on how high they're going to let us at this time. It's already established that you're not gonna get but so far.	4	2	4	It's hard. I'm not really going to go any further. I've hit, in terms of management level, as far as I'm going to go. So, I'm saying, I'm there.
Covert discrimination*	1	1	0		11	10	9	
Encountering overt hostility from whites	6	5	5	I have black patients and they're sweet. They'll come and sit with you. White people [are more likely to say] "Hey! Hey" ... "Don't touch this! Don't touch that!"	0	0	0	

Category							Example
Name calling	1	4	3	0	0	0	The Caucasians will call us directly to our face "nigger this, nigger that." But we won't to them. It's not right to build up to their level and do the same thing their doing. *So you got to go around* that too.
Overt prejudice*	7	9	8	0	0	0	
Issues around being one of few blacks	2	0	0	6	7	9	There was this one situation when there were only 2 black males and like 40 white males. And so any time an incident would happen in the paper they come and ask you "What's your opinion?" You have to explain for any incident happen with somebody. / You walk into any of these corporations and you're maybe one of two or three. I've been in all these meetings in different organizations and I could probably count on my hands the meetings where there was another black face across the table from me. I know you've all seen it. When you have a point to make, it's like, people stop because first they want to see if you can put together a logical statement.
Encountering stereotypes about	5	3	2	2	1	2	In delivering mail, if you go upstairs and the woman is white and she looks through her peep hole and she should see a black brother ... right away she thinks "Oh, that can't be a letter carrier. He's out to mug me." So, therefore, she won't open the door and you're stuck with a package. And, you've wasted your time.
Subtle prejudice*	7	3	2	8	8	11	Orienting children towards race and race relations.

Table I. Continued

	Blue-collar groups				White-collar groups				
	1	2	3	Example	4	5	6	Example
Tries to teach child not to be biased in attitudes	6	3	3	I talk to them [children] about there's good and bad in all races. There's bad in all people period. So, you got to weed out and judge for yourself.	2	3	3	My husband strongly believes in teaching our kids street sense. He says a lot of his street smarts that he learned from hanging out with the brothers have helped him in the corporate world today. So we try to do a similar thing with our son. We have him in acourse at Essex Community College because we want him to start knowing the guys from Newark and some of these less fortunate kids.
Tries to teach child to treat everyone equal	3	7	6	I teach my kid to enjoy each and everyone. And everyone's a human being regardless of what color skin they are. Try to have fun with each and every person.	0	0	0	
Teaches cultural equivalence*	9	10	9		2	3	3	
Tries to teach child street knowledge	9	5	3	I also try to teach my kid street knowledge, you know? That's very important because in school they don't give you that type of education. They give you a lot of bull crap and really that's not helping in dealing with real life, with reality.	2	3	2	
Tries to protect child	6	2	0	I try to teach my child everything he				

Category				Example				Example
from the streets				needs to know to deal with the streets. And that's one of the hardest things todo. Cause the streets will change your child. So I try to make sure everything's safe for him.				
Teaching to negotiate the street*	15	7	3		1	0	1	I tell her, you know, people are gonna try to get in your way— to tell you you can't do what you think you can. Cause, you know, … and you just have to go around that, maneuver around it. Cause otherwise it's gonna hold you up, get in your way.
Teaches child about "going around"	1	2	2	I teach my daughter that there's gonna be people that's coming along that's gonna try to play games with her. And, she has to be aware of what's gonna happen. I teach her that she's got to know how to dodge obstacles that comes towards her because it's not always gonna be straight up.				
Teaches child he has to be better than whites	0	0	0		5	8	4	My won children, I tell them, you know, life's just not fair. And what I try to instill in my children is that they have to be better.
Teaches child about racial bias against blacks	4	3	4	I try to let my children know about racial bias. Its really not an, um, racist thing—actually pointing towards black and white. So, I try to let them know that also.	4	5	5	
Teaching to negotiate white environments*	5	5	6		10	13	10	I tell [my daughter] there's gonna be people out there who are going to dislike you—gonna think they're better than you—because of the color of your skin. She'll have to work that. But it's gonna happen.
	10							

Table I. Continued

	Blue-collar groups				White-collar groups			
	1	2	3	Example	4	5	6	Example
Exposes child to black culture	2	1	1	We go to the Shaumberg, Black expo, things like that.	5	3	4	We have books that we read them. We tell them about our culture and we do different things like Kwanza.
Teaching black history	2	3	2	I find myself thinking about entering the Muslim religion just so my son can get force fed what I didn't get and what he hasn't got yet. But he needs to get what only the Muslim religion can give him: Understanding of our history and pride in the black man.	5	4	4	I try to reinforce what the school does. Cause they do a lot around Dr. Martin Luther King and so-on. I tell him stories about the white water fountains, Rosa Parks. We're constantly taking about it.
Enhancing positive black identity	3	2	2	I teach my daughter we come from royalty. I teach her to be proud of her blackness. Cause we come from royalty. And if they [whites] don't see that, that's on them.	5	4	6	I'm constantly talking to them about building their self-esteem, getting them to feel comfortable with their features.
Teaching positive orientation towards black culture*	7	6	5		15	11	14	

*a*Rows marked with an asterisk summarize first-level codes.

racial bias were mentioned by multiple participants across both blue-collar and white-collar groups. Thus, this first level of coding permitted us to identify recurrent themes in participants' descriptive statements within and across groups.

An overarching goal in coding descriptive statements was not simply to count the number of times a specific theme emerged but rather to build an image of how African Americans perceive their race as influencing their roles as workers and parents. To facilitate this goal, first-level descriptive codes were grouped into a smaller number of overarching constructs, a process Miles and Huberman (1984) referred to as "pattern coding." Pattern coding requires that researchers go beneath the surface of descriptive codes, identifying subtle commonalities so as to reduce data yet amplify its meaning. In essence, the researcher must look for higher order threads that connect descriptive codes.

Pattern codes developed to summarize first-level descriptive codes are shown in the rows marked with an asterisk in Table I, again for the purposes of illustration; these pattern codes summarize a large volume of data using a small number of constructs which seem to adequately represent it. Further, pattern codes highlight general gestalts governing participants' descriptive statements. In particular, they highlight the differences between blue-collar and white-collar focus groups in the constructs underlying their common knowledge. For instance, pattern codes suggest that descriptions of work environments that are overtly discriminatory, antagonistic interracial contact, and parenting strategies that emphasize cultural equivalence and the importance of street knowledge were more common in blue-collar than in the white-collar focus groups. Descriptions of covert prejudice and discrimination at work, along with of parenting strategies that emphasize positive ethnic group orientation, were more common in white-collar than in blue-collar focus groups.

Stories

Stories are a narrative form through which individuals reconstruct particular events that took place at a particular time in the past, involving particular actors and particular settings (Polanyi, 1985). They are a central medium through which people reconstruct and interpret their experiences and are a primary channel for the transmission of cultural knowledge (Bruner, 1991; Howard, 1991; Mair, 1988; Plas, 1986; Polanyi, 1985). Stories are a fundamental element of social interaction and, in the focus groups described here, were used often by participants to achieve a variety of ends. For instance, participants used stories to amuse, inform, illustrate, and explain perspectives that were most readily justified by way of concrete examples.

The coding of participants' stories proceeded in a manner similar to that outlined for coding descriptive statements. That is, to identify patterns and redundancies (e.g., common knowledge), stories were grouped into first-level codes according to their surface content. The first-level coding categories were labeled with words that were close to the events participants described (e.g., "different rules for blacks," "stereotypes," "teaching children to respect all races"). Then, as in the coding of descriptive statements, pattern codes were generated to group first-level codes into a smaller number of themes, using the strategies that have been described.

Although the coding of participants' stories paralleled the coding of their descriptive statements, stories provided unique information. While descriptive statements provided access to the content of participants' common knowledge, stories elucidated the discrete events that shaped them. Thus, events described in stories seemed to be the basis upon which participants generated descriptive statements. For instance, consistent with descriptive statements, which suggest that blue-collar workers' common knowledge included recognition of overt discrimination and interracial hostility, 70% of the stories told across the blue-collar focus group indexed overt interracial hostility. Only one of the stories across the white-collar focus groups indexed such overt interracial hostility. In contrast, most of the stories in white-collar focus groups referenced more subtle forms of interpersonal racism such as ignorance about, as well as insensitivity to, black cultural phenomenon. Of the stories in the blue-collar focus groups 20% indexed subtle interpersonal racism. Thus, participants' stories and descriptive statements tend to converge around similar themes.

Stories not only illustrate specific events shaping participants' descriptive statements but also prompt participants to compare and contrast their experiences. The data produced by such comparisons were the initial impetus for the development of shared knowledge within a group and can only be garnered using methods that rely on group interaction (Morgan & Spanish, 1984). More specifically, comparisons prompt participants to synthesize the knowledge present in stories and then to elaborate more abstract summaries of their experiences and perspectives (Morgan, 1988; Morgan & Spanish, 1984). In terms of the conceptualization of knowledge previously described, stories facilitated the translation of common knowledge displayed by individuals into shared knowledge that was elaborated consensually by the group. This process is illustrated using a segment from one of our focus group transcripts. In this segment, the moderator is probing participants for descriptions of their perspective on race and race relations:

Example 1.

1 M: Have you ever experienced racism or prejudice at your
       workplace?
2 R1: No, not in the workplace. I have experienced it elsewhere
        though.
3 M: Where else? Where at?
4 R1: I was stopped ... I went into the service at 19 and by 21 I had me
        a car that was fairly brand new, about a year old. I was always
        pulled over by the cops. I was young, I was black, and I was in
        a poor neighborhood, South Bronx, with a car. And I guess they
        pulled me over—I know they pulled me over—cause they know
        I didn't make this by earning it, you know. Why they pulled me
        over was: "this guy dealing drugs or he know somebody but he
        stole this car."
5 R2: [If you're white] You're allowed to have a car. They pulled over
        Branford Marsalis with his BMW.
6 R3: Right!
7 R4: I was riding with a girl who was white and the cop stopped me.
        I had a new car. He wanted the registration and insurance and
        everything else. I said, "Well, what's the problem? Why did you
        stop me?"
8 R3: [Me], my father and a white kid one time going down town. The
        cops pull us over. Spread eagle ... the whole nines. He [father]
        said, like, "What's this all about?" [The police said] "Uh, we got
        a report. Two black guys and a white guy robbed."
9 R5: I was frisked up. I was in the car with my mom before and they
        like, you know, I just had problems.
10 R6: Yeah, I've experienced that. Now what's the problem officer?
         "We just got a report ..."
11 R3: Yeah!
12 R1: That's part of being a black man in NYC.
13 R4: Right!

In this segment participants describe their perception that different rules are applied to African Americans than to white Americans. Being pulled over by the authorities was a familiar and shared experience. Each story was less fully elaborated than the next, suggesting that focus group participants could draw on their common knowledge to complete each story themselves. Such a phenomenon could not be detected using individual-level data collection methods.

Of particular interest in this segment, and in the many others like it which appear in the focus group transcripts, is the pattern of emerging consensus within the group regarding the meaning of being African American for one's social experiences. The story told in Exchange 4 is the initial stimulus that prompts participants to interpret their experiences within the context of the experiences of other group members. Participants' recognition of their shared experiences begins to emerge in Exchange 6, via consensus statements (e.g., Right; I've been through that). By Exchange 12, participants begin to focus less on individual circumstances and actual events and more on patterned experiences of African American men. Thus, by comparing their experiences, participants extract general principles that can explain their common experiences.

Abstract Generalizations

Abstract generalizations are summary statements describing principals that participants have extracted from their own and other group members' common experiences. Like descriptive statements, they are characterized by durative clauses which depict ongoing states of affairs. However, abstract generalizations have several characteristics that distinguish them from descriptive statements. Rather than describing particular individuals, participants describe classes of people. Rather than using singular pronouns such as "I" or "my kids," participants use plural pronouns such as "we" or "our kids." Rather than describing particular people, places, or things participants describe larger patterns of behavior and general ways of perceiving and responding to the social environment.

An additional distinguishing characteristic of abstract generalizations is that they emerge in a context that is inherently synergistic: Participants build upon each others statements, complete each others sentences, and collectively represent ideas. Thus, abstract generalizations are more prevalent in the latter parts of each focus group session, when the nucleus of the focus group discussion is located in group dialogue rather than in exchanges between each participant and the moderator. The segment of text presented below illustrates the structure of such abstract statements.

Example 2.

1 M: Do you think there are things that black parents deal with when raising children that white parents don't have to deal with?
2 R1: Our kids may not have access to, you know, the updated materials, books, the computers ...
3 R2: Yeah! Computers in the school.
4 R3: Touché!
5 R1: White folks have it all, you know, and that's a big problem because you're hindering this child's education. And he already has a strike against him because he's black.
5 R5: Because he's black!
6 R3: Touché!

7 R2: So, we're always playing catch up.
8 R3: They got more tools. They got more tools.
9 R4: It never evens out.
10 R3: It can't! We're playing on a slanted field.
11 R2: It may even out. But, I tell myself ... you gotta be aware of what's happening, and when ... and they got the ball. It's their ball in their court, you know what I'm saying. And they don't want to play? They take the ball and go home. And you just gotta realize that and then when you ... then you can play the game better. When you realize it ain't gonna be a fair game, when you got loaded dice, then you play.
12 R1: Yeah! It's a steady uphill climb for us being black and that's the way it's gonna be for the kids.

In contrast to the segment presented in the discussion of stories, the dialogue in this segment is characterized by a series of statements which reflect a broader model of intergroup relations. These statements do not refer to particular individuals but rather to social units (e.g., "our kids," "white folks," "us being black," "the kids"). Statements contain nonspecific referents, suggesting that the principals described are the same regardless of the particular actors or the particular place and time.

Like descriptive statements and stories, participants' abstract generalizations could conceivably be coded using first-level codes and pattern codes that group statements according to similarities in their surface and implicit content. However, the most useful information contained in abstract generalizations is held in their connection to other abstract generalizations. Thus, coding such generalizations acontextually can obscure much of their meaning. In this regard, it is especially noteworthy that the cognitive models embedded in participants' abstract generalizations tend to be collectively supported within the group. That is, these models are group rather than individual-level phenomena. For instance, the segment presented above is organized around a series of semantic structures that link one participant's statement to another's. Five of the 12 exchanges contain a consensus statement (e.g., "touché" "right"). Many of the exchanges also contain isomorphic metaphors, such as "playing catch-up," "slanted field," "loaded dice," and "uphill climb," which underscore the similarities in participants' world views and which reference structural inequities that participants perceive as characterizing intergroup relations between African Americans and whites.

To the extent that similar abstract generalizations are put forth across two or more focus groups, they facilitate researchers access to the shared cognitive models that groups develop to interpret and give-meaning to their experiences. They can also facilitate researchers' identification of between-group differences in these cognitive models, although such differences did not emerge in this study.

Contributions of Enhanced Understanding to Culturally Anchored Research

Thus far, the description of the research example has highlighted the structure of focus group transcripts and how they can be organized to facilitate an understanding of participants' common and shared knowledge. In this section, the discussion shifts to a consideration of how an understanding of such knowledge can contribute to the development of a culturally anchored quantitative study.

One important contribution of such an understanding is that it enables researchers to evaluate and challenge their a priori conceptualization of a phenomenon within a model. A priori conceptualizations may reflect the researchers ideas about what processes are important and how they operate more so than they reflect the social realities experienced by the target population (Morgan, 1988). In the present research, this was an important function of the focus group sessions. More specifically, the common knowledge identified in participants' descriptive statements and stories highlighted limitations in the conceptualization of racial job stressors, which was a construct of central importance to the study.

Based primarily on studies of white-collar African American workers (e.g., Alderfer, Alderfer, Tucker, & Tucker, 1980; Davis & Watson, 1982; McAdoo, 1982; Quinn & Staines, 1979; Work, 1980) the initial conceptualization included four constructs. These were (a) structurally induced bias in wages, benefits, job quality, and opportunities for advancements (institutional discrimination); (b) racial bias in interpersonal interactions (interpersonal racism); (c) demands for adaptation of culturally based behaviors and affective styles (cultural discordance); and (d) detachment from work-based social networks (social isolation). It was hypothesized that variation on these constructs would predict different patterns of racial socialization. However, an additional dimension of racial job stress emerged from the focus transcripts. Both descriptive statements and stories suggested that participants' jobs varied in the extent of exposure to overt versus covert racism and discrimination. In fact, the distinction between overt and covert racial job stressors differentiated the descriptive statements and stories emergent in blue-collar and white-collar focus groups. Had we overlooked this distinction, important differences in the experiences of blue-collar and white-collar workers may have been masked. Thus, the focus groups highlighted important gaps in the conceptualization of a central construct.

Focus groups can also identify constructs that have been omitted completely from a conceptual framework but that are important to a group's experiences. Such omissions constitute a form of model misspecification, which can undermine the validity of research findings and can distort the social realities of a group (Blalock, 1982). In our focus groups, several such constructs were identified based on the interpretations of participants' descriptive statements, stories, and abstract generalizations. For example, encounters with subtle and overt discrimination and racism outside of the work environment were mentioned repeatedly in both blue-collar and white-collar focus groups but were omitted from the initial conceptual model. Such encounters were referred to as frequently within each group as were similar work-based encounters. Insofar as such encounters, in turn, influence racial socialization practices, omission of the construct could result in a biased estimate of relationships between racial job stressors and racial socialization. In a multiple regression framework, the influence of racism and discrimination outside of work on dimensions of racial socialization would be relegated to the error term for relationships between racial job stressors and racial socialization, and the power to detect relationships of interest would be reduced.

It is also important to note that an understanding of participants' common and shared knowledge may help researchers interpret data from a quantitative study, although this possibility has not yet been evaluated in the research described here. However, it is not uncommon for contradictory or anomalous findings to emerge in any research endeavor. An understanding of culturally based world views and perspectives may equip researchers with the tools to make sense of such findings. Moreover, the contributions to conceptual and theoretical aspects of the study illustrate both the limitations of implementing a quantitative study without adequate understanding of participants experiences and how understanding obtained from focus group sessions can contribute to the development of a more useful conceptual model.

REVISION OF THE SURVEY INSTRUMENT

In the research program described here, a second objective in conducting focus groups was to develop items to assess race relations at work and racial socialization. To our knowledge, established measures for adequately assessing these constructs were not available in the published empirical literature. Thus, evaluating and refining the items developed to assess them was a central aim of the focus group study. In this section, examples are used to illustrate how focus groups contributed to the development of the survey instrument.

Developing Additional Survey Items

Focus groups can serve important functions when researchers have identified the relevant constructs to be measured but have not identified the specific items that will be used to assess them, as is often the case when little is known about the central research question. Most notably, participants' descriptions of their experiences and perspectives can provide concrete materials from which to generate survey items.

One example of how the focus groups for this study contributed to the development of the survey instrument comes from our development of items to assess "interpersonal racism," a component of racial job stress. The conceptualization of racial job stressors was based on the literature on African American white-collar workers. The conceptualization reflected a corporate model in which subtle racial biases, such as expectations for failure and ethnocentrism, were important concerns. In reviewing the focus group transcripts, however, it became evident that these items did not adequately cover the universe of experiences that were relevant to the construct. For example, the items primarily covered interactions that occur within an organizational setting. However, many participants described exposure to individual racial bias in encounters with clients or the general public—exposures that occurred outside of the work group and would not have been captured using the initial item pool. In addition, items assessing blatant interpersonal racism (e.g., overtly antagonistic interracial conflict, use of racial slurs and derogatory terms, and blatant disrespect for African Americans) were conspicuously absent from the index. Yet, these sorts of interactions were mentioned frequently in the context of the focus group discussions. Finally, many of items reflected the experiences of African Americans who worked in predominantly white work environments. Consequently, they did not adequately reflect the experiences of those who worked in predominantly black environments or in clerical/technical occupations.

Thus, the focus groups prompted the development of additional items to assess interpersonal racism that more adequately represented a broad range of experiences. The words participants used provided a basis upon which to generate these items. Examples of items generated based on participants descriptions are: "On my job, I sometimes deal with people who treat me badly because I am black" and "On my job, I see racial bias in how people are treated day to day."

Revision of Item Wording

Focus groups, like other in-depth interviews, can contribute to questionnaire development by providing the researcher with direct access to the language participants use to think and talk about their experiences. Such access enables researchers to gauge the appropriateness of item wording for a specified population. For example, by listening to the words participants use and the way they speak, researchers may be better able to bridge the gap between their own language and that used by the population of interest.

In the focus groups for this study, participants used much simpler language than that contained in the original item pool. For instance, they referred to African Americans as blacks rather than as African Americans. In our revisions, all items were changed to reflect this use of language. Participants also used simple words and spoke in short sentences. We revised many questionnaire items to reduce the number of words and syllables in contained in them. As an example, the item "Have you ever done something to prepare your child for the possibility that s/he might experience racism or discrimination in his/her childhood" was changed to read "Have you ever told your child that some people might treat him/her badly because s/he is black." Thus, the focus groups highlighted differences in the language commonly used by the focus group participants and that typically used by academic scholars.

Evaluating the Clarity and Relevancy of Existing Items

A final contribution of the focus groups to the development of the survey instrument was that it enabled us to evaluate the clarity of items that had been generated a priori and to gauge their relevancy to group participants. The set of items to assess racial job stressors and racial socialization were distributed to participants at the close of each focus group session. Participants were asked to identify items that were irrelevant to their experiences, awkward, or unclear.

For the most part, participants' responses to the survey items increased our confidence in the items that had been developed. Comments participants made while completing the questionnaire suggested that most items were clear and relevant (e.g, "Yeah, you getting to the nitty gritty with these questions"; "You hitting the nail on the head with these questions." Thus, feedback from participants suggested that items were appropriate and clearly understood. However, participant feedback also cued us to certain questions that participants misinterpreted or misunderstood. For example, several participants questioned the item "Have you ever told your child that race is not important," an item generated to assess racial socialization. For example, one participants words capture the confusion this item caused: "I don't know how to take that because you're asking about racism and then how could you tell her that race is not important." Another item,

"Have you ever told your child that s/he cannot behave in certain ways because s/he is Black," which was generated to assess adaptive strategies parents use to protect children from racial bias, was consistently misinterpreted by participants. For example, one participants said: "That's absurd! I think this question is a little off. I think my child is very well behaved. I never have to tell her that."

SUMMARY AND DISCUSSION

In this article, focus groups were described as a tool for facilitating research that is grounded in the experiences and perspectives of a particular population. More specifically, it was argued that focus groups can facilitate a rich understanding of particular phenomena and can provide the raw materials with which to develop instruments that are appropriate to a particular problem or population. Focus groups achieve this end by (a) emphasizing participants' own perspectives and experiences regarding the phenomenon of interest and (b) providing a mechanism by which researchers can observe social interaction among group members around issues the researcher specifies. Each of these can help facilitate culturally anchored research.

The qualitative and unstructured nature of focus group interviews gives researchers access to *how* participants think and talk about issues that are of interest to the researcher (Morgan & Krueger, 1993; O'Brien, 1993). As in other qualitative interviews, participants are able to respond to questions in their own terms rather than terms provided by the moderator, providing for a more grounded approach to the development of constructs and theories. Although ethnographic interviews may offer similar opportunities, the dialogue that takes place among participants from similar sociocultural backgrounds may more textured, less formal, and less regulated than that between an interviewer and a respondent. For instance, a trained interviewer is less likely to disagree with or challenge a respondents' point of view or recollection of an experience than is another focus group participant.

Related to this, group interaction may also yield data that are less readily available using individual-level data collection methods. For one, group dialogue inherently fosters agreement and disagreement among participants, encouraging them to clarify or justify their statements. The within-group homogeneity that characterizes most focus group research facilitates self-disclosure, and thereby, the elaboration of experiences and perspectives that may be less readily available to the researcher in one-on-one situations. Most important, however, group interaction prompts comparative processes within focus groups that prompt participants to elaborate more abstract models of the phenomenon of interest, providing researchers with access to consensual models that underlie participants' experiences and perspectives.

The example presented here, based on a program of research among African American dual-earner families, provides a concrete illustration of how focus groups can contribute to culturally anchored research. It was argued that focus group dialogues contain distinct narrative structures that facilitate the identification of cultural knowledge. Descriptive statements, describing enduring states of affairs, enable researchers to identify recurrent themes that emerge within and across groups, termed common knowledge. Identification of recurrent themes can facilitate the development of a relevant conceptual framework that is rooted in the social realities of a group. Moreover, rather than imposing a framework on participants' experiences, descriptive statements permit a framework to emerge from participants' own dialogue. Although in-depth individual interviews can also facilitate the emergence of such a framework, the focus group format can provide more depth and texture in this regard. In the focus groups described here, participants moved discussions of race-related issues in directions that facilitated the research objectives, suggesting that the discussion reflects participants' world views rather than just the researcher's. This dynamic is more likely to occur in a group than in an individual in-depth interview, since the interviewer's control over the discussion is diffused (Morgan, 1988).

Stories, describing discrete events, facilitated an understanding of participants' common knowledge regarding race relations by elucidating the concrete events that shape participants' descriptive statements. They also prompt participants to compare and contrast their experiences and, thereby, to extract more general information from the commonalities across their experiences. In this regard, it should be emphasized that the coding scheme developed to categorize participants' stories in the present study did not fully capture the information contained within them. Although some stories were embedded in lengthy monologues, many were immediately followed by other participants' similar stories, as the example presented suggests. The give-and-take of these sorts of transactions provided information about the commonalities participants themselves recognize, information that cannot be garnered by simply counting redundant themes within and across groups.

Abstract generalizations can be an important source of information on group members' schematic representations of the phenomenon of interest. They provide a context for interpreting earlier narratives and gave them both texture and meaning. In addition, to the extent that abstract generalizations are embedded in larger consensual models that are agreed upon by the group, they can facilitate researchers' identification of shared knowledge that governs the members' experiences and perspectives. In the present focus groups, multiple focus group sessions among different segments of the population proved to be especially useful. Though participants each describe unique situations and their own individual stories, the shared knowledge that emerged within each of the focus group sessions tended to be remarkably similar across groups.

Thus, focus groups have many strengths that make them particularly useful for facilitating a culturally anchored quantitative study. However, it is important to note that focus groups can be designed in a variety of ways to facilitate insights into cross-cultural and intracultural phenomenon. As described here, they may be used during the planning stages of a larger study to identify relevant constructs, to generate conceptual frameworks, and to develop adequate question wording and response categories for questionnaire items (e.g., Joseph et al., 1984; O'Brien, 1993). They may be conducted in conjunction with other methods to triangulate information on a phenomenon of interest (e.g., de Vries et al., 1992; Gottlieb et al., 1992; Hugentobler, Israel, & Schurman, 1992). They may be used as a follow up to a quantitative study to clarify and amplify study findings (e.g., Wolff et al., 1993) or they may stand on their own as explorations into the norms, phenomenology, and experiences of a group of participants (e.g., Lengua et al., 1992; Morgan, 1989; Morgan & Spanish, 1984; Pramualratana, Havanon, & Knodel, 1985; Wolff et al., 1993).

While the strengths of focus groups may facilitate a rich understanding of phenomena, it is important to recognize that they also have limitations. For example, they are expensive and time-consuming. Incentives for hard-to-reach populations, moderator fees, transcription fees, room rental fees, and costs for refreshments can consume a large portion of a research budget. In addition, coding and analysis of group dialogue is tedious and time-consuming. Although computer programs may speed the process of organizing data, they are not capable of interpreting it. In addition, it is important to recognize that the structure imposed on the group by the moderator may threaten the ecological validity of the interaction the researcher is able to observe. More specifically, interaction that is generated in a formal environment around research questions specified by an investigator may differ in unknown ways from the interaction one might observe in more naturalistic settings. Thus, in choosing the focus group method, the researcher compromises the ecological validity of observations in favor of control over the topic of discussion. Finally, focus group samples are typically small and nonrepresentative. Although groups can be organized to represent the diversity of experiences within a population, findings from a focus group study cannot be generalized to a larger population. Thus, focus groups more readily facilitate exploration rather than hypothesis testing.

However, we have argued that focus groups can be ideally suited to increase researcher's knowledge or understanding, to rethink how problems are framed and how to interpret data, and to provide the researcher with a broader and richer understanding of phenomenon. Each of these may facilitate the development of more culturally anchored research.

ACKNOWLEDGMENTS

The writing of this manuscript was supported in part by grants from the National Science Foundation (#DBS-9154413) and The William T. Grant Foundation (92147692) awarded to the first author.

REFERENCES

Alderfer, C., Alderfer, C., Tucker, L., & Tucker, S. (1980). Diagnosing race problems in management. *Journal of Applied Behavior Science, 16*, 135–166.

Basch, C. E. (1987). Focus group interview: An under-utilized research technique for improving theory and practice in Health Education. *Health Education Quarterly, 14*, 411–448.

Blalock, H. M., Jr. (1982). *Concephialization and measurement in the social sciences.* Beverly Hills, CA: Sage.

Boykin, A. W. (1979). Black psychology and the research process: Keeping the baby but throwing out the bath water. In A. W. Boykin, A. J. Franklin, & J. F. Yates (Eds.), *Research directions of Black psychologists* (pp. 85–103). New York: Russell Sage.

Bronfenbrenner, U. (1979). *The ecology of human development.* Cambridge, MA: Harvard University Press.

Bruner, (1991). The narrative construction of reality. *Critical Inquiry, 18*, 1–21.

Crosby, F. J. (1987). *Spouse, parent, worker: On gender and multiple roles.* New Haven, CT: Yale University Press.

Davis, G., & Watson, G. (1982). *Black life in Corporate America.* New York: Doubleday.

de Vries, H., Weijts, W., Dijkstra, M., & Kok, G. (1992). The utilization of qualitative and quantitative data for health education program planning, implementation, and evaluation: A spiral approach. *Health Education Quarterly, 19*, 101–115.

Gottlieb, N. H., Lovato, C. Y., Weinstein, R., Green, L. W., & Eriksen, M. P. (1992). The implementation of a restrictive worksite smoking policy in a large decentralized organization. *Health Education Quarterly, 19*, 77–100.

Hecht, M. L., Collier, M. J., & Ribeau, S. A. (1993). *African American communication: Ethnic identity and cultural interpretation.* Newbury Park, CA: Sage.

Howard, G. S. (1991). Culture tales: A narrative approach to thinking, cross-cultural psychology, and psychotherapy. *American Psychologist, 46*, 187–197.

Howard, A., & Scott, R. A. (1981). The study of minority groups in complex societies. In R. H. Munroe, R. L. Munroe, & B. B. Whiting (Eds.), *Handbook of cross-cultural human development* (pp. 113–152). New York: Guilford.

Hugentobler, M. K., Israel, B. A., Schurman, S. J. (1992). An action research approach to workplace health: Integrating methods. *Health Education Quarterly, 19*, 55–76.

Hui, C. H., & Triandis, H. C. (1989). Effects of culture and response format on extreme response styles. *Journal of Cross-Cultural Psychology, 20*, 296–309.

Joseph, J. G., Emmors, CA., Kessler, R. C., Wortman, C. B., O'Brien, K., Hockev, W. T., & Schaefer, C. (1984). Coping with the threat of AIDS. An approach to psychosocial assessment. *American Psychologist, 39*, 1297–1302.

Knodel, J. (1993). The design and analysis of focus group studies: A practical approach. In D. L. Morgan (Ed.), *Successful focus groups: Advancing the state of the art* (pp. 35–50). Newbury Park, CA: Sage.

Kohn, M. L. (1969). *Class and conformity.* Homewood, IL: Dorsey.

Kohn, M. L. & Schooler, C. (1973). Occupational experience and psychological functioning: An assessment of reciprocal effects. *American Sociological Review, 38*, 97–118.

Kohn, M. L., & Schooler, C. (1978). The reciprocal effects of substantive complexity of work on intellectual flexibility: A longitudinal assessment. *American Journal of Sociology, 84*, 24–52.

Krippendorf, K. (1980). *Content analysis: An introduction to its methodology.* Beverly Hills: Sage.

Krueger, R. A. (1988). *Focus groups: A practical guide for applied research.* Newbury Park, CA: Sage.

Kreckel, M. (1981). *Communicative acts and shared knowledge in natural discourse.* New York: Academic Press.

Lengua, L. J., Roosa, M. W., Schupak-Newbery, E., Micheals, M. L., Berg, G. N., & Weschler, L. F. (1992). Using focus groups to guide the development of a parenting program for difficult-to-reach, high risk families. *Family Relations, 41*, 163–168.

Mair, M. (1988). Psychology as storytelling. *International Journal of Personal Construct Psychology, 1*, 125–138.

Marsella, A. J., & Kameoka, V. A. (1989). Ethnocultural issues in the assessment of psychopathology. In S. Wetzler (Ed.), *Measuring mental illness: Psychometric assessment for clinicians* (pp. 231–255). Washington, DC: American Psychiatric Press.

McAdoo, H. P. (1982). Patterns of upward mobility in Black families. In H. P. McAdoo (Ed.), *Black families.* Beverly Hills, CA: Sage.

Miles, M. B., & Huberman, A. M. (1984). *Qualitative data analysis: A sourcebook of new methods.* Newbury Park, CA: Sage.

Mohler, P. P., & Zull, C. (1984). *TEXTPACK Version V. Release 2.* Mannheim: ZUMA.

Morgan, D. L. (1988). *Focus groups as qualitative research.* Newbury Park, CA: Sage.

Morgan, D. L. (1989). Adjusting to widowhood: Do social networks really make it easier? *Gerontologist, 29*, 101–107.

Morgan, D. L. (1993). *Successful focus groups: Advancing the state of the art.* Newbury Park, CA: Sage.

Morgan, D. L., & Krueger, A. (1993). When to use focus groups and why. In D. L. Morgan (Ed.), *Successful focus groups: Advancing the state of the art* (pp. 3–19). Newbury Park, CA: Sage.

Morgan, D. L., & Spanish, M. T. (1984). Focus groups: A new tool for qualitative research. *Qualitative Sociology, 7*, 253–270.

O'Brien, K. O. (1993). Improving survey questionnaires through focus groups. In D. L. Morgan (Ed.), *Successful focus groups: Advancing the state of the art* (pp. 105–117). Newbury Park, CA: Sage.

Piotrkowski, C. S. (1979). *Work and the family system: A naturalistic study of working-class and lower-middle-class families.* New York: The Free Press.

Plas, J. M. (1986). *Systems psychology in the schools.* New York: Pergamon.

Polanyi, L. (1985). *Telling the American story: A structural and cultural analysis of conversational storytelling.* Norwood, NJ: Ablex.

Popko, E. S. (1980). *Key-word-in-context bibliographic indexing: Release 4.0 users manual.* Cambridge, MA: Harvard University Laboratory for Computer Graphics and Spatial Analysis.

Pramualratana, A., Havanon, N., & Knodel, J. (1985). Exploring the normative age at marriage in Thailand. An example from focus group research. *Journal of Marriage and the Family, 47*, 203–210.

Quinn, R. P., & Staines, G. L. (1979). *The 1977 quality of employment survey: Descriptive statistics with comparison data from 1969–70 and 1972–73 surveys.* Ann Arbor, MI: Institute for Social Research.

Seidel, J. V., Kjolseth, R., & Seymour, E. (1988). *The ethnograph: A user's guide.* Littleton, CO: Qualis Research Associates.

Shweder, R. A., & LeVine, R. A. (1984). *Culture theory: Essays on mind, self, and emotion.* New York: Cambridge University Press.

Stewart. D. W., & Shamdasani, P. N. (1990). *Focus groups: Theory and practice.* Newbury Park, CA: Sage.

Voydanoff, P. (1980). Work roles as stressors in corporate families. *Family Relations, 2 9*, 489–494.

Weber, R. P. (1985). *Basic content analysis.* Beverly Hills: Sage.

Wolff, B., Knodel, J., & Sittitrai, W. (1993). Focus groups and surveys as complementary research methods: A case example. In D. L. Morgan (Ed.), *Successful focus groups: Advancing the state of the art* (pp. 118–138). Newbury Park, CA: Sage.

Work, J. (1980). Management blacks and the international labor market: Answers to a questionnaire. *Human Resource Management* (Fall), 16–22.

11

The Structure of Problem and Positive Behavior among American Indian Adolescents: Gender and Community Differences

Christina M. Mitchell and Janette Beals

Using Problem-Behavior Theory as a framework, the latent structure of problem and positive behaviors was examined within a sample of 1,894 American Indian adolescents. Support was found for a two-factor second-order structure in which problem behaviors (antisocial behavior, alcohol use, drug use, and risky sexual behavior) and positive behaviors (school success, cultural activities, competencies, and community-mindedness) represented two relatively uncorrelated aspects of behavior. Hierarchical multiple regressions demonstrated that the positive behaviors construct contributed significant incremental construct validity in the statistical prediction of psychosocial outcomes, over and above the problem behaviors. In addition, the fit of the structure was examined across gender and the four participating communities. The importance of the inclusion of positive behaviors is discussed from the standpoint of both prevention/promotion activities and the communities' perceptions. Further recommendations are made for deeper understandings of community concerns and strengths in conducting preventive/promotive research efforts.

Originally published in the *American Journal of Community Psychology*, 25(3) (1997): 257–288.

Ecological Research to Promote Social Change: Methodological Advances from Community Psychology, edited by Tracey A. Revenson et al. Kluwer Academic/Plenum Publishers, New York, 2002.

In recent years, the problem and risk behaviors of American Indian adolescents have received considerable attention. For instance, American Indian youths have been reported to exhibit higher levels of serious problems such as depression and suicide, substance use, and school leaving (U.S. Congress, 1990). Blum, Harmon, Harris, Bergeisen, and Resnick (1992) reported that for the majority of the psychological and physical problems of concern during adolescence, American Indian youths showed higher levels than a comparison group of white youths. At the same time, these authors also noted "As is true for most teenagers throughout the United States, the majority of American Indian youths are not faced with significant health risks" (p. 1643). One area of research that has been prominent in exploring interrelationships among adolescents has been Problem-Behavior Theory (PBT); however, the relevance of PBT has not been examined to date with American Indian adolescents. Moreover, the positive aspects of adolescent behavior in general have received little systematic attention. To address these concerns, this study had four goals: (a) to attempt to raise the discussion of positive behaviors in research literature to a level comparable to that of problem behaviors; (b) to expand work on the construct validity of both problem and positive behaviors; (c) to test empirically whether problem and positive behaviors are endpoints of a single continuum or are instead two separate constructs; and (d) to extend work on the structure of problem and positive behaviors to American Indian adolescents and to begin to examine differences in these structures by gender and community. We discuss each of these goals below; however, we begin with a brief orientation to PBT.

PROBLEM-BEHAVIOR THEORY

A number of recent research endeavors have provided evidence that adolescent alcohol use, other drug use, delinquent behaviors, and sexual intercourse may be best understood as elements of a "syndrome" of adolescent problem behaviors (Donovan & Jessor, 1978; Donovan & Jessor, 1985; Donovan, Jessor, & Costa, 1988; Farrell, Danish, & Howard, 1992; Huba, Wingard, & Bentler, 1981a). Much of the work on problem behaviors has been conducted under the rubric of Problem-Behavior Theory, spearheaded by Jessor in the 1970s (Jessor & Jessor, 1977). Underlying PBT is the dimension of conventionality–unconventionality, conceptualized as summarizing "an orientation toward, commitment to, and involvement in the prevailing values, standards of behavior, and established institutions of the larger American society" (Donovan, Jessor, & Costa, 1991, p. 52). For example, problem behaviors are behaviors that have been defined as undesirable by society and that elicit some kind of social control response (Donovan et al.,

1991). At the other end of the underlying dimension, "conventional" behaviors—or, paralleling the term "problem behavior," *positive* behaviors—include behaviors that are considered appropriate for adolescents within their particular cultures or communities.

Moving from theory to operationalization, Jessor, Donovan, and their associates have reported that getting drunk, marijuana use, delinquent behavior, and precocious sexual intercourse constitute a syndrome of problem behaviors (Donovan & Jessor, 1985; Donovan et al., 1988). These four problem behaviors have correlated positively with each other and negatively with measures of positive behavior (e.g., church attendance, grades in school). These intercorrelations have been used as evidence for this single underlying factor of conventionality–unconventionality (Donovan, Jessor, & Costa, 1993; Jessor & Jessor, 1977).

POSITIVE BEHAVIORS

To date, the most detailed research efforts have emphasized problem behaviors almost exclusively, neglecting the positive end of the dimension (Donovan & Jessor, 1985; Donovan et al., 1988; Farrell et al., 1992; Gillmore, Hawkins, Catalano, & Day, 1991; McGee & Newcomb, 1992). PBT is not alone in this oversight of positive or adaptive outcomes, though. Overall, research on positive behaviors such as competence remains a much less mature "sibling" of the older and more thoroughly studied maladaptive outcomes or problem behaviors (Garmezy, 1993). However, the relevance and importance of adaptive developmental outcomes to prevention and promotion is undeniable: to assess the impact of prevention and promotion efforts, we should look not simply for a decrease in pathology, but also for the enhancement of a wide variety of positive outcomes such as social and instrumental competence, community involvement, and religiosity or spirituality. In addition to a general optimism reflected in this construct, it can also suggest avenues for interventions that are more likely both to be embraced by the community and to have cost-effective and enduring impacts. As a result, we need to turn our attention to quantifying these positive outcomes so that we can begin to uncover the important *predictors* of such adaptive development. Thus, the first goal of this study was to attempt to raise the discussion of positive behaviors to a level comparable to that of problem behaviors.

Construct Validity

Most researchers who have explored the structure of problem and positive behaviors have relied on a relatively limited number of items to represent the construct. For instance, Donovan and his associates (Donovan & Jessor, 1985; Donovan et al., 1988) typically utilized only four measures: an antisocial behavior scale score, past-month's marijuana use, "number of times drunk in past month," and "ever had sex." A few researchers expanded slightly on this set (Farrell et al., 1992; Gillmore et al., 1991; Resnicow, Ross-Gaddy, & Vaughan, 1995). Items representing positive behaviors have been even more restricted, though. In Donovan and Jessor's work, at most one item of "academic achievement" and/or one item of "church attendance" have been utilized. Resnicow et al. (1995) selected five items to represent a general positive behaviors construct: attended church, read about African American history, did something fun with adult you live with, accomplished something you were proud of, and exercise or play sports. Farrell et al. (1992) utilized three items—church attendance, grade-point average, and school attendance—and a composite scale score of "eight positive behaviors (e.g., 'spent time studying for a test' and 'helped out around the house') ... selected to represent appropriate activities relevant to the target population" (p. 706).

While such efforts are important first steps, concern arises surrounding the construct validity of the operationalizations to date. In general, construct validity requires that a measure sample from the universe of relevant observed variables as widely as theory and resources allow (Messick, 1995). Thus, the item sampling to date may not have adequately represented the universe of construct-relevant behaviors that truly make up the constructs of problem behaviors and positive behaviors. Thus, a second goal of this research was to expand work on construct validity in two ways: (a) sampling a more diverse set of both problem and positive behaviors, and examining the underlying factor structure of this expanded set of items measuring problem and positive behaviors; and (b) assessing the importance of including both problem and positive behaviors in understanding adaptive and maladaptive processes among adolescents.

MODEL TESTING

General Approach

The fit of a one-factor model of problem behaviors, or problem and positive behaviors together, has rarely been tested against competing models that might also—and perhaps, *better*—explain the relationships among these variables. The strongest test would be to compare a model of a single underlying problem/positive behaviors construct to one with separate problem and positive behaviors constructs. Only a few authors have included a sufficient number of positive behaviors for such a test (e.g., Farrell et al., 1992; Resnicow et al., 1995); none has rigorously tested a two-factor structure against a one-factor structure. However, the correlations reported in these studies indeed suggest that problem and positive behaviors are not simply two endpoints of a single dimension. Thus, a third goal of this research was to test explicitly a one-factor latent structure against a two-factor latent structure using the expanded set of problem and positive items, to examine the assumption of a single underlying dimension of unconventionality and the importance of considering *both* problem and positive behaviors.

Ethnic Differences

Although early thinking about PBT arose from work with mostly white, middle-class youths, later testing has expanded to include other ethnicities (Donovan & Jessor, 1985; Donovan et al., 1988; Farrell et al., 1992; Gillmore et al., 1991; McGee & Newcomb, 1992; Resnicow et al., 1995). While some have reported solid support for the syndrome of problem behaviors (Farrell et al., 1992), others suggest that a more complex structure may underlie problem behaviors (Gillmore et al., 1991; McGee & Newcomb, 1992; Resnicow et al., 1995). To date, though, none has included American Indian adolescents as a particular focus. The universality of PBT for American Indian youths is especially suspect, given some of our own work with these populations. For instance, we have found that among Indian adolescents, the use of alcohol has strong "conventional" or normative aspects in addition to its unconventional aspects. More generally, we would expect that the "unconventionality" of alcohol use may vary to some degree across a number of key groups: for example, by *history*, to the extent that alcohol use is differentially associated with some adolescent behaviors, and then with others, in different historical periods; by *ethnicity*, to the extent that alcohol use is incorporated differently in different sociocultural traditions; and by *gender*, to the extent that drinking may be more normative for males than for females (Mitchell et al., 1996; O'Nell & Mitchell, 1996).

Moreover, while a proposed model may fit adequately across a heterogeneous sample, one should not assume that that structure necessarily fits equally well for subgroups such as ethnicity or gender. To date, ethnic differences in structure or meaning for problem and positive behaviors across subsamples have not been examined. Yet, especially among Indian nations, both historical and ongoing experiences of disruption and oppression from mainstream groups have differed dramatically across various culture groups; in addition, sociocultural integration can vary widely across tribe (Kunitz & Levy, 1994; Levy & Kunitz, 1974; May, 1982). Thus, one might anticipate differences in both the meaning and the structure of unconventionality–conventionally as well as problem and positive behaviors.

Gender Differences

Although ethnic subgroups have not been examined at all, a few studies have attempted to look at gender differences. Donovan and Jessor (1985) explicitly reported gender differences in only one study, and then only in a brief footnote: a "lack of fit with the single-factor model in three of the four male subsamples and in one of the female subsamples... suggests that the conforming behaviors may constitute a correlated second factor for the men" (p. 902). Farrell et al. (1992) looked at age-by-gender differences in structure, finding that a model that fit seventh-grade males and females and ninth-grade females did not fit ninth-grade males quite as well. The limited exploration of possible gender differences in problem and positive behaviors is surprising, given commonly reported gender differences in areas such as internalizing/externalizing (Chenbach & Edelbrock, 1987), school success (Cobb, 1992; Henderson & Dweck, 1990), and sexuality (Brooks-Gunn & Paikoff, 1993). Thus, a fourth goal of this research was twofold: to extend work on the structure of problem and positive behaviors to an American Indian sample and to utilize multisample confirmatory factor analyses to explore two sets of subgroup differences—gender and community.

METHOD

Sample

Communities

In working with Indian communities, protection of the confidentiality of the tribes is considered as important as that of the individual participants. Therefore, these tribal and cultural groups are described generally as South Central, Northern Plain, Southwestern, and Pueblo, consistent with the culture groups they represent. The South Central group originated on the east coast of the United States but was transferred to the southern Midwest in the 1800s. They have a small land-base, and tribal members' ties to this land-base are often more tenuous than those of other groups in the sample. The students from this community all attended a tribally administered school in the tribal nation's capital; 63% were boarders. The

Northern Plains adolescents come from a tribe that lives in relative isolation as well as considerable poverty, and has remained closely identified with their home reservation. Of the culture groups included in this sample, the Northern Plains tribes historically placed greatest emphasis on individuality and self-sufficiency. The Southwestern group represents a pastoral tradition. Currently they have a large land-base and experience unemployment rates lower than those of the Northern Plains group. Finally, the Pueblo group comprises several tribes living in the Southwest. Historically, these people had an agrarian economy and a tight-knit, community-oriented social structure. While certainly not representative of all Indian groups in the United States today, these four tribal groups allow a unique opportunity to reflect and demonstrate the differential life experiences of Indian adolescents.

Participants

Data for this study were drawn from the first full wave of the Voices of Indian Teens Project (VOICES), an ongoing longitudinal effort involving collaboration with 10 high schools located in five American Indian communities west of the Mississippi. In Fall 1993, a total of 2,804 youths completed self-report surveys, representing 74% of those students reported by the school to be enrolled as of "count week"—the date in early October at which total enrollment figures are reported to funding agencies for determination of federal educational monies.[1] Of these, 2,583 (92.2%) self-identified as being Indian and were therefore included in the sample for this study.

In addition to the exclusion of non-Indian adolescents, two other exclusion criteria were enforced. First, several of the schools included in the full sample were excluded because they are viewed locally and nationally as semitreatment facilities for youths experiencing either learning or emotional problems. This exclusion was considered important because these youths ($n = 431$) were clearly not representative of American Indian adolescents more generally and might bias the results. Second, we used only those youths with complete data ($n = 1,622$) to avoid the difficulties with statistical instability that can be introduced when using pairwise deletion.

To determine whether these exclusions introduced a bias, we used one-way ANOVAs to compare those included in the analyses to those who were excluded because of missing data ($n = 530$) on the variables involved in

---

[1] During the 4 to 6 weeks between this reporting period and the data collection period, a number of schools dropped students from their rolls, due to chronic absenteeism or transfer; as a result, the participation rate noted here is conservative.

these analyses. Of the 33 problem and positive behavior variables, 10 of the 33 were significantly different, and in directions one might anticipate (e.g., those with missing data reported doing less well in school, using marijuana more often, starting a fist fight more often, having more negative consequences after drinking). However, given the sample size, the power of the ANOVAs was quite high. In fact, the average ω^2 across the 10 significant differences was only .0035—the differences between the two groups on average accounted for less than 0.4% of the variance. Thus, any bias introduced by using only those with complete data is likely to have been minimal.

Procedures

Parents of all youths at each school were sent a letter explaining the study; those wanting more information or refusing permission for their children to participate returned the enclosed letter signifying such in a self-addressed stamped envelope.[2] (Only 2% of the parents refused.) School-based data collection consisted of one scheduled testing day, with a follow-up day approximately 1 week later for absentees. On the day of testing in school, youths actively agreed to participate by providing informed, written assent. Youths completing the survey received compensation worth $5 (e.g., a $5 money order or gift certificate). In school, surveys were administered within one class period, lasting approximately 45 to 50 minutes. Members of the research staff were on hand at each school to facilitate administration, answer questions, and ensure confidentiality of student responses. Additionally, 2 to 3 months of community-based follow-up, conducted by research staff who were members of each community, then focused on finding those youths who could not be contacted in the schools.

Measures

Extensive focus group work within the communities helped guide the selection and modification of the measures discussed here. In addition, because of classroom time constraints, the VOICES measures underwent extensive pilot-testing to permit measure reduction prior to the commencement of the full study; measures that were shortened during this process are noted below. Means and standard deviations of both problem

---

[2] This procedure of "active refusal" was approved in advance at many levels, including the home institution's Institutional Review Board, consortium institutions' Institutional Review Boards, and each participating school and community.

Table I. Item-Level Statistics, Full Sample (N = 1,622)

Item	Range	M	SD
Started a fist fight	1–5	1.75	1.14
Shoplifted from a store	1–5	1.55	1.11
Damaged property	1–5	1.44	1.02
Stayed out all night	1–5	2.12	1.48
Lied to parents or dorm aides	1–5	2.29	1.51
Quantity/frequency of alcohol use (z score)	−.78–2.51	−0.04	0.81
Negative consequences of alcohol use	1–4	1.17	0.36
Problem drinking behavior	1–4	1.45	0.63
No. of times used marijuana in the past month	0–31	4.05	7.96
No. of times used inhalants in the past month	0–31	0.55	2.67
No. of drugs ever tried	0–7	1.22	1.42
No. of drugs used in past month	0–7	0.91	1.25
Ever had sexual intercourse	0–1	0.51	0.50
Had sexual intrercourse in past month	0–1	0.30	0.46
No. of times used condom in past month	1–4	0.90	1.42
No. of times used other birth control in past month	1–4	1.03	1.56
Grade-point average	1–4	2.67	0.77
How well do you do in school	1–5	3.30	0.74
Do schoolwork carefully	1–4	2.81	0.89
Live by the Indian way	1–4	2.92	0.92
Speak tribal language	1–4	2.70	0.95
Participate in traditional activities	1–4	2.88	1.01
Make other kids feel comfortable	1–4	2.84	0.89
Find lots of fun things to do in free time	1–4	2.79	0.91
Good at creative things	1–4	2.49	1.04
Make others laugh	1–4	2.72	0.97
Good at sports and athletic games	1–4	2.62	1.01
Make friends with people	1–4	3.07	0.87
Visit older relatives	1–4	2.39	0.91
Try to help others	1–4	2.53	0.88
Please the elders in the community	1–4	2.43	0.95
Visit elders	1–4	2.19	0.94
Volunteer to help elders	1–4	1.98	0.93

and positive behavior variables are presented in Table I. In addition, to explore the importance of considering both problem and positive behaviors, we also identified six psychosocial variables—representing both maladaptive and adaptive psychological functioning—that were theorized to have differential relationships with problem and conventional behaviors. All variables were computed as average-item scale scores; when item metrics differed within a scale, individual items were converted to z scores prior to the computation of the average-item scale score.

Problem Behaviors

Antisocial Behavior. Five items were selected from Donovan et al.'s (1988) 10-item general deviance scale. The 10 items were grouped into five pairs: aggression, stealing, vandalism, lying, and acting without permission; within each pair, that question reflecting the more serious behavior was selected. Asking about the past 6 months, the 5 final items ($\alpha = .73$) were "started a fist fight or shoving match," "shoplifted from a store," "damaged or marked up public or private property," "stayed out all night without permission," and "lied to your parents, grandparents, or dorm aides about where you had been or whom you were with." Responses ranged from 1 (*never*) to 5 (*5 or more times*).

Alcohol Use. Items representing alcohol use included quantity/frequency items as well as items measuring negative consequences following drinking and commonly utilized indicators of serious problem drinking. Six questions were included concerning the level of the youth's use of alcohol during the previous month: (a) number of days the youth drank; (b) the usual number of drinks when drinking; (c) the greatest number of drinks at one time; (d) the number of times drunk; (e) self-perception of drinking (light, moderate, or heavy drinker); and (f) experience of drinking binges (yes or no). On the basis of earlier pilot work noted above (Mitchell et al., 1993), 14 items of the 25-item alcohol subscale of the Diagnostic Interview Schedule for Children (DISC-2.1, Shaffer et al., 1993) were selected to tap both negative consequences and indicators of serious problem drinking. The format was altered from a verbal administration format to a self-administered measure; response categories ranged from 1 (*rarely or never*) to 4 (*almost always*). Two additional questions were created to reflect problems with family and friends, due to drinking. We utilized all of the above items in a three-component structure of alcohol use (Mitchell et al., 1996): quantity/frequency, negative consequences following drinking, and problem drinking behaviors ($\alpha = .87$).

Drug Use. Four indicators of drug use ($\alpha = .76$) were utilized. Two were single items: "number of times used marijuana in the past month" and "number of times used inhalants in the past month"; response sets for both questions ranged from 0 to 31 times. In addition to these two drugs, youths were asked about use of five other groups of substances: crack or cocaine, solvents, amphetamines or speed, barbiturates or downers, and other drugs. Using all seven groups, two composite variables were created to represent the breadth of drug experimentation and use: "number of drugs *ever* used" was calculated by counting the number of drugs the youth had endorsed as having ever used; "number of drugs used during the past month" counted only those endorsed as used in the past month.

Sexual Behavior. Four indicators ($\alpha = .88$) of sexual behavior were included. "Ever had sexual intercourse" and "had sexual intercourse during the past month" were both yes/no questions. "Number of times used condoms in the past month" and "number of times used *other* birth control in the past month" were answered from 1 (*almost always*) to 4 (*never*). All items were coded so that higher response categories represented more risky sexual behavior. Answers of those who reported never having had sex or not having had sex in the past month were recoded to 0.

Positive Behaviors

School Success. Indicators of school success included three items ($\alpha = .66$): self-reported grade-point average, rated from 1 (*mostly Ds and Fs*) to 4 (*mostly As*); "Compared with your classmates, how well do you do in school?," rated from 1 (*much below average*) to 5 (*much above average*); and "I do my schoolwork carefully," rated from 1 (*rarely or never*) to 4 (*almost always*).

Cultural Activities. In earlier work, "church attendance" has served as a proxy for positive behaviors; however, our earlier work within these Indian communities suggested that the idea of church attendance as a proxy for spirituality is not generally appropriate. More appropriate is the idea of participating in cultural activities in the community. Three items ($\alpha = .73$) concerning Indian cultural activities were utilized: "Do you live by or follow the Indian way," "Do you speak your tribal language," and "Do you participate in traditional practices"—all rated from 1 (*not at all*) to 4 (*a lot*).

Competencies. Competencies are almost by definition an important aspect of positive behaviors. Adapted from a measure created for the Adolescent Pathways Project (Seidman, Aber, Allen, & Mitchell, 1994), questions tapped six social and instrumental competencies ($\alpha = .82$): making other kids feel comfortable, finding fun things to do in free time, being good at creative things, making others laugh, being good at sports and athletic games, and making friends with people. All responses ranged from 1 (*rarely or never*) to 4 (*almost always*).

Community-Mindedness. Being involved in community activities is an important aspect of life in many Indian communities (Mitchell, 1997). We included five items ($\alpha = .87$) to measure this construct: the frequency of visiting older relatives, trying to help others, pleasing the elders in the community, visiting elders, and volunteering to help the elders. Response categories ranged from 1 (*rarely or never*) to 4 (*almost always*).

Psychosocial Variables

Anxiety. Anxiety has been shown to have some relationship to problem behaviors, such as substance use. For example, Orive and Gerard (1980) found that lower anxiety was correlated to greater substance use; Swaim, Oetting, Edwards, and Beauvais (1989) found a positive zero-order correlation, as well as a strong indirect path to drug use, mediated by anger and peer drug associations. This study used nine stem items ($\alpha = .78$) of the Anxiety module of the DISC 2.1 (Shaffer et al., 1993), which asked about having a variety of feelings in the past 6 months; responses were either yes (1) or no (0).

Depression. Depression may be a cause or a result—or both—of problem behaviors. It may also represent a "turning in" or internalization in contrast to the "acting-out" or externalization of problem behaviors (Achenbach & Edelbrock, 1987; Harlow, Newcomb, & Bentler, 1986; Hartka et al., 1991). In this study, depression was measured using the 7-item "depressed affect" subscale of the Center for Epidemiologic Studies Depression Scale (CES-D; Radloff, 1977). This subscale of the CES-D has demonstrated the greatest concurrent validity of the CES-D subscales with a diagnosis of depression; it has also been shown to be robust in Indian (Beals, Manson, Keane, & Dick, 1991) and other samples (Golding & Aneshensel, 1989; Radloff, 1977, 1991). Responses asked about the past week and ranged from 0 (*rarely or none of the time*) to 4 (*most or all of the time*); internal consistency was high ($\alpha = .89$).

Sensation-Seeking. In viewing problem behaviors as risky behaviors, sensation-seeking has been implicated as an important correlate among teens (Huba, Newcomb, & Bentler, 1981b). We utilized six items adapted from Zuckerman's (1979) measure, as shortened for an adolescent sample by Huba et al. (1981b), including such items as "I like wild parties" and "I would like to try parachute jumping" ($\alpha = .74$). Responses ranged from 1 (*disagree*) to 5 (*agree*).

Self-Esteem. Although self-esteem has demonstrated inconsistent relationships with problem behaviors, it is commonly considered an important marker of satisfactory development. We utilized six items of the Rosenberg (1979) Self-Esteem Scale ($\alpha = .79$); the response set ranged from 1 (*disagree*) to 5 (*agree*).

Personal Mastery. Within Euro-American samples, personal mastery or internal locus of control has been related to more positive outcomes (e.g., Pearlin & Schooler, 1978). This measure was a composite of Pearlin and Schooler's mastery scale and Levenson's (1981) internality items ($\alpha = .69$); the response set ranged from 1 (*disagree*) to 5 (*agree*).

Social Support. Support from peers and family has been found to predict problem behaviors—especially in instances where family support is low and peer support is high (e.g., Wills & Vaughan, 1989). We selected six items ($\alpha = .85$) from the Multidimensional Scale of Perceived Social Support (Zimet, Dahlem, Zimet, & Farley, 1988): two items asked about support from a special person; two from family; and two from a friend. Responses ranged from 1 (*disagree*) to 5 (*agree*).

ETHNOGRAPHIC COMPONENT

In addition to the quantitative aspects of this study, two anthropologists conducted ethnographic investigations in the two largest communities. Through repeated use of both adolescent and adult key informants, the anthropologists worked to understand the local meanings of problem and positive behaviors among adolescents within the community. As a result, the anthropologists were able to inform important aspects of the quantitative study. For example, they were able to provide feedback throughout the measure development period, from initial construct selection to specific wording of individual items. They also reviewed results for interpretability and, when necessary, consulted their key informants to help with particular interpretations and implications of the quantitative results.

RESULTS

We assume that the reader has a general understanding of the basics of confirmatory factor analyses and structural equation modeling; for those who are less familiar with *multisample* confirmatory factor analyses using structural equations, we present a summary in the Appendix. In this study, we first used confirmatory factor analysis (CFA) within the full sample to test an expanded second-order two-factor model, using nested models to examine the question of the unidimensionality of problem and positive behaviors. With a set of hierarchical regression analyses, we next examined the incremental validity (Sechrest, 1963) of positive behaviors in conjunction with problem behaviors in predicting psychosocial adaptation and maladaptation. We then conducted two sets of multisample CFAs, to explore the goodness-of-fit for this expanded two-factor model across gender and community.

Full-Sample Confirmatory Factor Analysis

Figure 1 shows the fit and loadings for the two-factor structure of the expanded problem and positive behavior constructs. This bidimensional

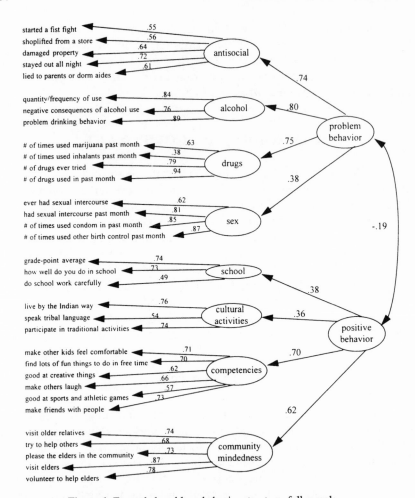

Figure 1. Expanded problem–behavior structure: full sample.

factor model represented a significant improvement in the fit over a one-factor (i.e., unidimensional) model, $\Delta\chi^2(1) = 50.17$; $p < .05$. The comparative
fit index (cfi) met the standard cutoff criterion of .90, suggesting that the
structure provided a satisfactory fit for the observed data. (More precisely,
the fit of the second-order structure need not be rejected.)[3] All first-order

---

[3] Some authors suggest that a nonsignificant χ^2 statistic indicates an appropriate model fit.
However, χ^2 statistics are related to sample size; as a result, χ^2 statistics based on large samples
are often significant even in the face of very small differences between observed and expected
matrices (Hoyle, 1995). Thus, although the χ^2 tests are presented, we discuss only comparative
fit indices, as providing discriminating guidance about goodness-of-fit with large samples.

factor loadings were statistically significant, although Inhalants had a loading (.38) quite a bit lower than the other loadings on the first-order Drug Use factor. Second-order loadings were all significant, as well. However, the loading for Sexual Intercourse (.38) was lower than the other loadings on problem behavior; School Success (.38) and Cultural Activities (.35) also loaded quite a bit lower on positive behaviors. Finally, the correlation between the two second-order factors was significant, but very small (−.19).

Validity Analyses

The results of the CFAs reported above supported a two-factor structure underlying problem and positive behaviors; however, if maintaining two separate components provides no significant and meaningful discrimination, the utility of two separate factors is questionable. To examine this issue, we first standardized all variables to adjust for different response metrics; we then created unit-weighted, average-item scale scores for each of the six problem and positive behavior constructs. We then examined the extent to which the positive behaviors added predictive utility above and beyond the problem behaviors in concurrent prediction of measures of psychosocial adaptation and maladaptation. Using hierarchical multiple regression, scale scores for those constructs typically utilized in PBT—antisocial behavior, alcohol use, drug use, and sexual behavior—were entered as a first block, followed by the scale scores of the positive behaviors of school success, cultural activities, competencies, and community-mindedness as a second block. As shown in Table II, the problem behavior variables in the first block provided a significant increment in the R^2 for each equation; however, in every case, the second block of positive behaviors also explained statistically significant increments in variance—even *after* the problem behaviors had been accounted for. Moreover, in predicting the more adaptive psychosocial outcomes (self-esteem, personal mastery, social support), the positive behaviors explained more than twice as much of the variance as did the problem behaviors. It should be noted that although these constructs provided support for the possible importance of both problem and positive behaviors, these relationships were all concurrent, and therefore do not necessarily carry information about *causal* relationships.

MULTISAMPLE CONFIRMATORY FACTOR ANALYSES

Given the satisfactory fit of the two-factor second-order structure, and the apparent utility of including both problem and positive behaviors, we

Table II. Validity Analyses: Hierarchical Multiple Regression

Criterion variable	Block 1					Block 2				
	R^2	Antisocial behavior[a]	Alcohol use	Drug use	Sexual behavior	R^2	School success	Cultural activities	Competence	Community-mindedness
Anxiety	$.05^b$	$.21^b$	$.08^b$	$-.01$	$-.03$	$.02^b$	$.08^b$	$.03$	$-.14^b$	$.02$
Depression	$.09^b$	$.17^b$	$.15^b$	$.02$	$.03$	$.01^b$	$-.06$	$-.04$	$-.09^b$	$-.01$
Sensation-seeking	$.15^b$	$.16^b$	$.12^b$	$.15^b$	$.07^b$	$.02^b$	$-.01$	$.02$	$.17^b$	$.04$
Self-esteem	$.01^b$	$-.03$	$-.09^b$	$.02$	$.06^b$	$.09^b$	$.18^b$	$-.03$	$.19^b$	$-.03$
Personal mastery	$.06^b$	$-.07^b$	$-.17^b$	$.01$	$.03$	$.16^b$	$.16^b$	$-.04$	$.29^b$	$.06^b$
Social support	$.03^b$	$-.06^b$	$-.06^b$	$-.04$	$.06^b$	$.14^b$	$.11^b$	$.02$	$.24^b$	$.19^b$

[a] β at last step.
[b] $p < .05$.

then turned to an examination of differences in the factor structure that might exist within two demographic subgroups: gender and community.

Gender

The multisample CFA across gender provides a first example of the multisample CFA.[4] As summarized in Table III, seven constraints were released. (In this table, those loadings that were *not* significantly different across the groups have a numerical entry in the Constrained B column; one then interprets the columns entitled Unconstrained B, with a different B for each group.) Looking at the unconstrained Bs for those seven constraints, both "shoplifted" and "damaged property" loaded higher for males on the first-order Antisocial Behavior construct. On the first-order Alcohol Use construct, females had a slightly lower loading of "negative consequences of alcohol use" and a slightly higher loading of "problem drinking" behavior. Males had a higher loading of "past-month marijuana use" on the first-order Drug Use construct. Females had a slightly higher loading of "careful schoolwork" on the first-order "School Success construct." Finally, the first-order construct of Sexual Intercourse was more strongly related to the second-order Problem Behavior construct for males than for females.[5]

Communities

Not surprisingly, moving from a two-group analysis to a four-group analysis introduces much greater complexity. In all, 21 cross-group equality constraints were suggested as problematic. The constraints to be released fell into four groups. First, first-order constraints for two items were released across *all* communities: "problem drinking," on the first-order construct of Alcohol Use, and "past-month's marijuana use," on the first-order Drug Use construct. Clearly, these two items represented the most

---

[4] In the multisample analyses, the cfi approached but did not quite reach the .90 criterion. The inclusion of correlated errors among correlated items increases this criterion above .91; however, such an activity may capitalize on chance variation within this sample. As a result, we have not included such parameters to be estimated and instead draw inferences concerning the fit of the model across the samples from $\Delta\chi^2$ tests.

[5] This analysis demonstrates the potential differential interpretation of βs and Bs. If one interpreted only βs, "past-month's marijuana use" would appear to be similar across gender; "careful schoolwork" would make males appear to be *more* related to the latent construct of School Behavior.

Table III. Final Multisample Test: Gender

Item	Constrained B	Unconstrained B		β	
		M	F	M	F
Started a fist fight	1.00			.51	.54
Shoplifted from a store	—[a]	1.19	0.82	.62	.45
Damaged property	—[a]	1.28	0.89	.66	.55
Stayed out all night	1.84			.74	.70
Lied to parents or dorm aides	1.60			.68	.59
Quantity/frequency of use	1.00			.84	.84
Negative consequences of alcohol use	—[a]	0.42	0.37	.75	.76
Problem drinking behavior	—[a]	0.80	0.86	.91	.89
No. of times used marijuana past month	—[a]	4.58	3.84	.62	.62
No. of times used inhalants past month	0.81			.40	.36
No. of drugs ever tried	0.99			.83	.75
No. of drugs used in past month	1.00			.96	.94
Ever had sexual intercourse	0.25			.59	.64
Had sexual intercourse past month	0.30			.75	.87
No. of times used condom past month	1.00			.83	.88
No. of times used other birth control past month	1.10			.83	.90
Grade-point average	1.00			.66	.77
How well do you do in school	0.96			.65	.75
Do schoolwork carefully		1.05	1.20	.58	.47
Live by the Indian way	1.00			.78	.75
Speak tribal language	0.73			.55	.53
Participate in traditional activities	1.06			.75	.72
Make other kids feel comfortable	1.00			.72	.71
Find fun things to do in free time	1.00			.71	.68
Good at creative things	1.01			.64	.61
Make others laugh	1.01			.70	.47
Good at sports and athletic games	0.91			.61	.63

[a] Loadings significantly different across groups.

consistent differences across the communities. As shown in Table IV, youths from the Pueblo communities had the highest loading of "problem-drinking" on the Alcohol Use construct, followed by those from the Southwestern, Northern Plains, and finally South Central communities. With "past-month marijuana use," Southwestern youths had the highest loading, followed by Northern Plains, Pueblo, and South Central youths.

Second, *second*-order factor loadings for five items were released across just two communities: Southwestern and Pueblo. For Pueblo youth, Antisocial Behavior was more strongly related to problem behaviors, and Drug Use was slightly less strongly related to problem behaviors, than in the other sites. In addition, Cultural Activities was less related to positive

Table IV. Expanded Problem-Behavior Structure, Final Multisample Test: Community

Item	Constrained B	Unconstrained B				β			
		SC	NP	S	P	SC	NP	S	P
Started a fist fight	1.00					.55	.47	.51	.62
Shoplifted from a store	0.99					.51	.51	.55	.62
Damaged property	0.98					.50	.59	.66	.65
Stayed out all night	—[a]	1.80	1.80	1.80	1.52	.76	.67	.70	.72
Lied to parents or dorm aides	1.48					.63	.56	.57	.68
Quantity/frequency of use	1.00					.85	.82	.81	.84
Negative consequences of alcohol use	0.39					.73	.79	.74	.74
Problem drinking behavior	—[a]	0.70	0.82	0.87	0.93	.86	.91	.92	.90
No. of times used marijuana past month	—[a]	2.92	4.46	4.64	4.25	.58	.60	.66	.63
No. of times used inhalants past month	—[a]	0.46	0.93	0.46	1.08	.37	.39	.30	.40
No. of drugs ever tried	0.97					.78	.79	.80	.85
No. of drugs used in past month	1.00					.96	.94	.96	.96
Ever had sexual intercourse	—[a]	0.19	0.19	0.37	0.25	.60	.54	.68	.65
Had sexual intercourse past month	1.00	0.31	0.31	0.38	0.27	.83	.83	.84	.78
No. of times used condom past month	—[a]					.88	.82	.82	.87
No. of times used other birth control past month	1.00	1.08	1.08	1.37	1.08	.86	.85	.88	.89
Grade-point average	1.00					.71	.77	.78	.73
How well do you do in school	0.94					.70	.74	.73	.70
Do schoolwork carefully	0.74					.49	.48	.50	.46
Live by the Indian way	1.00					.71	.63	.81	.72
Speak tribal language	—[a]	0.86	0.86	0.55	0.86	.65	.54	.51	.55
Participate in traditional activities	1.07					.67	.64	.79	.71
Make other kids feel comfortable	1.00					.75	.70	.71	.67
Find fun things to do in free time	1.02					.69	.71	.74	.66
Good at creative things	1.03					.62	.61	.64	.59
Make others laugh	1.03					.69	.65	.68	.63
Good at sports and athletic games	0.94					.58	.58	.60	.55
Make friends with people	1.02					.75	.75	.73	.71

[a] Loadings significantly different across groups.

behaviors among Pueblo youths. For Southwestern youths, Alcohol Use, Sexual Intercourse, and Drug Use were less strongly related to problem behaviors than for any of the other communities.

Finally, the remaining constraints were quite community-specific. With "past-month's use of contraception other than condoms," Southwestern youths were higher than the other sites, and "speaking the tribal language" was least related to Cultural Activities among Southwestern youths. For Southwestern youths, "ever had sexual intercourse" was most strongly related to the Sexual Intercourse construct; Pueblo youths were slightly lower; South Central and Northern Plains youths had the lowest loadings. Southwestern youths had the highest loading of "past-month's sexual intercourse," with Northern Plains and South Central slightly lower, and Pueblo youths the lowest. For Pueblo youths, "stayed out all night" was less strongly related to other items on the Antisocial Behavior construct. Finally, for both Pueblo and Northern Plains youths, "past-month's inhalant use" was more strongly related to other aspects of Drug Use than for the other two communities.

DISCUSSION

The Structure of Problem and Positive Behaviors

Most of the goals of this study focused on various approaches to expanding and extending the utility of PBT, focusing on the construct validity of the problem and positive behavior constructs. We accomplished this in several ways: (a) utilizing multiple measures of the four most commonly utilized problem behavior constructs (antisocial behavior, alcohol use, drug use, and sexual behavior); (b) including multiple measures of four age- and population-appropriate positive behavior constructs (school success, cultural activities, competencies, and community-mindedness); (c) testing nested unidimensional and bidimensional models of the underlying structure of problem and positive behaviors; (d) exploring the additional predictive power that might accompany the inclusion of both problem and positive behaviors in understanding psychosocial adaptation; and (e) examining these issues within a new sample. A series of confirmatory factor analyses provided support for a two-factor second-order structure, in which items loaded on individual first-order problem- and positive-behavior constructs. These first-order constructs loaded in turn on one of two second-order constructs of problem or positive behaviors, which were not strongly related to each other. Finally, positive behaviors—which have been too often overlooked in both PBT and the broader psychological literature—added unique and important information in predicting measures of psychosocial adaptation.

From these analyses, we drew three conclusions that have direct implications for PBT and the operationalization of problem and positive behaviors. First, a broader sampling of both problem and positive behaviors does not contraindicate a latent structure of problem and positive behaviors, *providing a sufficiently complex latent structure is permitted.* In other words, both a first- and second-order level of constructs are necessary to explain both the variance that is *shared* within individual problem and positive behaviors and the variance that is *unique* to the individual problem and positive behaviors. Second, contrary to one of PBT's basic suppositions, positive and problem behaviors do not appear to fall at opposite ends of the single dimension stretching from conventionality to unconventionality. While the correlation between the two second-order constructs was statistically significant, it was extremely small—accounting for less than 4% of the total variance. In effect, these adolescents were neither "good" kids nor "bad" kids; as a group, they represented a complex mixture of both problem and positive behaviors. Finally, as we move toward prevention and promotion efforts, we will clearly miss important aspects of adaptation if we focus only on problem behaviors. With a richer approach to measurement that includes both problem behavior and positive behaviors, we are much better positioned to understand processes underlying not only maladaptive behavior but also those that lead to adaptive outcomes.

Subgroup Analyses

Another goal of this study was to explore the structure of problem and positive behaviors within gender and community subgroups. However, little quantitative work in the structure of problem and positive behaviors has been conducted in American Indian communities. Thus, while the findings of gender differences have some precedence in the broader developmental literature, we leave that comfort as we move to a discussion of community-level differences.

Gender Differences

While seven significant differences emerged across gender, the most interesting differences occurred with alcohol use, school success, and sexual activity. First, for girls, "problem drinking" was more closely related to the second-order alcohol use factor than it was for boys. This may reflect others' findings that girls are generally more attuned to internal signals

(e.g., drinking more than one intended or feeling hung over) whether referring to psychological symptomatology, such as depression or anxiety, or
alcohol use. On the other hand, "negative consequences following drinking" was more strongly related to the second-order alcohol use factor for
boys than for girls. In the same vein, then, perhaps the boys connect more
external signs—such as fighting with friends or school grades dropping—
with higher levels of drinking (Achenbach & Edelbrock, 1987). Second,
"do schoolwork carefully" was more closely related to school success for
girls than for boys. Others have reported that girls tend to attribute their
successes in school to their own hard work whereas boys tend to attribute
their school successes to greater intellectual ability (Cobb, 1992;
Henderson & Dweck, 1990). Finally, the second-order loading of sexual
behavior on problem behaviors for girls was lower than for boys. This difference may reflect the different meanings given to boys and girls about
sexual intercourse. For example, Brooks-Gunn and Paikoff (1993) noted
that "Sexual desire is seen as paramount for boys and is ignored for girls"
(p. 187). Also, since the sexual behavior construct is made up primarily of
risky sexual behaviors (e.g., not using birth control), this lower relationship
with other problem behaviors among girls may reflect the fact that the
consequences of unprotected sexual intercourse are far higher for girls than
for boys—and for a girl, engaging in other problem behaviors is motivated
differently than is putting oneself at risk for a pregnancy.

Community Differences

Here, we note interesting differences and speculate about what might
underlie the observed community differences in three areas: substance use,
sexual behavior, and cultural activities.

Substance Use. The South Central youth had lower loadings of problem drinking, marijuana use, and inhalant use on the respective first-order
constructs than did the other three communities. It may be that the
processes that lead to a youth's attending this school—the majority of
whom are boarders, living away from their families—may operate in some
way to make these three items less related to other issues of substance
use than at the other three communities. A second hypothesis focuses on
the possible impact of a substance use treatment facility that is located on
the campus of the South Central high school: while the youths may not be
affected *directly* by the presence of that facility, the constant presence of a
treatment facility may indirectly influence the substance use behavior of
the youths at that site.

Sexual Behavior. The responses of the Southwestern youths were more
consistent on the four items representing sexual behavior than were those

of the other three sites. Although not presented here, item-level means show that fewer youths in the Southwestern community reported high endorsements of any of these four items. Most dramatic is the fact that while over one third of the youths in the other three communities reported having had sexual intercourse in the past month, only 17% of the Southwestern youth had done so. As a result, the internal consistency of the items among Southwestern youths may have been a result of the greater number of "none" answers among these youths. (In general, it should be noted that either high or low endorsements of items can result in lower loadings, due to truncated variance.) Moreover, at the second-order level, sexual activity was less strongly related to the underlying problem-behavior construct in the Southwestern community than in the other three communities—perhaps as a result of the less widespread occurrence of sexual intercourse.

Cultural Activities. Among the Southwestern youths, "speaking your tribal language" was less integrally related to other involvements in Indian culture than it was for youths in the other communities. The pattern of means was different for this community: In the other three communities, the two nonlanguage "cultural activities" items had means similar to each other, whereas "speaking your tribal language" had the lowest mean; among the Southwestern youths, all of the means were similar. However, these findings may be better explained by looking at characteristics of the community. For instance, the tribal language of the Southwestern community is widely spoken throughout the community—by young and old alike. This situation is quite unique to this community; as a result, given that a wide range of youths speak the language, that activity may be less related to other cultural activities than it is in the other communities. Similarly, Cultural Activities was less strongly related to the other positive behaviors for the Pueblo youths than for the other three communities. In this community, much attention focuses on community-wide feast days for celebration and solidarity. In effect, everyone in the community becomes involved in the celebratory activities. Thus, as with the greater exposure to the spoken tribal language in the Southwestern community, a wider variety of adolescents participate in cultural activities in general in the Pueblo communities, thus lessening the link between that construct and other more general positive behaviors.

To this point, we have focused on differences across samples. However, it is even more important to note that the four communities appear to have much more in common than they have differences: roughly 75% (25) of the 33 *item*-level equality constraints were not rejected for *any* community. In general, the South Central and Northern Plains were most like each other: only three first-order loadings—and none of the second-order loadings—were different across those two communities. The majority of the differences lay with the Southwestern and Pueblo communities. The Southwestern youths' second-order loadings for problem behaviors were consistently the lowest, implying that problem behaviors tend to be less clustered for these youths than for the youths in the other communities. Finally, practically no differences appeared across communities in the *positive* behaviors—at either the first- or second-order levels. This may imply that similarities exist across these communities in the messages adolescents receive about appropriate ways to act. The community differences existed almost without exception in ways in which adolescents were acting out. By this, we do not mean to imply any sort of "universal" structure among positive behaviors; indeed, the "culture" of these communities is made up of a number of important "subcultures," such as traditional customs and macrosystem influences such as television and radio (Bronfenbrenner, 1977). However, the similarities among the positive behaviors are striking—especially when contrasted with the differences among problem behaviors. Clearly, we need to move back to the individual communities with ethnographic investigations of valid interpretations of the findings.

LIMITATIONS

A discussion of limitations helps to put this study in its appropriate context. First, while the sample drew on youths from four diverse Indian communities—and included youths from more than 50 difference tribes— they still represent only a small portion of the diversity among Indian nations. Moreover, most of the youths were living on or near their reservations; thus, issues surrounding Indian youths living in more urban settings need to be addressed in the future, as well. In addition, we have treated the communities here as if they were homogeneous groups; as is true of any community, though, important subgroups are likely to exist within communities, as well. For instance, not all adolescents are likely to identify equally strongly with the traditions and customs of their culture groups; thus, the structure of problem and positive behaviors might differ by ethnic identity. In general, though, other researchers need to replicate the more complex model supported here within other cultural groups. Furthermore, while this effort represents an attempt to sample more broadly from the universe of potential measures of positive and problem behaviors, other important domains still remain untapped. Moreover, the indicators chosen for the communities in this research may not necessarily be the behaviors of great concern to other communities or cultural groups; thus, the universe of items is likely to vary somewhat by culture.

Second, as with Jessor and Donovan's efforts, the data in this study were all youth self-report. As a next step, other sources of information about a youth's behavior, such as parent or teacher reports and academic records, could be helpful. We also did not examine possible interactions between community and gender, due to several small subgroups; however, it is possible that this structure might also vary by gender within community. In addition, the utility of these more fully operationalized cross-sectional relationships need to be examined in longitudinal designs, such as those of McGee and Newcomb (1992) and Osgood, Johnston, O'Malley, and Bachman (1988). Finally, we found a number of differences across samples; however, the enhanced statistical power that accompanies a large sample such as the one in this study could result in interpreting differences across samples that are *statistically* significant but not necessarily important or meaningful in the real world.

CONCLUSIONS

This work raises four central issues that need continuing attention. First, a key point of PBT has been that problem behaviors such as adolescent substance use, risky sexual behavior, and antisocial behavior are socially defined—that is, they depart from social and legal norms and are negatively sanctioned by systems of authority (Mitchell et al., 1996). Implicit in this idea is the importance of understanding the culture within which the problem and positive behaviors occur. Yet the empirical work around PBT to date has ignored the sociocultural context within whichthe problem and positive behaviors exist. For instance, PBT's emphasis on "unconventionality," dysfunction, and deviance casts teens who use substances as "distressed actors" whose patterns of substance use reflect a universal "tension-reducing" response to stress and distress—ignoring cultural variation in definitions of normal and pathological uses of alcohol. In sharp contrast, our ethnographic work points to the fact that the meaning of substance use lies much more with aspects of social convention than in individual psychological factors. As O'Nell and Mitchell (1996) pointed out, such a conclusion is "tantamount to locating the non-emotive styles of Euro-American males (or conversely, the emotive styles of Euro-American females) in cultural conventions of gender, rather than in pathological psychological functioning or differential social stresses. Thus, if women talk more about feelings, it does not mean that women are more stressed or unable to cope than men who talk less about their feelings" (p. 567). Clearly, researchers need to explore systematically the culture(s) within which they are conducting their research. And we need to ascertain not only the relevance of key constructs for the populations of interest—we must also search for constructs that may have local relevance but that have been overlooked thus far in the empirical literature (O'Nell & Mitchell, 1996).

Second, we need to include both problem and positive behaviors in any research effort—either in basic research studying adolescent development or in applied research working hand in hand with preventive and promotive interventions. Although most communities are well aware of problems among their adolescents, they also know that many of their teens are succeeding. Community members want to understand not only how to circumvent the processes that result in maladaptive outcomes but also—and just as important—how to support the processes that underlie the development of successful adolescents as well. Unless researchers begin to develop reliable and valid measures of the positive outcomes, we cannot help in this effort, and we do the communities with which we collaborate a serious disservice. Along the same lines, the low correlation between positive and problem behaviors implies that prevention and promotion activities should not necessarily operate on a "hydraulic" or "see-saw" model of behavior change: The fact that an intervention might effectively prevent problem behaviors does not necessarily mean that positive behaviors will automatically begin to increase. Similarly, promotion efforts that focus only on enhancing positive behaviors may find that any increase does not necessarily result in a lowering of the frequency of problem behaviors. Instead, in light of the low interrelationships between positive and problem behaviors, the inclusion of *both* promotive and preventive efforts in any intervention would be wise.

Third, researchers need to be in close touch with members of the communities they are working with in order to be able to pinpoint those problem and positive behaviors that are of most interest—and concern—to them. This is especially important for those in Community Psychology. Given our interest in diversity and strengths, the importance of working within local understandings of both problem and positive behaviors cannot be overestimated. One way to accomplish this is to develop Community Advisory Committees, who are partners with the researchers from the beginning conceptualizations and the development of measures through the interpretation and dissemination of findings and the generation of recommendations for further research and intervention.

Finally, how are problem behaviors and positive behaviors configured similarly or differently across cultures? For instance, in this research, the Southwestern adolescents appeared to be quite different from those in the other three communities in the area of risky sexual behavior. Does this quantitative difference make sense *within* the community? One can only know this by returning to the community, presenting the findings, and getting the feedback of the important "actors" or "stakeholders." As noted above, one way to accomplish this is to engage community members through a Community Advisory Committee. A second powerful approach is to team quantitative researchers with ethnographers who work in the communities. In this way, many of the often artificial restrictions surrounding quantitative work can be placed within the context of a rich, community-specific understanding that can arise only from solid ethnographic work. Ethnographers can also identify ambiguities and further questions to be explored within the context of the communities. In addition, ethnographic work can highlight areas of investigation that are important from the community perspective but that may never emerge from the more main-stream research and theoretical literature. Without such collaborations, quantitatively oriented researchers risk restricting themselves to a world of numbers and numerical relations that includes at best only cursory attempts to capture community concerns.

APPENDIX

A brief discussion of one basic aspect of structural equation modeling—multisample confirmatory factor analysis (CFA)—may be useful. We assume that readers have a general understanding of the logic involved in a single-sample CFA; readers desiring a more introductory level discussion are referred to any number of good basic references (Byrne, 1994; Dunn, Everitt, & Pickles, 1993). Here, we utilized the EQS/PC program (version 3.0, Bentler, 1992); the specific steps involved in other packages (such as LISREL) may vary.

Typically, research samples are made up of subsamples which may have underlying structural differences that are of theoretical interest (e.g., boys vs. girls, Puerto Rican vs. Dominican women, younger vs. older parents). Most researchers have tested the fit of a proposed model across subsamples by fitting the model in question sequentially on each group and attempting to determine if differences exist in fit (e.g., Donovan & Jessor, 1985; Farrell et al., 1992; McGee & Newcomb, 1992). However, a *multi*-sample CFA addresses the issue of subgroup differences simultaneously, directly, and powerfully. One begins first by specifying the parameters or "paths" of the model to be tested, as in a single-sample CFA; one also specifies which paths should also be required or "constrained" to be equal across the groups. While *all* paths can be constrained across groups, such a test is an extremely stringent, and often theoretically meaningless, test for understanding the factor structure across groups. For example, does one's theory really specify that all error variances as well as factor loadings must be equal for the groups? In most cases, the answer is "No." In general, for such questions, one tests only whether the first- and, if relevant, second-order factor loadings are equal, by constraining only the factor loading paths to be equal across groups. In some instances, one might also be interested in examining a second level of equality across groups, as well—the equality of the latent factor variances and covariances (Byrne, 1994). For simplicity's sake, though, we here demonstrate only this first level of testing; however, one would follow the same steps at the second level, as well.

While the basic steps used in a single-sample analysis apply to a multisample analysis, one additional step is required for a multisample analysis. One first tests a *loadings-constrained model*, where all first- and second-order factor loadings are constrained to be equal across all groups. In EQS, the program then provides a single estimate for each constrained variable which best fits all groups. The multivariate Lagrange Multiplier test identifies those constraints which are not appropriate—that is, those for which forcing equality across subsamples is lessening the fit of the model.[6] One then reruns the analysis releasing those identified constraints; that analysis provides the *partially constrained model*, representing the minimum number of parameters that need to be estimated separately across groups—that is, those points of the structure where the groups differ significantly. One can then interpret those individually estimated parameters to begin to explore the subgroup differences in structure.

Two final points specific to multisample analyses should be made. First, any CFA must meet the requirements of mathematical identification.[7] Mathematically, one is simply unable to estimate both a factor's variance and all of its loadings. Instead, one must determine the scale of an unmeasured, latent factor in one of two ways: (a) standardize or fix underlying factor variances to be 1.0 (thereby *not* estimating those variances), and instead estimate all factor loadings on each factor with reference to this "standardized" latent factor; or (b) fix one loading (a "marker" variable) on each first-order factor to be 1.0. Either approach will establish a scale for the unmeasured latent factor; and in a single-sample analysis, one can choose based on the questions one wants to address. When dealing with multisample analyses, though, the better choice is always the latter—establishing a marker variable for each first-order factor. If one were instead to set the factor variances to 1.0, one has in effect standardized *within* each group (in effect, adjusting differently by group); this procedure removes the information carried by group-specific standard deviations—which may differ significantly—from the determination of the fit across groups. In addition, if one fixes the factor variances to 1.0, one cannot subsequently examine the equality of these factor variances and covariances across groups at a second level of testing, should that be of interest.

Second, a similar problem occurs with the conventions of reporting and interpreting factor loadings. In single-sample analyses, one commonly reports standardized regression coefficients (the β coefficients) to discuss differences in the relative importance of the loadings within the sample. However, βs are calculated by dividing each unadjusted regression coefficient (the B coefficient) by its standard deviation. If one interprets only the βs in a multisample analysis, one has again removed the information carried by the group-level standard deviations from any interpretations. Thus, the βs may appear more intuitively interpretable in a multisample analysis and can help in looking at patterns within a subgroup; however, they

---

[6] In EQS, this can be found in the multivariate Lagrange Multiplier test; those with a significance level $p < .05$ are those targeted for release.

[7] Identification is a complex topic, which is difficult to describe in nontechnical terms. In general, though, it is the process of determining whether the parameters of the model can be estimated. It focuses on the number of variances and covariances and the number of parameters which must be estimated. One must have at least as many variances and covariances as one has parameters to be estimated. This is parallel to solving for "unknowns" in algebraic equations. In algebra, if you have more unknowns (i.e., variables to be solved for) than you have equations containing those unknowns, an infinite number of solutions is possible, and the unknowns cannot be uniquely determined. In structural equation modeling, a model with fewer variances and covariances than it has parameters is called "underidentified." If one has exactly as many variances and covariances as one has parameters to be estimated, a unique solution can be found. Such a model is called "just-identified"; and although it produces a unique solution, it is not particularly interesting because it has no degrees of freedom available to test the fit of the model. To test the fit of the model, one needs to have at least 1 more covariance than one has parameters to be estimated; such a model is "overidentified" (Kenny, 1979).

may also lead to incorrect interpretations concerning across-group differences. For the same reason as noted above—possibly different standard deviations across groups—one is better advised to utilize the Bs for comparisons of relative differences across groups (Bollen, 1989). In the tables presented here, we have reported both B and β for all multisample analyses; however, in the text, we discuss only the Bs.

ACKNOWLEDGMENTS

The preparation of this paper was supported by NIAAA Grant R01-AA08474 and NIDA R01-DA10039. In addition, we deeply appreciate the time and contribution of the community schools and the research participants, without whom this study could not have been conducted.

REFERENCES

Achenbach, T. M., & Edelbrock, C. (1987). *Manual for the Youth Self-Report and Profile.* Burlington: University of Vermont Department of Psychiatry.

Beals, J., Manson, S. M., Keane, E. M., & Dick, R. W. (1991). Factorial structure of the Center for Epidemiologic Studies: Depression scale among American Indian college students. *Psychological Assessment, 3,* 623–627.

Bentler, P. M. (1992). *EQS: Structural equations program manual.* Los Angeles: BMDP Statistical Software.

Blum, R. W., Harmon, B., Harris, L., Bergeisen, L., & Resnick, M. D. (1992). American Indian—Alaska Native youth health. *Journal of the American Medical Association, 267,* 1637–1644.

Bollen, K. A. (1989). *Structural equations with latent variables.* New York: Wiley.

Bronfenbrenner, U. (1977). Toward an experimental ecology of human development. *American Psychologist, 32,* 513–531.

Brooks-Gunn, J., & Paikoff, R. L. (1993). "Sex is a gamble, kissing is a game": Adolescent sexuality and health promotion. In S. G. Millstein, A. C. Petersen, & E. O. Nightingale (Eds.), *Promoting the health of adolescents: New directions for the twenty-first century.* New York: Oxford University Press.

Byrne, B. M. (1994). *Structural equation modeling with EQS and EQS/Windows.* Thousand Oaks, CA: Sage.

Cobb, N. J. (1992). *Adolescence: Continuity, change, and diversity.* Mountain View, CA: Mayfield.

Donovan, J. E., & Jessor, R. (1978). Adolescent problem drinking: Psychosocial correlates in a national sample study. *Journal of Studies on Alcohol, 39,* 1506–1524.

Donovan, J. E., & Jessor, R. (1985). Structure of problem behavior in adolescence and young adulthood. *Journal of Consulting and Clinical Psychology, 53,* 890–904.

Donovan, J. E., Jessor, R., & Costa, F. M. (1988). Syndrome of problem behavior in adolescence: A replication. *Journal of Consulting and Clinical Psychology, 56,* 762–765.

Donovan, J. E., Jessor, R., & Costa, F. M. (1991). Adolescent health behavior and conventionality–unconventionality: An extension of Problem-Behavior Theory. *Health Psychology, 10,* 52–61.

Donovan, J. E., Jessor, R., & Costa, F. M. (1993). Structure of health-enhancing behavior in adolescence: A latent-variable approach. *Journal of Health and Social Behavior, 34,* 346–362.

Dunn, G., Everitt, B., & Pickles, A. (1993). *Modelling covariances and latent variables using EQS.* London: Chapman & Hall.

Farrell, A. D., Danish, S. J., & Howard, C. W. (1992). Relationship between drug use and other problem behaviors in urban adolescents. *Journal of Consulting and Clinical Psychology, 60,* 705–712.

Garmezy, N. (1993). Children in poverty: Resilience despite risk. *Psychiatry, 56,* 127–136.

Gillmore, M. R., Hawkins, J. D., Catalano, R. F., & Day, E. (1991). Structure of problem behaviors in preadolescence. *Journal of Consulting and Clinical Psychology, 59,* 499–506.

Golding, J. M., & Aneshensel, C. S. (1989). Factor structure of the Center for Epidemiologic Studies Depression scale among Mexican Americans and Non-Hispanic whites. *Psychological Assessment, 1,* 163–168.

Harlow, L., Newcomb, M., & Bentler, P. (1986). Depression, self-derogation, substance use, and suicide ideation: Lack of purpose in life as a mediational factor. *Journal of Clinical Psychology, 42,* 5–21.

Hartka, E., Johnstone, B., Leino, E. V., Motoyoshi, M., Temple, M. T., & Fillmore, K. M. (1991). A meta-analysis of depressive symptomatology and alcohol consumption over time. *British Journal of Addiction, 86,* 1283–1298.

Henderson, V. L., & Dweck, C. S. (1990). Motivation and achievement. In S. S. Feldman & G. R. Elliott (Eds.), *At the threshold: The developing adolescent.* Cambridge, MA: Harvard University Press.

Hoyle, R. H. (1995). *Structural equation modeling: Concepts, issues, and applications.* Thousand Oaks, CA: Sage.

Huba, G., Wingard, J., & Bentler, P. (1981a). A comparison of two latent variable causal models for adolescent drug use. *Journal of Personality and Social Psychology, 40,* 180–193.

Huba, G. J., Newcomb, M. D., & Bentler, P. M. (1981b). Comparison of canonical correlation and interbattery factor analysis on sensation seeking and drug use domains. *Applied Psychological Measurement, 5,* 291–306.

Jessor, R., & Jessor, S. (1977). *Problem behavior and psychosocial development: A longitudinal study of youth.* New York: Academic Press.

Kenny, D. A. (1979). *Correlation and causality.* New York: Wiley.

Kunitz, S. J., & Levy, J. E. (1994). *Drinking careers: A 25-year study of three Navajo populations.* New Haven, CT: Yale University Press.

Levenson, H. (1981). Differentiating among internality, powerful others, and chance. In H. M. Lefcourt (Ed.), *Research with the locus of control constructs: Vol. 1. Assessment methods.* New York: Academic Press.

Levy, J. E., & Kunitz, S. J. (1974). *Indian drinking: Navajo practices and Anglo-American theories.* New York: Wiley.

May, P. A. (1982). Substance abuse and American Indians: prevalence and susceptibility. *International Journal of the Addictions, 17,* 1185–1209.

McGee, L., & Newcomb, M. D. (1992). General deviance syndrome: Expanded hierarchical evaluations at four ages from early adolescence to adulthood. *Journal of Consulting and Clinical Psychology, 60,* 766–776.

Messick, S. (1995). Validity of psychological assessment: Validity of inferences from persons' responses and performance as scientific inquiry into score meaning. *American Psychologist, 50,* 741–749.

Mitchell, C. M. (1997). Interventions with ethnic minority adolescents: Before the beginning. In S. Rieger & L. DiLalla (Eds.), *Assessment and intervention issues across the life span.* Hillsdale, NJ: Erlbaum.

Mitchell, C. M., O'Nell, T. D., Beals, J., Dick, R. W., Keane, E., & Manson, S. M. (1996). Dimensionality of alcohol use among American Indian adolescents: Latent structure, construct validity, and implications for developmental research. *Journal of Research on Adolescence, 6,* 151–180.

Mitchell, C. M., & the Scientific Advisory Committee of the Voices of Indian Teens Project. (1993). *Designing, refining and implementing longitudinal research with American Indian communities: The Voices of Indian Teens Project.* Unpublished manuscript, National Center for American Indian and Alaska Native Mental Health Research.

O'Nell, T. D., & Mitchell, C. M. (1996). Alcohol use among American Indian adolescents: The role of culture in pathological drinking. *Social Science and Medicine, 42,* 565–578.

Orive, R., & Gerard, H. (1980). Personality, attitudinal, and social correlates of drug use. *International Journal of the Addictions, 15,* 869–881.

Osgood, D. W., Johnston, L. D., O'Malley, P. M., & Bachman, J. G. (1988). The generality of deviance in late adolescence and early adulthood. *American Sociological Review, 53,* 81–93.

Pearlin, L. I., & Schooler, C. (1978). The structure of coping. *Journal of Health and Social Behavior, 19,* 2–21.

Radloff, L. S. (1977). The CES-D scale: A self-report depression scale for research in the general population. *Applied Psychological Measurement, 1,* 385–401.

Radloff, L. S. (1991). The use of the Center for Epidemiologic Studies Depression Scale in adolescents and young adults. *Journal of Youth and Adolescence, 20,* 149–166.

Resnicow, K., Ross-Gaddy, D., & Vaughan, R. D. (1995). Structure of problem and positive behaviors in African American youth. *Journal of Consulting and Clinical Psychology, 63,* 594–603.

Sechrest, L. (1963). Incremental validity: A recommendation. *Educational and Psychological Measurement, 23,* 153–158.

Seidman, E., Aber, J. L., Allen, L., & Mitchell, C. M. (1994). The impact of school transitions in early adolescence on the self-system and perceived social context of poor urban youth. *Child Development, 65,* 507–522.

Shaffer, D., Schwab-Stone, M., Fisher, P., Cohen, P., Piacentini, J., Davies, M., Conners, C. K., & Regier, D. (1993). The Diagnostic Interview Schedule for Children-Revised Version: I. Preparation, field testing, interrater reliability, and acceptability. *Journal of the American Academy of Child and Adolescent Psychiatry, 32,* 643–650.

Swaim, R. C., Oetting, E. R., Edwards, R. W., & Beauvais, F. (1989). Links from emotional distress to adolescent drug use: A path model. *Journal of Consulting and Clinical Psychology, 57,* 227–231.

U.S. Congress (1990). *Indian adolescent mental health.* Washington, DC: U.S. Government Printing Office.

Wills, T. A., & Vaughan, R. (1989). Social support and substance use in early adolescence. *Journal of Behavioral Medicine, 12,* 321–339.

Zimet, G., Dahlem, S., Zimet, S., & Farley, G. (1988). The multidimensional scale of perceived social support. *Journal of Personality Assessment, 52,* 30–41.

Zuckerman, M. (1979). *Sensation seeking: Beyond the optimal level of stimulation.* Hillsdale, NJ: Erlbaum.

About the Editors

Tracey A. Revenson (Senior Editor) is Associate Professor of Psychology at the Graduate Center of the City University of New York, where she is the former director of the Health Psychology Concentration. In addition to this volume and its companion (*Ecological Research to Promote Social Change: Methodological Advances from Community Psychology*, Kluwer Academic/Plenum Publications, 2002), Revenson is the co-author or co-editor of three other books: *The Handbook of Health Psychology* (Erlbaum, 2001), *Understanding Rheumatoid Arthritis* (Routledge, 1996), and *A Piaget Primer: How a Child Thinks* (revised edition, Penguin, 1996). From 1995–1999, Dr. Revenson was the founding Editor-in-Chief of the journal, *Women's Health: Research on Gender, Behavior and Policy*, and has served on the Editorial Board of *AJCP*. Her primary research interests include stress and coping processes among individuals, couples, and families facing chronic physical illnesses and psychosocial aspects of women's health. Her current work examines long-term adaptation among breast cancer survivors and the interactive effects of gender, discrimination, and ethnic identity on smoking among African Americans.

Anthony R. D'Augelli is Professor of Human Development at The Pennsylvania State University. In 1999 he received the Distinguished Scientific Contribution Award from the Society for the Psychological Study of Lesbian, Gay, and Bisexual Issues (Division 44 of APA) and an award from the Society for Community Research and Action for Outstanding Contribution to Education and Training in Community Research and Action. He is currently on the Editorial Board of *AJCP*. He is co-editor of three books reviewing psychological research on sexual orientation: *Lesbian, Gay, and Bisexual Identities over the Lifespan* (1995), *Lesbian, Gay, and Bisexual Identities in Families* (1998), and *Lesbian, Gay, and Bisexual Identities and Adolescence* (2001), all published by Oxford University Press. His primary research interests concern sexual orientation and human development in community settings.

Sabine E. French is Assistant Professor of Psychology at the University of California, Riverside. She has conducted research on the development of racial and ethnic identity in ethnically diverse urban adolescents and its impact on self-esteem and academic achievement. Her current research includes longitudinal studies examining the development of racial and ethnic identity, racial socialization, experiences of discrimination, and adjustment to school after the transitions to senior high school and college.

Diane L. Hughes is Associate Professor of Psychology at New York University. She is an Associate of the MacArthur Network on Successful Mid-life Development, and Chair-elect of the Black Caucus of the Society for Research in Child Development and of the Council of Program Directors in Community Psychology. In 1997, she was a Visiting Scholar at the Russell Sage Foundation. She co-edited a special issue of *AJCP* on *Culturally Anchored Methods* (1993). Her continuing research has been in the areas of ecological influences on family processes and children's development, cultural diversity, and exposure to racial bias and race-related socialization among African American and Latino families. She received a grant from the Carnegie Corporation to improve intergroup relations among youth, and serves nationally as a peer reviewer of articles and grants related to minority youth and families. Her recent research focuses on how parents' and children's experiences with race-related prejudice and discrimination in workplaces and schools influence family process and psychosocial adjustment.

David Livert is a doctoral candidate in Social-Personality Psychology at the Graduate Center of the City University of New York and a Research Associate for the national impact evaluation of the Fighting Back program, sponsored by the Robert Wood Johnson Foundation. His research has examined attributional influences on support for public assistance, and social support processes among clinical psychologists. Current projects include a longitudinal study of friendship formation and intergroup attitudes, neighborhood influences on political attitudes and crime concerns, and physicians' age and gender stereotyping of patients.

Edward Seidman is Professor of Psychology at New York University. He has received international recognition as a Scholar in Residence at the Rockefeller Foundation's Bellagio Center (2001) and Senior Fulbright-Hays Research Scholar (1977), and is the recipient of several awards from the Society for Community Research and Action (SCRA), including Outstanding Contribution to Education and Training in Community Research and Action (1999), Distinguished Contribution to Theory and Research in Community Psychology (1990), and Ethnic Minority Mentoring (2001). He served as President of SCRA in 1998, as Associate Editor for Methodology of *AJCP* from 1988–1992, and co-editor for the special issue,

Culturally Anchored Methods (1993). He is co-editor with Julian Rapport, of the *Handbook of Community Psychology* (2000), *Redefining Social Problems* (1986), the *Handbook of Social Intervention* (1983), and the author of the forthcoming, *Risky School Transitions, Engagement, and Educational Reform* (Harvard University Press). His current research focuses on understanding developmental trajectories of economically at-risk urban adolescents and how these trajectories are altered by the social contexts of family, peer, school, neighborhood, and their interactions.

Marybeth Shinn is Professor of Psychology at New York University. She is a former president of the Society for Community Research and Action and received its awards for Distinguished Contributions to Theory and Research (1996) and for Ethnic Minority Mentoring (1997). She has co-authored several books on childcare, and edited or co-edited special issues of the *Journal of Social Issues (JSI)* and *AJCP* on *Institutions and Alternatives (JSI*, 1981), *Urban Homelessness (JSI*, 1990), and *Ecological Assessment (AJCP*, 1996). She has served two terms as Associate Editor of *AJCP*, and on various scientific and policy panels including the NIMH Child/Adolescent Risk and Prevention Review Committee, The NIMH Behavioral Science Task Force, and the Task Force on Integrating Behavioral/Social Science into Public Health for the New York City Department of Health. Her current research interests are in homelessness, welfare reform, and methods for assessing the social and policy contexts of people's lives.

Hirokazu Yoshikawa is Assistant Professor of Psychology at New York University. He received the award for best dissertation in community psychology from the Society for Community Research and Action in 1999 and the Louise Kidder Early Career Award from the Society for the Psychological Study of Social Issues and the APA Minority Fellowship Program Early Career Award in 2001. He co-authored, with Jane Knitzer, a monograph on mental health in Head Start, *Lessons from the Field: Head Start Mental Health Strategies to Meet Changing Needs* (1997). He is a member of the Committee on Family Work Policies of the Board on Children, Youth, and Families of the National Academy of Sciences. He has conducted research on long-term effects of early childhood programs, mental health, and family support in Head Start, and competence among urban adolescents in poverty. His current projects examine the effects of welfare and anti-poverty policies on children and families and community-based HIV prevention among Asian/Pacific Islander immigrants to the U.S.

Index